Lecture Notes in Computer Science 16392

The series Lecture Notes in Computer Science (LNCS), including its subseries Lecture Notes in Artificial Intelligence (LNAI) and Lecture Notes in Bioinformatics (LNBI), has established itself as a medium for the publication of new developments in computer science and information technology research, teaching, and education.

LNCS enjoys close cooperation with the computer science R & D community, the series counts many renowned academics among its volume editors and paper authors, and collaborates with prestigious societies. Its mission is to serve this international community by providing an invaluable service, mainly focused on the publication of conference and workshop proceedings and postproceedings. LNCS commenced publication in 1973.

Emil R. Kaburuan · Sam Goundar
Editors

Health Information Science

14th International Conference, HIS 2025
Bandung, Indonesia, December 2–4, 2025
Proceedings

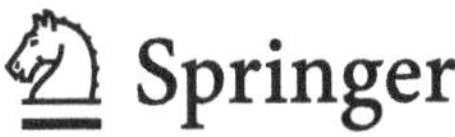

Editors
Emil R. Kaburuan
Mercu Buana University
Jakarta, Indonesia

Sam Goundar
University of Central Asia
Naryn, Kyrgyzstan

ISSN 0302-9743 ISSN 1611-3349 (electronic)
Lecture Notes in Computer Science
ISBN 978-981-95-6303-6 ISBN 978-981-95-6304-3 (eBook)
https://doi.org/10.1007/978-981-95-6304-3

This Springer imprint is published by the registered company Springer Nature Singapore Pte Ltd.
The registered company address is: 152 Beach Road, #21-01/04 Gateway East, Singapore 189721, Singapore

Preface

The International Conference Series on Health Information Science (HIS) provides a forum for disseminating and exchanging multidisciplinary research results in computer science/information technology and health science and services. It encompasses all facets of health information sciences and systems that facilitate health information management and health service provision. The 14th International Conference on Health Information Science (HIS 2025) occurred in Bandung, Indonesia, from December 2–4, 2025. Established in April 2012, the conference continues to expand to encompass an increasingly diverse range of activities.

The primary objective of these events is to establish international scientific platforms for researchers to exchange innovative ideas across various sectors, facilitating in-depth talks with global peers. The conference encompasses: (1) medical, health, and biomedicine information resources, including patient medical records, devices, equipment, software, and tools for capturing, storing, retrieving, processing, analysing, and optimizing health information; (2) data management, data mining, and knowledge discovery, which are essential for decision-making, public health management, standards examination, and addressing privacy and security concerns; (3) computer visualization and artificial intelligence for computer-aided diagnosis; and (4) the development of novel architectures and applications for health information systems.

The conference requested and collected technical research submissions pertaining to all facets of its scope. All submitted papers underwent single-blind review by a minimum of two worldwide experts selected from the Program Committee. Following the stringent peer-review procedure, 29 full papers out of 74 submissions were chosen for publication in the proceedings based on their originality, importance, and clarity. The authors hailed from Australia, China, Indonesia, Italy, Japan, Malaysia, and the Philippines. The program's exceptional quality, ensured by the involvement of numerous internationally acclaimed experts, is evident in the proceedings' content. The conference was a distinctive occasion, allowing guests to comprehend the latest findings in their area of expertise and gain supplementary knowledge in other domains.

The program was designed to promote interactions among participants from diverse scientific and geographical backgrounds, encompassing both academia and industry. We extend our gratitude to the host organization, IDEAS LAB Foundation, and Universitas Kristen Maranatha, Bandung, as well as our co-hosts: Bina Nusantara University, Bandung Institute of Science and Technology, and Pradita University. We recognize all individuals who contributed to the achievement of HIS 2025, while their names are not included here.

December 2025

Emil R. Kaburuan
Sam Goundar

Organization

General Chairs

Emil R. Kaburuan	Mercu Buana University, Indonesia
Yanchun Zhang	Zhejiang Normal University, China

Program Committee Co-chairs

Siuly Siuly	Victoria University, Australia
Yong Zhang	Tsinghua University, China
Abba Suganda Girsang	Bina Nusantara University, Indonesia
Qun Jin	Waseda University, Japan

Publicity Co-chairs

Muhammad Tariq Sadiq	University of Essex, UK
G. R. Sinha	GSFC University, India
Enamul Kabir	University of Southern Queensland, Australia
Shaofu Lin	Beijing University of Technology, China
Leonard Goeirmanto	Bandung Institute of Technology and Science, Indonesia

Industry Relationship Chairs

Zhisheng Huang	Vrije Universiteit Amsterdam, The Netherlands
Tianyong Hao	South China Normal University, China

Finance Chair

Monica Mayeni M.	Bandung Institute of Technology and Science, Indonesia

Publication Co-chair

Sam Goundar	University of Central Asia,Kyrgyzstan

Website Co-chairs

Mingshan You	Victoria University, Australia
Yosua Elwistio Malau	IDEAS LAB, Indonesia

Local Organization Co-chair

Cindrawaty	Universitas Kristen Maranatha, Indonesia

Coordination Chair

Hua Wang	Victoria University, Australia

HIS Steering Committee Representatives

Uwe Aickelin	University of Melbourne, Australia
Manik Sharma	DAV University, India
Yan Li	University of Southern Queensland, Australia
Agma Traina	University of São Paulo Institute of Mathematics and Statistics, Brazil

Program Committee

Nahida Afroz	University of Southern Queensland, Australia
Hesam Akbari	University of North Texas, USA
Ömer Faruk Alçin	Bingol Üniversitesi, Turkey
Jinli Cao	La Trobe University, Australia
Sven Casteleyn	Universitat Jaume I, Spain
Richard Chbeir	University of Pau and the Adour Region, France
Dario Colazzo	LAMSADE - Université Paris-Dauphine, France
Maria De Cola	IRCCS Centro Neurolesi Bonino-Pulejo, Italy
Yongfeng Ge	Victoria University, Australia

Allel Hadjali	LIAS/ENSMA, France
Umme Marzia Haque	University of Southern Queensland, Australia
Md. Rafiul Hassan	King Fahd University of Petroleum and Minerals, Saudi Arabia
Peiquan Jin	University of Science and Technology of China, China
Enamul Kabir	University of Southern Queensland, Australia
Eleanna Kafeza	Technology Innovation Institute, United Arab Emirates
Georgios Kambourakis	University of the Aegean, Greece
Verena Kantere	University of Ottawa, Canada
Taslima Khanam	Charles Darwin University, Australia
Smith Khare	Shri Ramdeobaba College of Engineering and Management, India
Anne Laurent	LIRMM — University of Montpellier, France
Xiaofan Li	Nanyang Technological University, Singapore
Kewen Liao	Deakin University, Australia
Guanfeng Liu	Macquarie University, Australia
Jiangang Ma	Federation University Australia, Australia
Santiago Melia	Universidad de Alicante, Spain
Sajib Mistry	Curtin University, Australia
Werner Retschitzegger	Johannes Kepler University Linz, Austria
Thomas Richter	Rhein-Waal University of Applied Sciences, Germany
Wieland Schwinger	Johannes Kepler University Linz, Austria
Supriya Supriya	Torrens University, Australia, Australia
Markel Vigo	University of Manchester, UK
Kate Wang	RMIT University, Australia
Hongzhi Wang	Harbin Institute of Technology, China
Jiao Yin	Victoria University, Australia
Mingshan You	Victoria University, Australia
Nicola Zannone	Eindhoven University of Technology, The Netherlands
Gefei Zhang	HTW Berlin, Germany
Wenjie Zhang	University of New South Wales, Australia
Rui Zhou	Swinburne University of Technology, Australia
Xiangmin Zhou	RMIT University, Australia

Additional Reviewers

Diykh, Mohammed
Sun, Lili
Jahan, Samsad
Wu, Junfeng
Xu, Puti
Quadri, Hakeem
Inan, Muhammad Sakib Khan

Organizer:

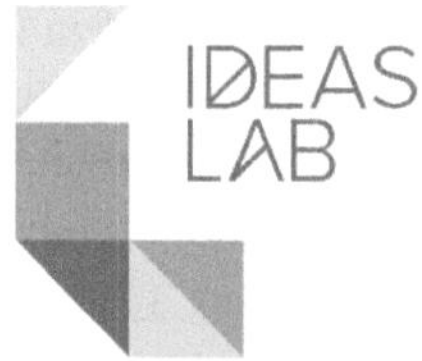

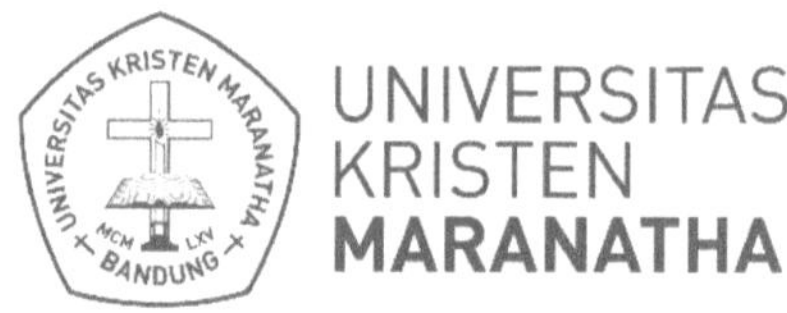

Co-organizer:

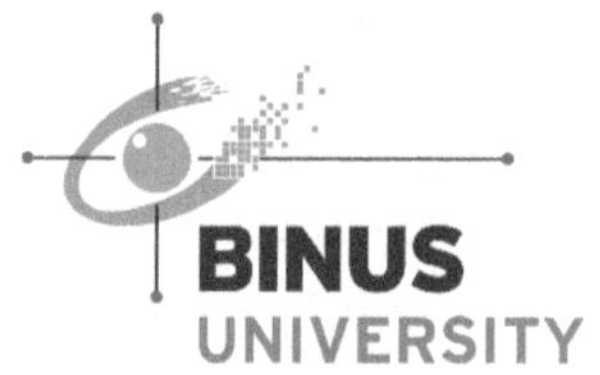

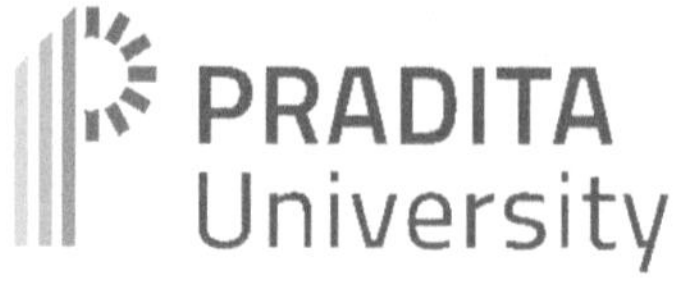

Contents

Equity by Design: Integrating Bias Audits and Fairness Mandates Into Healthcare AI Governance

Dulani Athukorala(✉), Khandakar Ahmed, and Raza Nowrozy

Victoria University, 295 Queen Street, Melbourne, VIC 3000, Australia
dulani.liyanaathukoralalage@live.vu.edu.au,
{Khandakar.Ahmed,Raza.Nowrozy}@vu.edu.au

Abstract. Artificial intelligence (AI) is reshaping healthcare, but without safeguards it can entrench disparities and erode trust. We advance an *Equity-by-Design* governance approach that embeds fairness audits, ethical oversight, and transparency across the AI lifecycle. Drawing on literature and regulation (e.g., EU AI Act, FDA GMLP) and two case studies, we show how continuous auditing, lifecycle checkpoints, institutional review, and post-deployment monitoring surface and mitigate demographic bias. We outline a practical architecture (metrics, dashboards, documentation) aligned with clinical workflows and regulatory duties, and conclude with policy and research actions to operationalize equity, accountability, and trustworthy deployment in diverse healthcare settings.

Keywords: AI governance · healthcare AI · algorithmic bias · equity-by-design

1 Introduction

Artificial intelligence (AI) is transforming healthcare by enhancing decision-making, predictive diagnostics, and workflow efficiency. Across radiology, pathology, genomics, and personalized medicine, machine and deep learning models now drive large-scale biomedical analysis [3,50,53,56,57,59,61,69,77,78]. These technologies improve diagnostic accuracy, reduce clinician workload, and strengthen healthcare delivery [52,54,58]. However, their integration raises ethical, regulatory, and sociotechnical challenges. Key issues include algorithmic bias, opacity, reduced autonomy, and unequal access to AI-assisted care [12,16,20,42]. Bias often arises from imbalanced datasets reflecting race, gender, or socioeconomic disparities, leading to inequitable outcomes [21,44,49,64]. Global oversight remains fragmented despite initiatives such as the EU AI Act and FDA Good Machine Learning Practice (GMLP) [1,13,26,66]. Standardized mechanisms for fairness, safety, and accountability are still limited [5,6,46]. Clinicians also question interpretability, liability, and reliance on opaque models [4,24,37], compounded by insufficient AI literacy and training [9,11,30,43].

E. R. Kaburuan and S. Goundar (Eds.): HIS 2025, LNCS 16392, pp. 1–12, 2026.
https://doi.org/10.1007/978-981-95-6304-3_1

Addressing these concerns requires collaboration among clinicians, data scientists, ethicists, regulators, and patients. Recent work promotes co-designed systems embedding fairness and transparency across the AI lifecycle [7,23,45,72]. Paradigms such as "ethics by design," "algorithmic stewardship," and "equity-by-design" aim to align AI with societal and health equity goals [27,31,38,63]. In response, this paper introduces an *Equity-by-Design* governance framework for healthcare AI. Drawing on interdisciplinary literature, regulatory standards, and case studies, it embeds fairness audits, ethical guardrails, and oversight throughout the AI lifecycle. The framework operationalizes measurable fairness metrics and bias monitoring within a scalable governance roadmap. Section 2 reviews algorithmic bias and governance models; Sect. 3 presents the framework; Sect. 4 evaluates case studies; Sect. 5 discusses policy implications; and Sect. 6 concludes with recommendations for equitable AI in healthcare.

2 Background and Methodology

AI systems in healthcare are often viewed as objective, yet they reproduce biases rooted in historical inequities and institutional disparities [16,29,32,33,42,47, 51,70]. Without safeguards, these biases distort diagnoses and reinforce unequal care. Within complex sociotechnical contexts, AI interacts with clinical workflows, regulations, and patient relations, amplifying bias in decision support and resource allocation [6,8,12,31,37,45]. Governance must thus progress beyond validation to achieve ethical, legal, and trust-based alignment.

A structured scoping review spanning computer science, medicine, ethics, law, and policy identified three core themes: (1) algorithmic bias and fairness mechanisms, (2) governance and regulatory frameworks, and (3) practical interventions such as audits and oversight bodies. Studies across radiology, genomics, and EHRs captured perspectives from clinicians, regulators, and patients in diverse contexts. Fairness metrics—including calibration, equal opportunity, and equalized odds—were used for multi-metric evaluation balancing equity and accuracy [13,20,63,66]. These findings inform the Equity-by-Design framework.

2.1 Algorithmic Bias and Fairness in Healthcare AI

Despite AI's promise of objectivity, biases persist due to underrepresentation and design limitations [2,16,25,29,47,51,70]. Examples include dermatology models misclassifying darker skin and risk scores encoding socioeconomic inequities through cost proxies [6,32,33,46,48,52]. Bias often arises from design choices—feature selection, optimization goals, or reliance on AUROC while neglecting fairness indicators [15,42,65]. Explainable AI (e.g., SHAP, saliency maps, counterfactuals) improves transparency but may trade off predictive performance [4,44,62,67]. Addressing such tensions requires human-centered, participatory design integrating contextual expertise [11,23,40,45,68]. Fairness therefore extends beyond computation to institutional accountability across data, design, validation, and oversight.

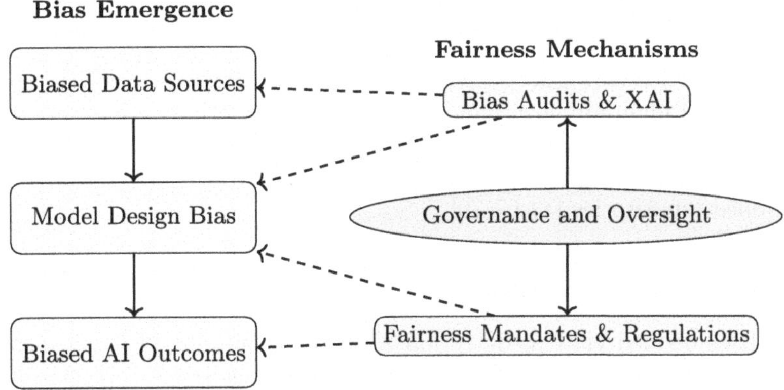

Fig. 1. Overview of bias and fairness checkpoints in healthcare AI.

2.2 Fairness Mandates and Governance in Healthcare AI

Fairness mandates aim to ensure transparency, accountability, and justice across the AI lifecycle [12,13,37,66]. The EU AI Act and WHO ethics guidelines classify healthcare AI as "high risk," mandating human oversight and ethical compliance [22,27,35]. Institutions increasingly establish ethics boards to review representativeness, fairness, explainability, and monitoring [23,26,45]. These frameworks adapt bioethical principles—beneficence, non-maleficence, autonomy, and justice—to algorithmic contexts [10,20,50]. Algorithmic management encourages continuous bias auditing and iterative validation, supported by regulatory sandboxes for pre-deployment testing [5,15,32,33,47,63]. Collectively, these mechanisms mark a shift from voluntary ethics codes to enforceable governance embedding fairness in design and deployment [1,42,46,70] (Fig. 1).

3 Equity-By-Design Governance Framework

AI has moved from experimentation to clinical use, yet persistent bias, opacity, and inequity reveal limits of reactive governance [9,16,45]. The Equity-by-Design framework promotes proactive, continuous oversight that embeds fairness, transparency, and accountability across the lifecycle, from data curation to post-market surveillance [12,13,66]. It treats bias as a sociotechnical issue requiring collaboration, ethical reflexivity, and auditability.

3.1 Core Principles

Four principles translate ethical intent into measurable actions:

1. **Continuous Bias Auditing:** Regular audits using calibration, equal opportunity, and parity ratio integrated into MLOps to sustain equity [16,28,79].

2. **Fairness Checkpoints:** Milestones across data, training, validation, and deployment with automated reports and human sign-offs [4,9,65].
3. **Institutional Oversight:** Multidisciplinary committees review logs, approve releases, and maintain governance registries [12,22,23].
4. **Transparency and Documentation:** Model Cards, Datasheets, and Impact Assessments capture rationales, risks, and intended use in version-controlled repositories [33,67,79].

3.2 Operational Architecture

Fairness is embedded via bias-detection APIs that compute TPR gaps, calibration slopes, and parity across gender, ethnicity, and age [16,34,71]. Dashboards visualize trends and trigger retraining when thresholds are exceeded. Explainability modules (SHAP, LIME) support clinical interpretation [4,28,67]. Audit outputs are versioned and mapped to the EU AI Act (Articles 9–15), FDA GMLP and SaMD guidance, and Australia's TGA and APPs [17,35,36,39,41,76] to ensure ethical and legal interoperability.

3.3 Lifecycle Integration

Accountability extends across five stages:

1. **Data Preparation:** Ensure demographic balance via inclusive sampling and federated learning [32,33].
2. **Model Development:** Integrate fairness objectives and bias probes; log experiments for review [16,65].
3. **Validation:** Use stratified testing and publish standardized fairness reports [9,47].
4. **Deployment:** Embed clinician feedback and bias alerts in workflows [22,73].
5. **Post-Market Surveillance:** Monitor fairness drift and recalibrate as needed [5,66].

Linking technical controls with institutional oversight and regulation makes equity an auditable, scalable property that advances clinical performance and social justice.

3.4 Governance Lifecycle Stages

Ethical intent is operationalized through checkpoints [5,13,27,46]:

1. **Data Preparation:** Inclusive pipelines with anomaly detection, provenance tagging, and consent tracing ensure representativeness and privacy [2,19,20,29,32,33].
2. **Model Development:** Apply fairness constraints (equal opportunity, calibration) and log results through governance APIs [6,8,16,30,38,65].

3. **Validation:** Stratified tests and bias-probe scripts feed dashboards for independent verification [4,25,28,47,48,67].
4. **Deployment:** Continuous monitoring triggers alerts; clinicians can flag anomalies or suspend models [9,11,24,45].
5. **Post-Market Surveillance:** Equity dashboards detect drift; retraining begins when fairness variance breaches thresholds [12,13,42,43,66,75].

This lifecycle embeds fairness as a traceable, data-driven process, strengthening reliability, transparency, and public trust.

4 Case Studies and Evaluation

Two case studies assess the Equity-by-Design framework's practical value, showing how lifecycle fairness interventions reduce real-world bias. The first examines bias from flawed proxies; the second addresses demographic underrepresentation in imaging. Each reports outcomes using δTPR, calibration shift, and allocation parity. A comparative analysis maps mitigation strategies and evaluation indicators across the pipeline.

4.1 Case Study 1: Biased Risk Scoring Algorithm

A commercial risk algorithm analyzed by Obermeyer et al. [60] showed racial bias. Using healthcare expenditure as a need proxy, structural inequities lowered recorded costs for Black patients despite higher burden, leading to systematic under-classification and fewer preventive services. The bias reflected a misaligned objective and absence of fairness audits or intersectional validation [5,6,16]. Replacing cost with clinical indicators (chronic conditions, labs) reduced the δTPR gap by over 80% and improved calibration parity, underscoring value-sensitive design and subgroup validation [37,65].

4.2 Case Study 2: Demographic Skew in Medical Imaging

In dermatology and radiology, AI often underperforms for racially diverse patients. Najjar et al. [48,55] found classifiers trained on light skin images had lower melanoma detection on darker skin due to underrepresentation and limited subgroup testing [25,33]. Mitigations included data augmentation, domain adaptation, and federated learning [32,38]. Reporting sensitivity by Fitzpatrick type and tracking δAUC improved parity; adding metadata on skin tone, ethnicity, and modality yielded further gains, linking fairness to representation and transparent evaluation.

4.3 Comparative Framework Analysis

Table 1 summarizes fairness interventions across the Equity-by-Design lifecycle, highlighting strengths, trade-offs, and applicability. Future studies should report both performance and fairness metrics (δTPR, δAUC, calibration error) to ensure clinical and ethical accountability. Algorithmic bias is systemic rather than isolated. The framework shows how proactive, metrics-based oversight embeds fairness auditing and ethical reflexivity, shifting governance from reactive fixes to sustained equity integration.

Table 1. Key fairness interventions across the healthcare AI lifecycle

Lifecycle Stage	Techniques	Notes/Impact
Data Sourcing	Representative sampling, inclusive datasets, federated learning [2,32,33]	Improves diversity and privacy; requires coordination and quality control.
Model Development	Fairness-aware loss, adversarial debiasing [6,16,65]	Embeds fairness early; possible accuracy trade-offs.
Validation	Stratified testing, external datasets [28,47,48]	Reveals subgroup bias; depends on annotated, diverse data.
Deployment	Feedback loops, clinician overrides [24,74]	Enables real-time oversight; needs clinician engagement.
Post-market	Drift tracking, equity dashboards, audits [13,43,66]	Monitors fairness over time; resource-intensive.

5 Discussion and Policy Implications

Equitable, trustworthy AI is a sociopolitical, ethical, and institutional challenge as much as a technical one. Effective fairness requires alignment of regulation, clinical workflows, and sociotechnical infrastructure. We examine regulatory coherence, adoption barriers, and social dynamics shaping healthcare AI governance.

5.1 Regulatory Alignment

Oversight for AI in healthcare is maturing but uneven. The EU AI Act classifies most healthcare AI as "high risk", requiring transparency, human oversight, and accountability [12,17,35], aligning with Equity-by-Design through lifecycle monitoring and documentation. The US FDA advances SaMD oversight via GMLP [36,54], though fairness and demographic accountability remain secondary [20,66]. Equity-by-Design maps to EU AI Act Articles 9–15, FDA GMLP and SaMD, and Australia's APP and TGA, linking ethical checkpoints to legal clauses for interoperable compliance [13,46].

5.2 Challenges in Clinical Adoption

Clinical adoption faces data inconsistency, EHR interoperability gaps, and costly retraining [10,48], especially in low-resource settings. Limited AI literacy fuels skepticism and underuse [24,37], while opacity restricts interpretability in high-stakes care [4,18,67]. Solutions include user-centered, explainable systems with embedded training. A pragmatic roadmap integrates audit and feedback within 8–12 weeks, offsetting costs via efficiency gains. Validation should assess accuracy, usability, workflow fit, and context [1,43].

5.3 Socio-Technical Considerations

AI operates within human and institutional ecosystems where equity, accountability, and fair outcomes are central [42,45]. Human-AI collaboration should emphasize augmentation that preserves clinician agency. Stakeholder roles include clinical AI translators, fairness auditors, data stewards, governance officers, legal experts, and patient representatives, each contributing at defined reviews [11,14,23]. Meaningful engagement with patients and marginalized communities through participatory design, consultation, and independent oversight strengthens legitimacy and reduces inequities [2,70]. Applied across regulatory, institutional, and technical domains, Equity-by-Design offers a scalable roadmap for equitable, transparent, socially responsible AI.

6 Conclusion and Future Work

AI is reshaping medicine through data-driven insights and decision support, yet without robust governance it can reinforce inequities and undermine trust. This paper presented the *Equity-by-Design* framework, a proactive lifecycle model embedding fairness, transparency, and accountability across data sourcing, development, validation, deployment, and monitoring. Bias is a systemic outcome of social and institutional imbalance, requiring mechanisms that promote justice, dignity, and contextual awareness. The framework urges co-design, adaptive auditing, and transparency structures that empower clinicians and patients.

Case studies showed that flawed proxies and underrepresented data perpetuate inequities and weaken credibility. Early fairness integration mitigates risks and bolsters reliability, safety, and public confidence.

To advance ethical AI in healthcare, we propose five priorities:

1. **Fairness Audits:** Embed adaptive audits within MLOps to reflect evolving clinical realities.
2. **Global Standards:** Harmonize regulations to promote equitable, trustworthy AI.
3. **Human-AI Collaboration:** Build user-centered systems that enhance clinical judgment.
4. **Continuous Oversight:** Maintain iterative governance and model refinement.

5. **Transparency for Trust:** Use model cards, impact assessments, and open reporting for accountability.

Sustaining equitable AI requires translating ethics into measurable practice. Future work should refine fairness metrics for real-world disparities, advance privacy-preserving models such as federated learning, and strengthen governance linking AI, institutions, and communities. Modular ethics-by-design toolkits and participatory co-design can enable responsible AI in resource-limited settings. The goal is systems that act fairly, transparently, and in service of health equity. Embedding equity as a design foundation reimagines digital healthcare as a driver of justice and inclusion. The Equity-by-Design framework offers a roadmap toward this vision, with longitudinal tracking of indicators (δTPR, δcalibration, cost-benefit ratios) essential for lasting ethical impact.

References

1. Ahuja, A.S.: The impact of artificial intelligence in medicine on the future role of the physician. PeerJ **7**, e7702 (2019)
2. Albahri, A.S., et al.: A systematic review of trustworthy and explainable artificial intelligence in healthcare: assessment of quality, bias risk, and data fusion. Inf. Fusion **96**, 156–191 (2023)
3. Almeida-Galárraga, D., Tirado-Espín, A.: Acceptability of ai in medical diagnostics: a discourse analysis. Commun. Appl. Technol. Proc. ICOMTA 2024 **427**, 383 (2025)
4. Amann, J., Blasimme, A., Vayena, E., Frey, D., Madai, V.I., Consortium, P.: Explainability for artificial intelligence in healthcare: a multidisciplinary perspective. BMC Med. Inform. Decis. Mak. **20**, 1–9 (2020)
5. Mennella, C., et al.: Anonymous: ethical and regulatory challenges of ai technologies in healthcare. Heliyon **10**(4) (2024). https://doi.org/10.1016/j.heliyon.2024.e26297
6. Arnold, M.: Teasing out artificial intelligence in medicine: an ethical critique of artificial intelligence and machine learning in medicine. J. Bioeth. Inq **18**(1), 121–139 (2021)
7. Bartoletti, I.: AI in healthcare: ethical and privacy challenges. In: Riaño, D., Wilk, S., ten Teije, A. (eds.) AIME 2019. LNCS (LNAI), vol. 11526, pp. 7–10. Springer, Cham (2019). https://doi.org/10.1007/978-3-030-21642-9_2
8. Beam, A.L., Drazen, J.M., Kohane, I.S., Leong, T.Y., Manrai, A.K., Rubin, E.J.: Artificial intelligence in medicine (2023)
9. Bekbolatova, M., Mayer, J., Ong, C.W., Toma, M.: Transformative potential of ai in healthcare: definitions, applications, and navigating the ethical landscape and public perspectives. Healthc. **12**(125) (2024). https://doi.org/10.3390/healthcare12020125
10. Bekbolatova, M., Mayer, J., Ong, C.W., Toma, M.: Transformative potential of ai in healthcare: definitions, applications, and navigating the ethical landscape and public perspectives. In: Healthcare, vol. 12, p. 125. MDPI (2024)
11. Blease, C., Kaptchuk, T.J., Bernstein, M.H., Mandl, K.D., Halamka, J.D., DesRoches, C.M.: Artificial intelligence and the future of primary care: exploratory qualitative study of uk general practitioners' views. J. Med. Internet Res. **21**(3), e12802 (2019)

12. Bouderhem, R.: Shaping the future of ai in healthcare through ethics and governance. Humanit. Soc. Sci. Commun. **11**(1), 1–12 (2024)
13. Char, D.S., Abràmoff, M.D., Feudtner, C.: Identifying ethical considerations for machine learning healthcare applications. Am. J. Bioeth. **20**(11), 7–17 (2020)
14. Chauhan, C., Gullapalli, R.R.: Ethics of ai in pathology: current paradigms and emerging issues. Artif. Intell. Pathol. 159–180 (2025)
15. Chen, I.Y., Pierson, E., Rose, S., Joshi, S., Ferryman, K., Ghassemi, M.: Ethical machine learning in healthcare. Annual Rev. Biomed. Data Sci. **4**(1), 123–144 (2021)
16. Chen, R.J., Wang, J.J., Williamson, D.F., Chen, T.Y., Lipkova, J., Lu, M.Y., Sahai, S., Mahmood, F.: Algorithmic fairness in artificial intelligence for medicine and healthcare. Nat. Biomed. Engg. **7**(6), 719–742 (2023)
17. Corfmat, M., Martineau, J.T., Régis, C.: High-reward, high-risk technologies? an ethical and legal account of ai development in healthcare. BMC Med. Ethics **26**(1), 4 (2025)
18. Durán, J.M., Jongsma, K.R.: Who is afraid of black box algorithms? on the epistemological and ethical basis of trust in medical ai. J. Med. Ethics **47**(5), 329–335 (2021)
19. El-Sherif, D.M., Abouzid, M., Elzarif, M.T., Ahmed, A.A., Albakri, A., Alshehri, M.M.: Telehealth and artificial intelligence insights into healthcare during the covid-19 pandemic. In: Healthcare, vol. 10, p. 385. MDPI (2022)
20. Farhud, D.D., Zokaei, S.: Ethical issues of artificial intelligence in medicine and healthcare. Iran. J. Public Health **50**(11), i (2021)
21. Ganesan, S., Somasiri, N., et al.: Navigating the integration of machine learning in healthcare: challenges, strategies, and ethical considerations. J. Comput. Cognitive Engg. **4**(1), 8–23 (2024)
22. Geis, J.R., et al.: Ethics of artificial intelligence in radiology: summary of the joint european and north american multisociety statement. Radiology **293**(2), 436–440 (2019)
23. Goirand, M., Austin, E., Clay-Williams, R.: Implementing ethics in healthcare ai-based applications: a scoping review. Sci. Eng. Ethics **27**(5), 61 (2021)
24. Grunhut, J., Marques, O., Wyatt, A.T.: Needs, challenges, and applications of artificial intelligence in medical education curriculum. JMIR Med. Edu. **8**(2), e35587 (2022)
25. Grzybowski, A., Jin, K., Wu, H.: Challenges of artificial intelligence in medicine and dermatology. Clin. Dermatol. **42**(3), 210–215 (2024)
26. Habli, I., Lawton, T., Porter, Z.: Artificial intelligence in health care: accountability and safety. Bull. World Health Organ. **98**(4), 251 (2020)
27. Holmes, J., Sacchi, L., Bellazzi, R., et al.: Artificial intelligence in medicine. Ann. R. Coll. Surg. Engl. **86**, 334–8 (2004)
28. Hossain, M.I., Zamzmi, G., Mouton, P.R., Salekin, M.S., Sun, Y., Goldgof, D.: Explainable ai for medical data: current methods, limitations, and future directions. ACM Comput. Surv. **57**(6), 1–46 (2025)
29. Huynh, E., et al.: Artificial intelligence in radiation oncology. Nat. Rev. Clin. Oncol. **17**(12), 771–781 (2020)
30. Iqbal, M.J., et al.: Clinical applications of artificial intelligence and machine learning in cancer diagnosis: looking into the future. Cancer Cell Int. **21**(1), 270 (2021)
31. Jimma, B.L.: Artificial intelligence in healthcare: a bibliometric analysis. Telematics Inf. Rep. **9**, 100041 (2023)

32. Kaissis, G.A., Makowski, M.R., Rückert, D., Braren, R.F.: Secure, privacy-preserving and federated machine learning in medical imaging. Nat. Mach. Intell. **2**(6), 305–311 (2020)
33. Khalid, N., Qayyum, A., Bilal, M., Al-Fuqaha, A., Qadir, J.: Privacy-preserving artificial intelligence in healthcare: Techniques and applications. Comput. Biol. Med. **158**, 106848 (2023)
34. Koçak, B., et al.: Bias in artificial intelligence for medical imaging: fundamentals, detection, avoidance, mitigation, challenges, ethics, and prospects. Diagn. Interv. Radiol. **31**(2), 75 (2025)
35. Kotter, E., et al.: Guiding ai in radiology: Esr's recommendations for effective implementation of the european ai act. Insights Imaging **16**(1), 33 (2025)
36. Larson, D.B., Harvey, H., Rubin, D.L., Irani, N., Tse, J.R., Langlotz, C.P.: Regulatory frameworks for development and evaluation of artificial intelligence-based diagnostic imaging algorithms: summary and recommendations. J. Am. Coll. Radiol. **18**(3), 413–424 (2021)
37. Lee, E.E., et al.: Artificial intelligence for mental health care: clinical applications, barriers, facilitators, and artificial wisdom. Bio. Psychiatr. Cog. Neurosci. Neuroimaging **6**(9), 856–864 (2021)
38. Li, F., Ruijs, N., Lu, Y.: Ethics & ai: a systematic review on ethical concerns and related strategies for designing with ai in healthcare. Ai **4**(1), 28–53 (2022)
39. Lindsay, D.: An exploration of the conceptual basis of privacy and the implications for the future of australian privacy law. Melbourne Univ. Law Rev. **29**(1), 131–178 (2005)
40. Liu, P., Lu, L., Zhang, J., Huo, T., Liu, S., Ye, Z.: Application of artificial intelligence in medicine: an overview. Current Med. Sci. **41**(6), 1105–1115 (2021)
41. Mahler, M., Auza, C., Albesa, R., Melus, C., Wu, J.A.: Regulatory aspects of artificial intelligence and machine learning-enabled software as medical devices (samd). In: Precision Medicine and Artificial Intelligence, pp. 237–265. Elsevier (2021)
42. McCradden, M.D., Joshi, S., Mazwi, M., Anderson, J.A.: Ethical limitations of algorithmic fairness solutions in health care machine learning. Lancet Digital Health **2**(5), e221–e223 (2020)
43. Megerian, J.T., et al.: Evaluation of an artificial intelligence-based medical device for diagnosis of autism spectrum disorder. NPJ Digit. Med. **5**(1), 57 (2022)
44. Mishra, R., Satpathy, R., Pati, B.: Interpretable ai in medical imaging: enhancing diagnostic accuracy through human-computer interaction. J. Artif. Intell. Sys. **6**(1), 96–111 (2024)
45. Morley, J., et al.: The ethics of ai in health care: a mapping review. Soc. Sci. Med. **260**, 113172 (2020)
46. Murphy, K., et al.: Artificial intelligence for good health: a scoping review of the ethics literature. BMC Med. Ethics **22**, 1–17 (2021)
47. Najjar, R.: Redefining radiology: a review of artificial intelligence integration in medical imaging. Diagnostics **13**(2760), (2023). https://doi.org/10.3390/diagnostics13172760
48. Najjar, R.: Redefining radiology: a review of artificial intelligence integration in medical imaging. Diagnostics **13**(17), 2760 (2023)
49. Nanjundan, P., Indu, P., Thomas, L.: Navigating the ethical landscape of artificial intelligence: challenges, frameworks, and responsible deployment. In: Artificial Intelligence Technologies for Engineering Applications, pp. 1–13. CRC Press (2025)
50. Nasir, S., Khan, R.A., Bai, S.: Ethical framework for harnessing the power of ai in healthcare and beyond. IEEE Access **12**, 31014–31035 (2024)

51. Nazar, M., Alam, M.M., Yafi, E., Su'ud, M.M.: A systematic review of human–computer interaction and explainable artificial intelligence in healthcare with artificial intelligence techniques. IEEE Access **9**, 153316–153348 (2021)
52. Nowrozy, R., Ahmed, K.: A systematic survey on ai governance in healthcare. ACM Comput. Surv. (2024)
53. Nowrozy, R.: A security and privacy compliant data sharing solution for healthcare data ecosystems. Ph.D. Thesis, Victoria University (2024)
54. Nowrozy, R., Ahmed, K.: Enhancing health information systems security: an ontology model approach. In: International Conference on Health Information Science, pp. 91–100. Springer, Singapore (2023). https://doi.org/10.1007/978-981-99-7108-4_8
55. Nowrozy, R., Ahmed, K., Wang, H.: Artificial intelligence in enhancing electronic health record systems: a comprehensive survey. In: International Conference on Health Information Science, pp. 1–16. Springer, Singapore (2024). https://doi.org/10.1007/978-981-96-5597-7_1
56. Nowrozy, R., Ahmed, K., Wang, H.: Gpt, ontology, and caabac: a tripartite personalized access control model anchored by compliance, context and attribute. PLoS ONE **20**(1), e0310553 (2025)
57. Nowrozy, R., Ahmed, K., Wang, H., Mcintosh, T.: Towards a universal privacy model for electronic health record systems: an ontology and machine learning approach. In: Informatics, vol. 10, p. 60. MDPI (2023)
58. Nowrozy, R., et al.: A blockchain-based secure data sharing framework for healthcare. In: Blockchain for Cybersecurity and Privacy, pp. 219–241. CRC Press (2020)
59. Ntjamba, F.C., Ashipala, D.O.: Impact on and ethical considerations of artificial intelligence on human healthcare. In: AI Technologies and Advancements for Psychological Well-Being and Healthcare, pp. 1–36. IGI Global (2025)
60. Obermeyer, Z., Powers, B., Vogeli, C., Mullainathan, S.: Dissecting racial bias in an algorithm used to manage the health of populations. Sci. **366**(6464), 447–453 (2019)
61. Pantelopoulos, A., Bourbakis, N.G.: A survey on wearable sensor-based systems for health monitoring and prognosis. IEEE Trans. Sys. Man Cybern. Part C Appl. Rev. **40**(1), 1–12 (2009)
62. Patrício, C., Neves, J.C., Teixeira, L.F.: Explainable deep learning methods in medical image classification: a survey. ACM Comput. Surv. **56**(4), 1–41 (2023)
63. Petersson, L., et al.: Challenges to implementing artificial intelligence in healthcare: a qualitative interview study with healthcare leaders in sweden. BMC Health Serv. Res. **22**(1), 850 (2022)
64. Priyadarshi, R., Ranjan, R., Vishwakarma, A.K., Yang, T., Rathore, R.S.: Exploring the frontiers of unsupervised learning techniques for diagnosis of cardiovascular disorder: a systematic review. IEEE Access (2024)
65. Rasheed, K., Qayyum, A., Ghaly, M., Al-Fuqaha, A., Razi, A., Qadir, J.: Explainable, trustworthy, and ethical machine learning for healthcare: a survey. Comput. Biol. Med. **149**, 106043 (2022)
66. Reddy, S., Allan, S., Coghlan, S., Cooper, P.: A governance model for the application of ai in health care. J. Am. Med. Inform. Assoc. **27**(3), 491–497 (2020)
67. Reyes, M., et al.: On the interpretability of artificial intelligence in radiology: challenges and opportunities. Radiol. Artif. Intell. **2**(3), e190043 (2020)
68. Sand, M., Durán, J.M., Jongsma, K.R.: Responsibility beyond design: physicians' requirements for ethical medical ai. Bioeth. **36**(2), 162–169 (2022)

69. Shrotriya, V., Jain, M.A., Shrivastava, P., Sharma, P.: Exploring iot solutions for connecting and synchronizing various maternal health monitoring devices. Interdisciplinary Work of Science and Technology in Maternal and Child Care, p. 100 (2019)
70. Siala, H., Wang, Y.: Shifting artificial intelligence to be responsible in healthcare: a systematic review. Soc. Sci. Med. **296**, 114782 (2022)
71. Stogiannos, N., Georgiadou, E., Rarri, N., Malamateniou, C.: Ethical ai: a qualitative study exploring ethical challenges and solutions on the use of ai in medical imaging. Euro. J. Radiol. Artif. Intell. **1**, 100006 (2025)
72. Sun, T.Q., Medaglia, R.: Mapping the challenges of artificial intelligence in the public sector: evidence from public healthcare. Gov. Inf. Q. **36**(2), 368–383 (2019)
73. Theriault-Lauzier, P., et al.: A responsible framework for applying artificial intelligence on medical images and signals at the point-of-care: the pacs-ai platform. Canadian J. Cardiol. **40**(10), 1828–1840 (2024)
74. Thompson, R.F., et al.: Artificial intelligence in radiation oncology: a specialty-wide disruptive transformation? Radiother. Oncol. **129**(3), 421–426 (2018)
75. Vaisman, A., et al.: Artificial intelligence, diagnostic imaging and neglected tropical diseases: ethical implications. Bull. World Health Organ. **98**(4), 288 (2020)
76. Veale, M., Borgesius, F.Z.: Demystifying the draft Eu artificial intelligence act. arXiv preprint http://arxiv.org/abs/2107.03721arXiv:2107.03721 (2021)
77. Zahlan, A., Ranjan, R.P., Hayes, D.: Artificial intelligence innovation in healthcare: literature review, exploratory analysis, and future research. Technol. Soc. **74**, 102321 (2023)
78. Zangana, H.M., Sallow, Z.B., Salih, B.A.: The impact of artificial intelligence on healthcare: a systematic review of innovations, challenges, and ethical considerations. J. Comput. Digit. Bus. **4**(1), 1–9 (2025)
79. Zhang, J., Zhang, Z.: Ethics and governance of trustworthy medical artificial intelligence. BMC Med. Infor. Decis. Making. **23**(1), 7 (2023)

Work Performance: Perspectives from Social Media Use and Its Implications for Early Detection of Mental Health

Ramadhana Kusuma Adiputra, Fitriyah Rachmawati, Eka Agus Sanjaya, and Anita Maharani(✉)

Management Department, BINUS Business School Master Program, BINUS University, Jakarta, Indonesia
ramadhana.adiputra@binus.ac.id, anita.maharani@binus.edu

Abstract. Through this research, we explore the effect of social media use on employee performance. However, social media use is divided into two categories: work and personal, with work stress as a mediator. We collect data through online survey, from December 2024 to February 2025, resulting in 73 returned surveys from specific one construction company. To analyse the data, we utilize partial least squares structural equation modeling (PLS-SEM), in two-stage process, first initial validation of the measurement assesment, then structural assesment. Results indicated that both personal and professional social media use have a positive impact on employee performance. Findings showed the potential for social media interactions in the workplace to facilitate early detection of mental health issues and provide actionable implications for organizational strategies and initiatives to improve employee well-being.

Keywords: Social Media Use · Work Stress · Work Performance · Early Detection of Mental Health

1 Introduction

Social media existed within the society, and the effect of its existence might altering communication patterns, information dissemination, social interactions, and psychological health. Research showed its influence extends across multiple domains of daily life, and it redefines on how people connect, consume content, and experiencing emotional states [1]. Interesting fact, when in the workplace, social media is now unavoidable, and despite its effect, it has the possibility of influencing employee voice, transparency, and moreover engagement [2]. However, the use of social media also might raise concerns, particularly regarding mental health.

Excessive social media engagement during work hours, might related to physical conditions such as sleep deprivation, physical discomfort, and nonphysical that is psychological issues such as the phenomena of fear of missing out, superficial relationships, and reduced productivity [3]. Work-related social media use, however, can alleviate

E. R. Kaburuan and S. Goundar (Eds.): HIS 2025, LNCS 16392, pp. 13–21, 2026.
https://doi.org/10.1007/978-981-95-6304-3_2

psychological strain [4], and its dual nature, enhancing connectivity while threatening genuine social bonds [5] demands further exploration.

This study seeks to explore how social media use affects work performance, with work stress as a mediator. Additionally, it explores how early detection of mental health signals through social media could inform organizational strategies to enhance productivity and well-being.

2 Literature Review and Hypothesis Development

Excessive use of social media, specifically in working environment may become a significant predictor of job overload, which can ultimately have a negative impact not only emotionally but also on job performance [6]. However, if social media is utilized for work purposes, there is a possibility that it can affect work stress, and even strengthen the beneficial relationship between employees facing stress at work and of course their work performance [7].

Hypothesis 1: Work stress affected by social media use for work negatively

When social media is utilized for non-professional activities, it has the potential to cause problems [8]. The use of social media during work hours might related to a fear of missing out, then compulsive use, and ultimately there will be a potential decline in overall work performance [4].

Hypothesis 2: Work stress affected by social media use for personal purpose negatively

However, using social media at work may also be able to build stronger connections among employees and encourage the sharing of knowledge, ultimately leading to improved job performance [9]. Work oriented social media use might generate synergies that will benefit to improve team and employee performance [10].

Hypothesis 3: Work performance affected by social media use for work purpose positively

Social media platforms may be able to enhance the development of employee social capital and serve as conduits for knowledge sharing, thereby exerting a positive influence on work performance [9]. Technically, even using social media like Facebook® and KakaoTalk® in the workplace improves job performance [11].

Hypothesis 4: Work performance affected by social media use for personal purposes positively

Employees experiencing in stress when using social media are more likely to feel burnt out and anxious, which ultimately will weaken job performance [12]. Moreover, the overuse of social media overuse in workplace might negatively affects employee work performance through employee work stress [3].

Hypothesis 5: Work stress mediates the effect of social media use for work purpose to work performance.

Excessive social media use in the work environment may cause anxiety, depression, tension, and cognitive overload, impairing professional, personal connections and real-life interactions [13]. Excessive use of social media when someone in their work environment leads to exhaustion, which significantly reduces job performance [14].

Hypothesis 6: social media use for personal purposes has a negative effect on work performance through work stress.

High levels of stress in the workplace are associated with low job satisfaction, high absenteeism, low productivity, and high turnover rates [15]. Work stress negatively affects employee performance also found in Karim [16].

Hypothesis 7: Work stress have a negative effect on work performance.

3 Method

This research adopts a quantitative, deductive methodology, with minimal researcher involvement. Individuals are the analytical focus in this cross-sectional study. Probability sampling, specifically stratified random sampling, is used to select participants from the employee population. A response rate of at least 60%, as suggested by Fincham et al. [17], is targeted. Data collection relies on questionnaires, with variable measurements based on established studies: social media use [18]; work stress [19]; and work performance [20]. Partial least squares structural equation modeling (PLS-SEM) is the chosen data analysis technique, featuring measurement and structural model evaluation. To guarantee the relevance of measurement items, a pre-test is administered to 30 randomly chosen respondents outside the study's target group, aiming to establish face validity. The pre-test data undergoes reliability testing via factor analysis and validity testing using r-count.

4 Results and Discussions

4.1 Results

To ensure that all items used in this study can be used to measure the problems represented through the dynamics between variables, the researcher conducted a pre-test by distributing all respondent items to 30 respondents. The pre-test itself was carried out for five days from December 18, 2024 to December 23, 2024. Using the online formula, namely https://forms.gle/PXcjRvyDkWXfGBASA, the following reliability and validity test results were obtained.

When we conduct pre-test, we found out two items were not reliable since the result unable to fulfill the standar based on cronbach's alpha, the two items were from social media use for work purpose, and from work performance.

Based on Table 1., above, it is known that there are two unreliable items. If the item does not meet reliability, the researcher has the discretion not to use it at the stage of distributing the questionnaire which aims to test the hypothesis [21]. However, the researcher still could assess the quality of the data through a validity test, as follows.

Also, there are several invalid items, and the reason might be because the items intended to measure the variables are not really understood by the respondents, or sensitizing, therefore the effort that can be made is to revise the statement items. The non valid items are excluded since the result unable to fulfill alpha 0,05 (df = 30).

After the pre-test, the researcher then distributed data for the research hypothesis testing stage. Data distribution was carried out from January 17, 2025, to February 14, 2025, and resulted in 73 respondents. Based on the previously set respondent target, the number of 73 people has reached 66.07%, and referring to Fincham's view [17], it was stated that the number of responses that reached more than 60% of the target sample can be continued for the data analysis stage.

Based on the respondent profile, the results of this study will represent the above characteristic groups, where majority are within 26–35 years old, male, and believes social media use will be useful in the workplace.

The parameters used to decide whether the construct validity results are ideal or otherwise based on Hair et al. [18], the results must be able to meet criteria's, as follow: Cronbach's alpha > 0,7; Composite reliability rho_a > = 0,7; Composite reliability rho_c > = 0,7; Average variance extracted > = 0,5. From the table, it may conclude that all has met the requirements.

Then for the discriminant validity results, it has been fulfilled because based on the reference, the ideal HTMT value is < 0.900 and all diagonal correlations have been fulfilled and can be continued to the next stage of analysis, namely the fit model, and all criteria is based on Hair et al. [18].

Then, for the fit model, based on the parameters SRMS < 0.08, NFI > 0.90 [18], where for SRMR it is fulfilled while for NFI it is below the specified parameters, thus indicating that the model's suitability to the existing conditions has not been fulfilled, although it cannot be called bad either.

Finally, in this measurement model assessment, from R-Square, there is a potential of 43.3 percent of the phenomenon that refers to the independent variables in this study, namely social media use for work purposes and social media use for personal use to influence work performance with work stress as a mediator (Fig. 1).

After all stages in the measurement model assessment are completed, the next stage is the structural model assessment. This stage is also known as bootstrapping, the purpose of which is to test the hypothesis. In this stage, the researcher will make decisions related to the conclusion of the hypothesis based on the P-values and t-statistics, and it can be concluded that there are four unsupported hypotheses (H1, H5, H6, H7), and three others are supported (H2, H3, and H4). Therefore, the next stage is that the researcher will discuss each result of the hypothesis testing above (Fig. 2).

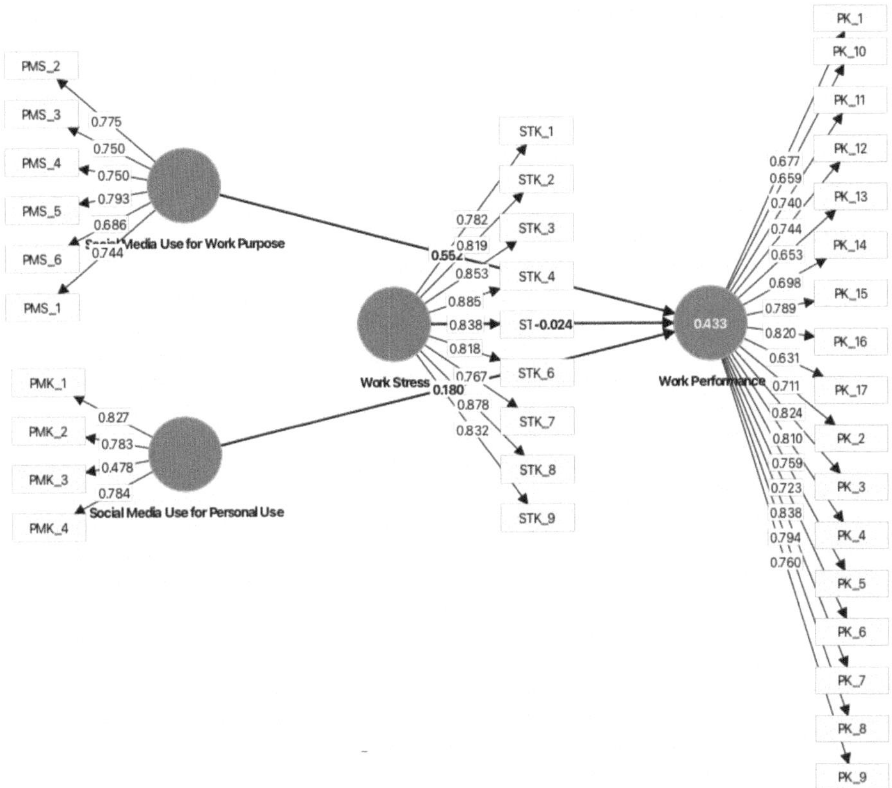

Fig. 1. Measurement Model Assessment Visual

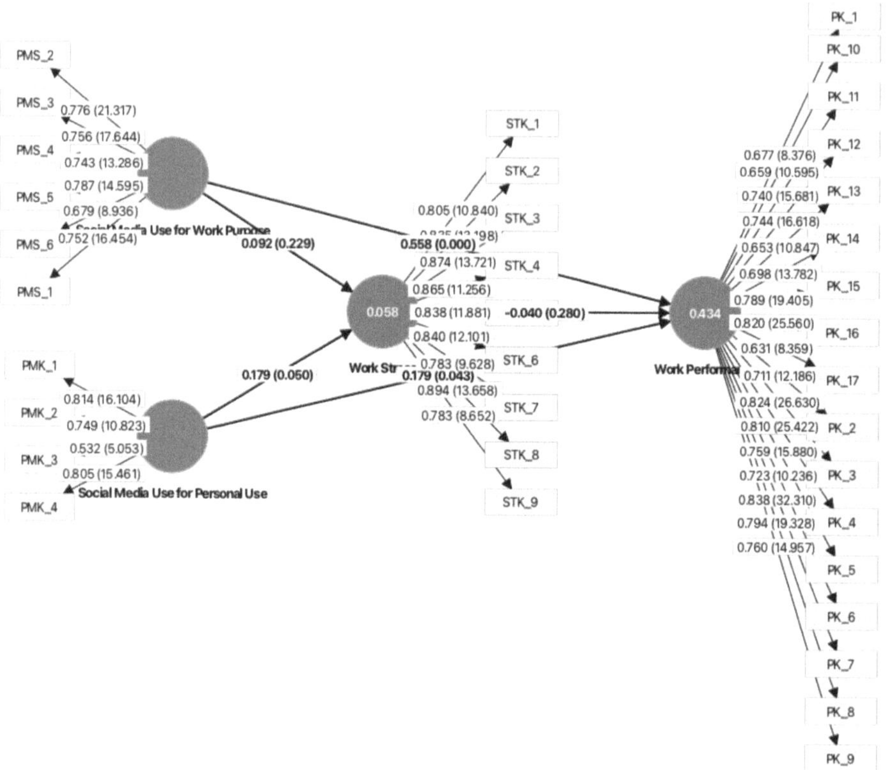

Fig. 2. Structural Model Assessment Visual

5 Discussions

From the results of the statistical tests above, of the seven hypotheses proposed, four hypotheses are not supported, and three others are supported. Several backgrounds can be associated with the unsupported hypothesis, among others, the impacts that are considered to exist can vary. In the context of this study, the research respondents also determine the direction of the results of this study.

Our proposed hypothesis one indicates that the use of social media in the workplace for work purposes does not cause increased stress in employees. This result is certainly contrary to previous studies [6, 7].

Then in hypothesis two indicates when employees use social media in the work environment, it has the possibility to lower work stress. In other words, the more social media is used in the work environment, the higher the stress a person will experience compared to those who do not use it, this could prove that the use of social media raises a number of psychological phenomena, that are fear of missing out and compulsive use [4, 8].

The results of this study show that the use of social media in the work environment for work purposes, can have a positive impact on employee performance. In this case, it supports previous research [9, 10]. Social media in principle is communicating using the internet, and where there is an exchange of information, ideas and so on. Therefore, with the support of this hypothesis, social media use in the workplace needs to be accompanied by the requirement, a form of sharing information and or ideas.

This study supports the proposed hypothesis and previous studies, namely that the use of social media in the workplace for personal purposes has a positive effect on employee work performance. This finding indicates that the wise use of social media for personal purposes can serve as a means of relaxation and stress relief for employees. Thus, employees can return to work with a fresher and more focused mind, which ultimately increases their productivity and performance, and social media, in this context, can be one form of effective rest.

Results of a study [12] showed that social stressors and technical stressors experienced by employees when using social media were related to fatigue and anxiety, but this research showed in contrary, which ultimately had a negative impact on their work performance. These findings highlight the complexity of the relationship between social media use, stress, and work performance. Further research is needed to identify other potentially relevant mediators, as well as to understand how different types of stressors (social, technical, and others) interact and affect performance. In addition, research with a longitudinal design can provide deeper insight into the direction of causality between these variables.

Research showed that excessive use of social media at work can cause anxiety, depression, tension, and cognitive overload, which ultimately interferes with professional, personal relationships, and real-world interactions, and this research is contrary with the previous study [13]. These findings do not support the proposed hypothesis, namely that the use of social media at work for personal purposes has a negative effect on employee job performance through the mediation of job stress. This indicates that other factors may play a role in explaining the relationship between social media use and decreased performance.

High levels of stress in the workplace are associated with low job satisfaction, high absenteeism, low productivity, and high employee turnover [15], but this research showed contrary. However, these findings do not support the proposed hypothesis, where employee's work stress have a negative effect on work performance. This indicates that other factors may play a role in explaining the relationship.

6 Conclusion, Suggestion, and Limitation

6.1 Conclusions

The consequences from this study show social media use for work purposes does not increase job stress, contrary to some previous studies; social media use for personal purposes increases job stress; social media use for work purposes increases job performance; social media use for personal purposes also increases job performance. In other words, overall, this study shows that the impact of social media use in the workplace is complex and depends on the purpose of use.

6.2 Suggestion

Organizations should implement adaptable social media policies that balance professional and personal usage. By clearly differentiating between work-related and private activities, companies can harness these platforms to enhance internal communication and teamwork while boosting productivity.

6.3 Limitations

This study claimed that the effects of workplace social media use are context-dependent, meaning findings may not apply universally. Although psychological concepts like *fear of missing out* and *compulsive use* were referenced, their measurement and analysis lacked depth, restricting a nuanced understanding of these phenomena.

7 Disclosure of Interests.

The is no competing interests.

Acknowledgments. This paper is part of co-hosting conferences participation from BINUS University. Ramadhana, Fitriyah, and Eka write concepts, and analysis, while Anita supervises the writing. Data may access through: https://drive.google.com/drive/folders/1CwCo4QjP4VhGhX4ij2k0h54SGnlYu8dK?usp=sharing.

References

1. Zhang, Y.: The impact of social media on all aspects of people. In: 3rd International Conference on Interdisciplinary Humanities and Communication Studies (2024)
2. Ghani, B., Malik, M.A.R.: Social Media and employee voice: a comprehensive literature review. Behav. Inf. Technol. **42**(14), 2407–2427 (2022). https://doi.org/10.1080/0144929X.2022.2126329
3. Priyadarshini, C., Dubey, R.K., Kumar, Y., Jha, R.R.: Impacts of social media addiction on employee's wellbeing and work productivity. Qual. Rep. **25**(1), 181–196 (2020). https://doi.org/10.46743/2160-3715/2020.4099
4. Tandon, A., Dhir, A., Islam, N., Talwar, S., Mantymaki, M.: Psychological and behavioral outcomes of social media-induced fear of missing out at the workplace. J. Bus. Res. **136**, 186–197 (2021). https://doi.org/10.1016/j.jbusres.2021.07.036
5. Sujon, Z., Dyer, H.T.: Understanding the social in a digital age. New Media Soc. **22**(7), 1125–1134 (2020). https://doi.org/10.1177/1461444820912531
6. Yu, L., Zhong, Y., Sun, Y.: The impact of excessive social media use at work: a usage of experience-stressor-strain perspective. Behav. Inf. Technol. **42**(7), 985–1004 (2021). https://doi.org/10.1080/0144929X.2022.2054358
7. Wu, S., Pitafi, A.H., Pitafi, S., Ren, M.: Investigating the consequences of the socio-instrumental use of enterprise social media on employee work efficiency: a work-stress environment. Front. Psychol. **12**, 738118 (2021). https://doi.org/10.3389/fpsyg.2021.738118
8. Cao, X., Yu, L.: Exploring the influence of excessive social media use at work: a three-dimension usage perspective. Int. J. Inf. Manag. **46**, 83–92 (2019). https://doi.org/10.1016/j.ijinfomgt.2018.11.019

9. Cao, X., Guo, X., Vogel, D., Zhang, X.: Exploring the influence of social media on employee work performance. Internet Res. **26**(2), 529–545 (2016). https://doi.org/10.1108/IntR-11-2014-0299
10. Song, Q., Wang, Y., Chen, Y., Benitez, J., Hu, J.: Impact of the usage of social media in the workplace on team and employee performance. Inf. Manag. **56**(8), 103160 (2019). https://doi.org/10.1016/J.IM.2019.04.003
11. Lee, S.Y., Lee, S.W.: Social Media use and job performance in the workplace: the effects of facebook and kakaotalk use on job performance in South Korea. Sustainability **12**(10), 4052 (2020). https://doi.org/10.3390/su12104052
12. Cao, X., Xu, C., Ali, A.: A socio-technical system perspective to exploring the negative effects of social media on work performance. Aslib J. Inf. Manag. **76**(2), 233–247 (2023). https://doi.org/10.1108/ajim-05-2022-0275
13. Stieger, S., Wunderl, S.: Associations between social media use and cognitive abilities: results from a large-scale study study of adolescents. Comput. Hum. Behav. **135**, 107358 (2022). https://doi.org/10.1016/j.chb.2022.107358
14. Yu, L., Cao, X., Liu, Z., Wang, J.: Excessive social media use at work: exploring the effects of social media overload on job performance. Inf. Technol. People **31**(6), 1091–1112 (2018). https://doi.org/10.1108/ITP-10-2016-0237
15. Shah, B.: Work stress and employee performance: analysis of work stress and its implication on employee performance. Int. J. Indian Psychol. **11**(4), 322–335 (2023). https://doi.org/10.56642/brdu.v03i04.023
16. Karim, K.: The effect of work stress on employee performance. Asean Int. J. Bus. **1**(1), 24–33 (2022). https://doi.org/10.54099/aijb.v1i1.68
17. Fincham, J.E.: Response rates and responsivess for surveys, standards, and the journal. Am. J. Pharm. Educ. **72**(2), 43 (2008). https://doi.org/10.5688/aj720243
18. Gonzales, E., Leidner, D., Riemenschneider, C., Koch, H.: The impact of internal social media usage on organizational socialization and commitment. In: International Conference on Information Systems (ICIS 2013) (2013)
19. Shukla, A., Srivastava, R.: Examining the effect of emotional intelligence on socio-demographic variable and job stress among retail employees. Cogent Bus. Manag. **3**(1), 1201905 (2016). https://doi.org/10.1080/23311975.2016.1201905
20. Ramos-Villagrasa, P.J., Barrada, J.R., Fernandez-del-Rio, E., Koopmans, L.: Assessing job performance using brief self-report scales: the case of the individual work performance questionnaire. J. Work Organ. Psychol. **35**(3), 195–205 (2019)
21. Sekaran, U., Bougie, R.: Research Methods for Business: A Skill Building Approach. John Wiley & Sons, Hoboken (2019)

Design of Integrated Machine Learning-Bidirectional LSTM Hybrid Model for Gastric Cancer Risk Prediction Driven by Multimodal Data

Jia-Yu Cao[1], Hua-Min Chen[1(✉)], Shaofu Lin[1], Biyu Yao[2], and Yan-Hua Sun[1]

[1] Beijing University of Technology, Pingleyuan 100, Chaoyang District, Beijing 100124, China
chenhuamin@bjut.edu.cn

[2] People's Hospital of Yuhuan, Taizhou 317600, Zhejiang, China

Abstract. Gastric cancer has become one of the major diseases that affect people's lives. Early and timely screening can effectively improve the survival rate of patients. However, the reality is that relying on a single type of data for prediction has a certain gap from the ideal level, and many prediction models ignore the connection of rich contextual signals in medical information. To address this challenge, this study proposes a hybrid model integrating machine learning and Bidirectional Long Short-Term Memory Network (Bi-LSTM) based on multimodal time series data, which fuses clinical laboratory test results and textual information of gastroscopy results at different times. In the proposed model, the Bi-LSTM module with residual connections is designed to effectively extract long-term dependencies in medical time-series data to generate high-dimensional feature vectors. The integrated machine learning module of XGBoost, LightGBM and CatBoost is employed to process data in parallel. Through dynamic weighting by the dual-head attention mechanism of features and models, the fusion prediction results become more accurate. The provided results approve that the prediction accuracy can reach 95.74%,the area under the curve (AUC) is 96.89%, and the F1 score is 93.23%. The designed hybrid model facilitates rational allocation of medical resources, thereby enhancing trust in patient-doctor relationships and efficiency in gastric cancer care.

Keywords: Gastric Cancer · Risk Prediction · Bidirectional LSTM · Integrated Machine Learning

1 Introduction

Gastric cancer is one of the major diseases threatening human health [1]. According to the latest research results from the International Agency for Research on Cancer (IARC), there were approximately 1.08 million new gastric cancer cases globally in 2020, ranking sixth among all cancers [2]. Joint calculations by the National Cancer Center and the International Agency for Research on Cancer show that China has 358,700 new gastric

E. R. Kaburuan and S. Goundar (Eds.): HIS 2025, LNCS 16392, pp. 22–33, 2026.
https://doi.org/10.1007/978-981-95-6304-3_3

cancer cases and 260,400 deaths from gastric cancer each year, with the death toll ranking third among all cancers. Influenced by genetic factors and dietary habits preferring high-salt and pickled foods, gastric cancer is highly prevalent in East Asia [3]. In contrast, the survival rates for gastric cancer in Japan and South Korea both exceed 60%, while China's survival rate is 35.9%. It is predicted that by 2030, China will have 550,000 gastric cancer patients, and the mortality rate will rank third among all cancers, becoming a major public health issue [4]. According to a joint study conducted by the World Economic Forum and Boston Consulting Group, the global medical generative AI market was valued at approximately 2 billion USD in 2023 and is projected to reach 22 billion USD by 2027. The Chinese medical AI market is likewise experiencing significant growth, driven by supportive government policies and increasing healthcare demand. With a market size of around 20 billion RMB in 2023, it is anticipated to expand to 180 billion RMB by 2031. Furthermore, the adoption rate of AI technologies in primary care hospitals is expected to surpass 50% by 2025.Therefore, gastric cancer screening and risk prediction based on AI technology are very necessary, but the research in this area is not very comprehensive and sufficient.

The main contribution of this paper is a hybrid model integrating multiple machine learning and Bidirectional Long Short-Term Memory Network (Bi-LSTM) is proposed, where in multi-dimensional medical features are extracted to construct a dynamic feature matrix from the longitudinal examination sequence of patients. Based on the XGBoost, LightGBM and CatBoost models, a dual-head attention mechanism of features and model contribution rates is designed to support dynamic weight allocation by sample level learning for end-to-end joint optimization.

The rest of this paper is organized as following. Related work up to now is summarized in Sect. 2. Section 3 gives the details of the core technical content, including framework overview, data preprocessing, the design of time-series features extraction module based on bidirectional LSTM and the design of integrated machine learning models based on dual - head attention mechanism. Corresponding experimental design and results analysis is presented in Sect. 4, followed by the drawn conclusion in Sect. 5.

2 Related Work

To systematically sort out the relevant studies, this study retrieved the literature in PubMed, Web of Science and China National Knowledge Infrastructure (CNKI) from January 2018 to June 2025. The search terms are "gastric cancer risk prediction" or "gastric cancer screening", and "machine learning" or "deep learning" or "long short-term memory network" or "multimodal data". The inclusion criteria for literature were to focus on gastric cancer prediction models, use at least one type of medical data, and report accuracy and other evaluation indicators. Non-research literature such as reviews, gastric cancer treatment response prediction models, and models with incomplete or unverified data were excluded. In recent years, in the field of gastric cancer risk prediction, researchers have proposed some models for gastric cancer risk prediction [5]. Most studies are based on pathological or imaging images for prediction. Several studies in recent years predict the risk of peritoneal recurrence and disease-free survival through preoperative CT images of gastric cancer patients [6]. Huo, J.J., Chen, F.J., Duan, Y.X et al. collected preoperative CT images and digital scan images of postoperative pathological films of patients with advanced gastric cancer and constructed multiple models such as automatic segmentation of gastric cancer tumor regions, preoperative grading, and pathological image recognition and classification, which is helpful to improve the accuracy of prognosis evaluation of gastric cancer [7]. Reference [8] utilized the endoscopic images and videos of patients. Through the analysis of these endoscopic image data, convolutional neural networks were employed to diagnose gastric cancer and predict the depth of invasion. Artificial intelligence deep learning models based on gastroscopy and radiological imaging provided a new auxiliary tool for the clinical diagnosis of gastritis [9].

However, it's quite expensive and time-waste to obtain such data in clinical diagnosis. In addition, the prediction accuracy relying on a single type of data will be affected. Some literature has proposed a survival prediction algorithm for gastric cancer patients based on multimodal and multi-instance learning, achieving information interaction among different modal data [10]. Textual information is extracted from admission records in electronic health records by leveraging pretrained language models and combined with multi-type heterogeneous data fusion for gastric cancer risk prediction [11]. Combining multimodal Transformer with multi-task learning can achieve survival prediction through multimodal data fusion and multi-task collaborative optimization [12]. Deep learning is a method to predict the degree of gastric cancer and gastritis [13]. Based on large-scale population retrospective data, machine learning is also a commonly used method [14], which can be used to screen key genes of gastric cancer and construct prediction models, showing great potential in prediction [15]. The machine learning model based on metabolomics has achieved accurate diagnosis and prognosis risk prediction for patients with gastric cancer [16]. Prediction based on multimodal time series is relatively less applied in the medical field, while it is more extensively utilized in the fields of finance and intelligent transportation [17]. The review of related work in this study has limitations, including language bias, restricted time scope and the lack of formal quality assessment for included studies.

3 Detail Design of Integrated Machine Learning-Bidirectional LSTM Hybrid Model

3.1 Framework Overview

One thing to be noted is the dataset used in this study was derived from Yuhuan County People's Hospital (Zhejiang Province), covering 32,318 gastric cancer screening records collected between 2019 and 2025, with the screened subjects being registered residents of Yuhuan City who participated in basic screening programs and those who underwent examinations at Yuhuan County People's Hospital. The dataset includes a complete system of variables, such as demographic characteristics (age and gender), clinical laboratory test results (Helicobacter pylori infection status, pepsinogen I, pepsinogen II, gastrin-17 level, pepsinogen ratio), and textual records of gastroscopy results at different time points, and these variables are denoted as $\{X_t\} = \{\mathcal{A}$ (age), $\mathcal{S}$ (gender), $\mathcal{G}$ (G-17), $\mathcal{P}$ (PGR), $\mathcal{P} - \mathcal{I}$ (pepsinogen I), $\mathcal{P} - \mathcal{II}$ (pepsinogen II), $\mathcal{H}$ (Helicobacter pylori infection status), and $\mathcal{T}$ (text information)$\}$ [18] [19].

The overall architecture of the proposed algorithm, as shown in Fig. 1, consists of three core modules: (1) Data preprocessing module: responsible for cleaning abnormal data and imputing missing values, ensuring the quality and availability of original data through technical means such as standardization and normalization; (2) Time-series feature extraction module based on Bi-LSTM: leveraging the unique bidirectional information flow structure of Bi-LSTM network, this module can deeply mine longitudinal medical data from both forward and reverse time dimensions simultaneously, effectively capturing complex temporal dependencies and dynamic change patterns in the data; (3) Dynamic weighted integrated machine learning model module: as the core innovation of the model, this module realizes adaptive optimization of base model weights through a dual-head attention mechanism of feature and model.

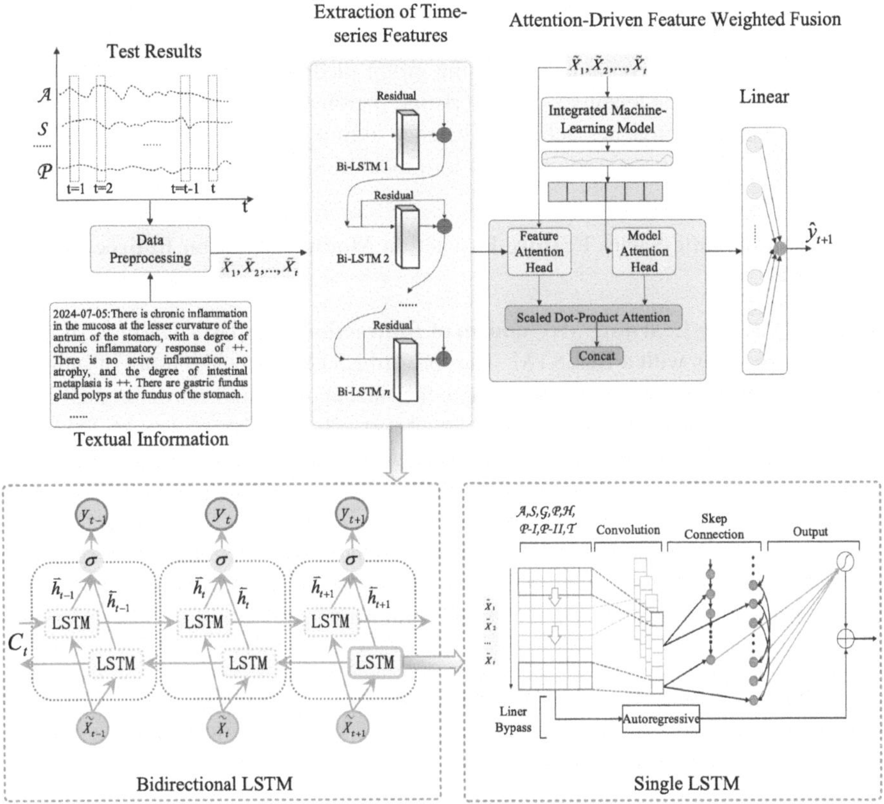

Fig. 1. Framework of the Integrated Machine Learning-LSTM Hybrid Model

3.2 Data Preprocessing

During the data cleaning phase, this study excluded personal privacy information such as patient names, hospitalization numbers, and ID card numbers from the original electronic medical records. To address issues like data redundancy and missing values, records and fields with excessively high missing rates are removed, and duplicate records are eliminated. The research extracts admission records, medical record homepages, and laboratory routine test records. Text extraction methods, including regular expressions and character matching, are used to process chief complaints and present illness histories, removing redundant characters such as spaces and line breaks. For laboratory test results data, box plots are employed to identify outliers. Given the significant variability in data distributions across different test items, outlier thresholds are set at Q3 + 10IQR and Q1 - 10IQR [20]. Manual verification is performed for test items with an outlier proportion exceeding 10% to prevent erroneous deletions. These processes result in 5,165 valid pathological datasets, comprising 2,565 gastric cancer patient records and 2,600 non-gastric cancer patient records.

To address the issue of missing data, this study adopts a tailor-made imputation strategy. For numerical data, the missing values are filled with within-group means after stratifying by gender and age, considering the distribution differences between subgroups and reducing the bias of unified normalization. For categorical demographic data such as gender and age, interpolation within the group medians is adopted to make them conform to their central tendency characteristics, thereby reflecting the true distribution accurately. These approaches achieve a balance among data completeness, statistical rigor, and the informational requirements for model training.

3.3 Design of Time-Series Feature Extraction Module Based on Bidirectional LSTM

Temporal Feature Learning Mechanism of Bidirectional LSTM. During extracting time-series features with a Bi-LSTM: The forward LSTM learns the trend of indicator changes from the early stage of the disease to the current moment in chronological order. As shown in the Bi-LSTM Network in the lower part of Fig. 1:The forward LSTM learns the trend of indicator changes from the early stage of the disease to the current moment in chronological order. The backward LSTM reversely mines the potential correlation between the current moment and subsequent disease progression. The LSTM lies in its unique gating mechanism design. Through the collaborative function of the forget gate, input gate, and output gate, it can selectively retain key historical information in long sequences, effectively addressing the gradient vanishing problem of ordinary recurrent neural networks.

The Gating Logic and Mathematical Expression of LSTM Units. Each LSTM unit achieves selective information flow through specific weight matrices and bias vectors, where the forget gate is used to filter out unimportant information.

$$f_t = \sigma \cdot (w_f \cdot \left(h_t + \pi_t\right) + b_f\right) \quad (1)$$

where f_t is the output of the forget gate, w_f is the weight matrix of the forget gate, σ is the sigmoid activation function, h_{t-1} is the hidden state of the previous time step, x_t is the input of the current time step, and b_f is the bias term.

The input gate is used to output the information retained by the input gate, determining which new information will be updated into the cell state. Its calculation process consists of two steps: first, a sigmoid layer is used to generate update information, and second, a *tanh* layer is employed to produce new candidate values $\widetilde{C}_t$. The output gate determines the output from the cell state to the hidden state and obtains the hidden state of the current time step. During the operation, the related parameters are determined as:

$$\begin{cases} O_t = \sigma \cdot \left(w_O \cdot \left[h_{t-1}, x_t\right] + b_t\right) \\ h_t = O_t * tanh(C_t) \end{cases} \tag{2}$$

where O_t is the output of the output gate, the update of the cell state C_t is jointly determined by the input gate and the forget gate, integrating past information and new candidate values; $*$ is element-wise multiplication, which refers to the multiplication of corresponding elements in two tensors of the same dimension (entry-wise multiplication). Correspondingly, the results C_t can be expressed as:

$$C_t = f_t * C_{t-1} + \sigma \cdot \left(w_i \cdot \left[h_{t-1}, x_t\right] + b_i\right) * \tilde{C}_t \tag{3}$$

Analysis of the Process and Structure of Temporal Feature extraction. The time-series feature extraction process, shown in the lower right half part of Fig. 1, is centered on a single LSTM network. The input$\{\tilde{X}\}$represents multi-dimensional time-series data. C_t is the "complete memory package to be output", and O_t is the "controller that determines how wide the memory package is opened and how much content is output". The two cooperate to enable LSTM to retain key information of long sequences. C_t orresponds to the horizontal line running through the unit in Fig. 1, and O_t corresponds to the output gate branch, intuitively reflecting the relationship of "the cell state carries memory, and the output gate regulates the output".

3.4 Design of Integrated Machine Learning Model Based on Dual - Head Attention Mechanism

The strategic integration of XGBoost, LightGBM, and CatBoost in gradient-boosting frameworks leverages their complementary algorithmic properties to address the multifaceted challenges in medical predictive modeling. High-precision tasks are effectively addressed by XGBoost through its second-order Taylor expansion and complex regularization, with overfitting being significantly alleviated. It is highlighted that LightGBM achieves unparalleled computational efficiency with histogram-based algorithms and leaf tree growth, thus making it an ideal choice for large-scale datasets. By aggregating models with different inductive biases, bias and variance are reduced, complex data patterns are captured, and sensitivity to noise is minimized at the same time.

This architecture processes two information streams in parallel: the feature attention head quantifies the importance of individual feature inputs, corresponding to the structured features and temporal features output by the multi-layer LSTM network in Fig. 1; while the model attention head evaluates the contribution of each base model to the final prediction, corresponding to the output by Integrated Machine-Learning Model in Fig. 1 (Fig. 2).

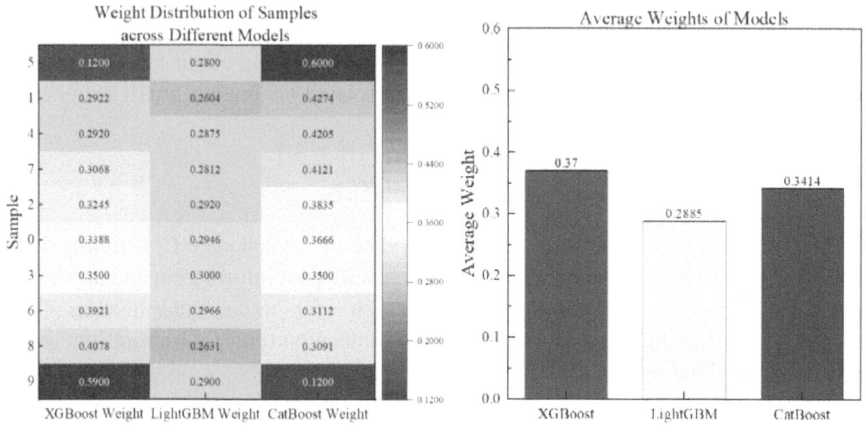

(a) Weight Distribution Heatmap (b) Average Weight Bar Chart

Fig. 2. Dynamic Weight Distribution Heatmap (a) and Average Weight Bar Chart (b) of Integrated Machine Learning Model

The importance of weights of features output by the feature attention head and the contribution weights of models generated by the model attention head are used as inputs. Internally, the fully connected layer performs linear combination on the inputs through a learnable weight matrix w_f and bias b_f. The fused features O_{F} are obtained as:

$$O_{\mathrm{F}} = ReLU \cdot \left(w_f \cdot \left[A_f, A_m\right] + b_f\right) \tag{4}$$

where $\left[A_f, A_m\right]$ is the concatenated vector of feature attention and model attention results, and the ReLU activation function introduces non-linearity. The final output O_{F} is added to the original input via a residual connection, forming a fused feature representation with dynamic weight information (Table 1).

Table 1. Implementation list for each life cycle stage of proposed model

Life cycle stage	Key task
Data input stage	Unification of multimodal data formats and Missing value filling Missing value filling
Feature extraction stage	Bi-LSTM network training and feature importance calculation
Model integration stage	Basic model training and dual-head attention weight learning
Prediction output	Dynamic weight fusion prediction and result visualization

4 Experimental Design and Results Analysis

4.1 Experimental Design

The experimental environment configuration in this paper is as follows. In terms of hardware, it is equipped with an NVIDIA RTX 5060 graphics card, an Intel Core i7–11700 processor, 32G of memory, and a 1TB hard disk. The software environment is based on Python 3.8.10 combined with the Py-Torch 2.4.0 deep learning framework, forming a complete operational environment for the experiments. The data set used for the experiment is divided into a training set, a validation set, and a test set at a ratio of 6:2:2. Each experiment uses five - fold cross - validation to ensure the stability of the experimental results.

The performance of the model is assessed in this paper using the evaluation metrics widely adopted in classification tasks, including Accuracy (A), Precision (P), Recall (R), F1-score ($F1$), and Area Under the Curve(AUC). The relevant metrics can be referenced as follows.

$$\begin{cases} A = \frac{T_{\mathrm{TP}}+T_{\mathrm{TN}}}{T_{\mathrm{TP}}+F_{\mathrm{FP}}+T_{\mathrm{TN}}+F_{\mathrm{FN}}} \\ P = \frac{T_{\mathrm{TP}}}{T_{\mathrm{TP}}+F_{\mathrm{FP}}} \\ R = \frac{T_{\mathrm{TP}}}{T_{\mathrm{TP}}+F_{\mathrm{FN}}} \\ F1 = \frac{2\times P\times}{}P + R \end{cases} \tag{5}$$

where T_{TP} is the number of correctly predicted positive examples; T_{TN} is the number of correctly predicted negative examples; F_{FP} is the number of incorrectly predicted positive examples; F_{FN} is the number of incorrectly predicted negative examples. AUC is a metric for evaluating binary classification models, representing the area under the receiver operating characteristic curve, reflecting the ability of a model to rank the predicted probabilities of positive samples higher than those of negative samples, with values ranging from 0 to 1 where a larger value indicates stronger capability to distinguish between positive and negative samples.

The Kaplan - Meier curve, also known as the Survival Curve, is a commonly - used visualization tool in survival analysis. It is used to show how the survival probability of research subjects changes over time. By conducting statistics on the survival data of two groups (low - risk and high - risk), it presents the changing trend of survival probability in a step. The horizontal axis is the time, and the vertical axis represents the survival probability (usually ranging from 0 to 1). The results can be calculated as:

$$S(t) = \prod\nolimits_{i=1}^{t}\left(1 - \frac{d_i}{n_i}\right) \tag{6}$$

where $S(t)$ represents the survival probability of the research subjects at time t, which is obtained by multiplying the survival probabilities of all previous time points.

4.2 Results Analysis

In Fig. 3, the bar charts of different colors represent the prediction accuracy of each model, where only pathological text descriptions and structured examination data are used, and these two types of data are integrated. It can be found from this figure that, except the CatBoost model, other models achieve better predictive performance when using fused data than a single type of data. One main reason, considering different types of data in medical records have their own unique information. Only by integrating more information can better prediction results be obtained. This further indicates that the use of multi-source heterogeneous data is helpful to improve the accuracy of gastric cancer prediction. Among different models, except the LSTM model, the prediction results based on text data are better than those based on structured data. One main reason is that the text records of patients contain more detailed and useful information, which partly indicates the importance of text records in the task of patient risk prediction. In conclusion, the model proposed in this paper achieves the best prediction performance for fused multimodal data.

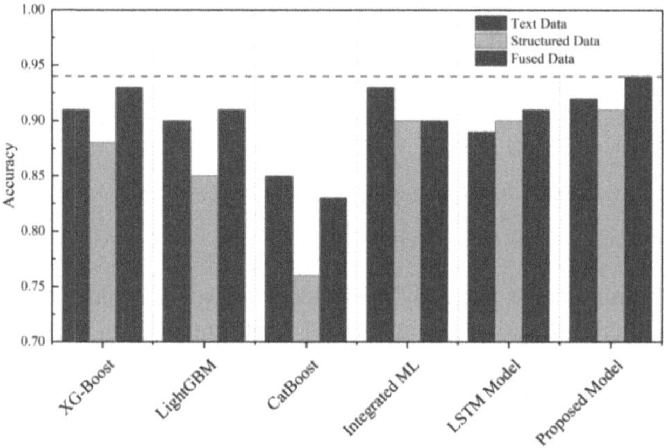

Fig. 3. Accuracy Comparison of Different Models under Different Conditions

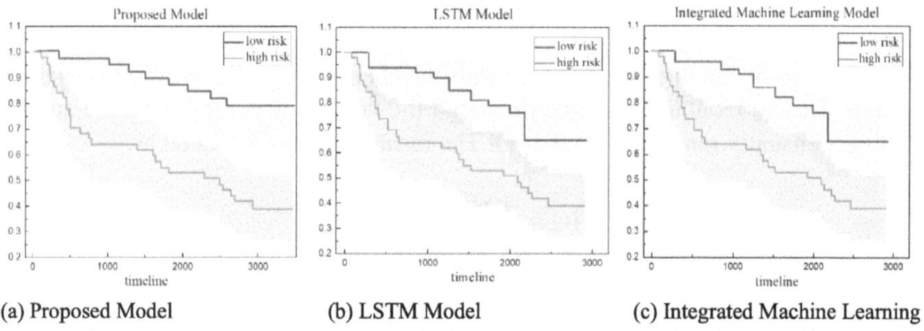

(a) Proposed Model (b) LSTM Model (c) Integrated Machine Learning

Fig. 4. Comparison of KM Curves Among Different Models

The stratification of low-risk patients and high-risk patients is shown on Fig. 4, where the data of low-risk patients and high-risk patients is represented by blue lines and orange lines, respectively. In contrast, the lines for the high-risk group show a more obvious downward trend, meaning that the survival probability of patients in this group decreases rapidly over time and is more strongly affected by risk factors. It can be seen from the figures that the proposed model in this paper has good classification ability and relatively good performance. The shaded area represents the confidence interval, which intuitively reflects the uncertainty range of the data.

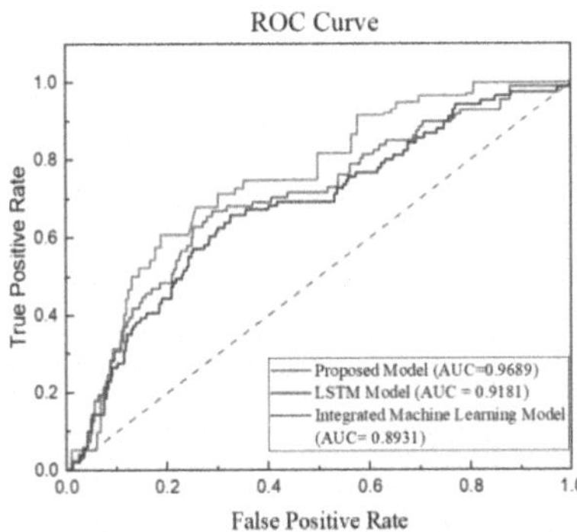

Fig. 5. Comparison of ROC Visualization Plots Among Different Models

Table 2. Comparison of Prediction Results from Different Models.

Model Name	Accuracy	Precision	Recall	F1	AUC
XG-Boost	0.8799	0.8612	0.8260	0.7954	0.8531
Light-GBM	0.8237	0.8679	0.8321	0.8641	0.8231
Cat-Boost	0.8595	0.8678	0.8321	0.8765	0.8631
Integrated Machine Learning	0.8789	0.8445	0.8944	0.9180	0.8931
LSTM Model	0.8863	0.9154	0.8340	0.8917	0.9181
Proposed Model	0.9574	0.9471	0.9286	0.9323	0.9689

Figure 5 compares ROC curves of different models. The horizontal axis represents the false positive rate, and the vertical axis represents the true positive rate. The AUC of the Proposed Model reaches 0.9689, which is higher than that of the LSTM Model (0.9181) and the Integrated Machine (0.8931). This indicates that the proposed model in this paper has a stronger ability to distinguish between positive and negative samples and is more accurate in prediction. The proposed model significantly outperforms all comparative models in all evaluation metrics, achieving an accuracy of 0.9574 (7% higher than the second-best LSTM model), and F1 score of 0.9323, and an AUC of 0.9689—all three core indicators reaching the highest values in Table 2. Its advantages lie in the deep fusion capability of multi-source data, demonstrating superior performance in balancing precision and recall compared to single models. High precision is more suitable for gastric cancer screening to reduce the waste of medical resources. In terms of the model's clinical impact, it reduces the number of unnecessary gastroscopies by 34.7%: among 5,165 valid cases, 1,283 patients who were originally recommended for gastroscopy by traditional methods were classified as low-risk by the model, and no gastric cancer was confirmed in these patients during the 12-month follow-up.

5 Conclusion

This paper proposes a hybrid model that integrates multiple machine learning and multi-layer Bi-LSTM. Our main work is to achieve dynamic weight distribution through a dual-head attention mechanism. On the one hand, the feature attention head quantifies the importance of the temporal features extracted by the bidirectional LSTM network and the features of the data itself. On the other hand, the model attention head adaptively assesses the contribution of basic models such as XGBoost, LightGBM, and CatBoost to the prediction, forming a dynamic correlation mapping of "feature-model". Experimental results show that the model performs excellently in the gastric cancer prediction task, with an AUC value of 94.64% and an accuracy of 92.58%. This result significantly outperforms the prediction effect of a single modal or a single model, effectively addressing the prediction bias issue caused by traditional methods ignoring the contextual associations among multimodal data. In the future, it will be necessary to make up for the lack of data by mining the correlations among different features and focus on the integration of high-dimensional and low-dimensional data to achieve more accurate predictions. The implementation pathway shall be defined in three phases—hospital piloting, public dataset construction, and regulatory standard formulation—to enhance the operability of actions and clarify the advancement timeline.

References

1. GBD Cause of death collaborators: Global, regional, and national age-sex-specific mortality for 282 causes of death in 195 countries and territories, 1980–2017: a systematic ana lysis for the global burden of disease study 2017. Lancet **392**, 1736–1788 (2018)
2. Wild, C.P., Weiderpass, E., Stewart, B.W. (eds.): World Cancer Research for Cancer Prevention (World Cancer Reports). International Agency for Research on Cancer (2020). ISBN-13: 978–92–832–0447–3, 978–92–832–0448–0
3. Van Eycken, L.J., Giannopoulos, E., Tittenbrun, Z., et al.: Future of population-based cancer registries: a global perspective-A survey of population-based cancer registries. Int. J. Cancer (2025). https://doi.org/10.1002/ijc.35516. PMID: 40490886
4. Zhou, J., Zheng, R., Zhang, S., et al.: Gastric and esophageal cancer in China 2000 to 2030: recent trends and short-term predictions of the future burden. Cancer Med. **11**(8), 1902–1912 (2022). https://doi.org/10.1002/cam4.4586. Epub 2022 Feb 11
5. Xu, L., Lyu, J., Zheng, X., Wang, A.: Risk prediction models for gastric cancer: a scoping review. J. Multidiscip. Healthc. **17**, 4337–4352 (2024). https://doi.org/10.2147/JMDH.S479699
6. Jiang, Y., Zhang, Z., Yuan, Q., et al.: Predicting peritoneal recurrence and disease-free survival from CT images in gastric cancer with multitask deep learning: a retrospective study. Lancet Digit Health. **4**(5), e340–e350 (2022). https://doi.org/10.1016/S2589-7500(22)00040-1

7. Huo, J.J., Chen, F.J., Duan, Y.X., et al.: Construction of a predictive model for efficacy of neoadjuvant immunotherapy combined with chemotherapy in gastric cancer based on CT radiomics. Chin. J. Clin. Oncol. **52**(1), 16–23 (2025). https://doi.org/10.12354/j.issn.1000-8179.2025.20241317
8. Xie, F., Zhang, K., Li, F., et al.: Diagnostic accuracy of convolutional neural network-based endoscopic image analysis in diagnosing gastric cancer and predicting its invasion depth: a systematic review and meta-analysis. Gastrointest. Endosc. **95**(4), 599-609.e7 (2022). https://doi.org/10.1016/j.gie.2021.12.021. Epub 2021 Dec 31
9. Turtoi, D.C., Brata, V.D., Incze, V., et al.: Artificial intelligence for the automatic diagnosis of gastritis: a systematic review. J. Clin. Med. **13**(16), 4818 (2024). https://doi.org/10.3390/jcm13164818
10. Jin, H.P., Tao, Y.Q., Li, Z.H., et al.: A survival prediction algorithm for gastric cancer patients based on multimodal multiple instance learning. J. Comput.-Aided Des. Comput. Graph. **37**(2), 349–360 (2025)
11. Chen, X.L., Jia, Y.Z., An, Y., et al.: Gastric cancer risk prediction model integrating multiple types of data. Comput. Eng. **48**(9), 254–261 (2022)
12. Cui, J.Q., Xu, Y.Y., Zheng, H.C., et al.: HMT: a hybrid multi-modal transformer with multi-task learning for survival prediction in head and neck cancer. IEEE Trans. Radiat. Plasma Med. Sci. (2025). https://doi.org/10.1109/TRPMS.2025.3539739
13. Huang, L., Li, Y.X., Wu, L.L., et al.: Artificial intelligence assisted diagnosis system of benign and malignant gastric ulcer based on deep learning. Chin. J. Digest. Endosc. **37**(7), 476–480 (2020)
14. Ke, X., Cai, X.; Bian, B., et al.: Predicting early gastric cancer risk using machine learning: a population-based retrospective study. Digit Health **10**, 20552076241240904 (2024). https://doi.org/10.1177/20552076241240905
15. Ke, X., Cai, X., Bian, B., et al.: Predicting early gastric cancer risk using machine learning: s population-based retrospective study. Digit Health **10**, 20552076241240904 (2024). https://doi.org/10.1177/20552076241240905
16. Chen, Y., Wang, B., Zhao, Y., et al.: Metabolomic machine learning predictor for diagnosis and prognosis of gastric cancer. Nat. Commun. **15**, 1657 (2024). https://doi.org/10.1038/s41467-024-46043-y
17. Jiang, Y., Yu, W., Lee, G., et al.: Explainable Multi-modal Time Series Prediction with LLM-in-the-Loop. arXiv:2503.01013. https://doi.org/10.48550/arXiv.2503.01013
18. Huang, M., Liu, X.: Correlations between pathological changes and Helicobacter pylori infection, pepsinogen, gastrin-17 in chronic atrophic gastritis. J. Pract. Med. **36**(20), 2838–2842 (2020)
19. Wu, L., Xu, J.: Research progress of serum gastrin G-17 in the diagnosis of chronic atrophic gastritis. Chin. J. Gastroenterol. Hepatol. **24**(1), 9–11 (2015). https://doi.org/10.3969/j.issn.1673-534X.2015.01.009
20. Tukey, J.W.: Exploratory data analysis. In: The Concise Encyclopedia of Statistics. Springer, New York (1993). https://doi.org/10.1007/978-0-387-32833-1_136

DiT-Dep: A Diffusion with Transformers-Based Framework for Depression Detection and Neuroimaging Biomarkers Identification

Yufu Huo[1,2], Ruitao Xie[1,3], and Yunpeng Cai[1(✉)]

[1] Shenzhen Institutes of Advanced Technology, Chinese Academy of Sciences, Shenzhen 518055, China
yp.cai@siat.ac.cn
[2] University of Chinese Academy of Sciences, Beijing 100049, China
[3] Faculty of Computer Science and Control Engineering, Shenzhen University of Advanced Technology, Shenzhen, China

Abstract. Depression presents a significant public health challenge, with recent advancements highlighting the need to investigate potential neuroimaging biomarkers underlying its complex neurobiological effects. This paper introduces Diffusion with Transformers for Depression (DiT-Dep), an innovative framework that utilizes DiT for effective depression detection and biomarkers identification. By modeling neuroimaging data as graphs, DiT-Dep optimizes the classification performance through a dual-objective training strategy. Moreover, a novel entropy-based attention refinement mechanism is introduced to enhance the model's ability to learn discriminative features, coupled with perturbation-based post hoc explanation methods that clarify the relationships between functional brain networks and depression. Evaluations across multiple datasets reveal that DiT-Dep significantly outperforms leading baselines, achieving superior detection performance while also providing meaningful insights into the replicable and verifiable neuroimaging biomarkers associated with depression, thereby underscoring the promise of using advanced AI methodologies for scientific research in psychiatry. The code is available at: https://github.com/RosalindFok/DiT-Dep.git.

Keywords: Depression Detection · Neuroimaging Biomarker · Diffusion with Transformers · Explainable AI · AI for Science

1 Introduction

Depression is a prevalent mental disorder and a major risk factor for suicide. Among juveniles aged 10 to 19 years, it is the leading cause of disability worldwide [1]. Furthermore, postpartum depression affects 12–20% of primiparous

E. R. Kaburuan and S. Goundar (Eds.): HIS 2025, LNCS 16392, pp. 34–45, 2026.
https://doi.org/10.1007/978-981-95-6304-3_4

women [2], while in the elderly, depression is the most common comorbid condition [3]. The current mainstream approach to diagnosing depression primarily relies on a clinical evaluation process conducted by psychologists and structured psychological assessment scales, such as Hamilton Depression Scale (HAMD) as well as Beck Depression Inventory (BDI) [4]. However, the inherent subjectivity in clinician assessments, coupled with patients' tendencies to underreport or exaggerate symptoms, substantially compromises diagnostic accuracy.

Recent advances in non-invasive neuroimaging techniques have paved the way for investigating the complex structural and functional changes in brain regions associated with depression. Among the most widely used modalities is magnetic resonance imaging (MRI), which includes structural MRI (sMRI) for characterizing brain anatomy and functional MRI (fMRI). Notably, resting-state fMRI (rs-fMRI) captures low-frequency fluctuations in the blood-oxygenation-level-dependent (BOLD) signal acquired from subjects in a task-free resting state, reflecting brain activity alterations and regional interactions [5].

In parallel, advanced deep learning algorithms, owing to their powerful pattern recognition capabilities, have attracted significant attention across diverse domains. For neuroimaging-based depression detection, deep learning approaches have been applied to reveal subtle differences in imaging data between depression patients (DPs) and healthy controls (HCs) that are typically indiscernible to the naked eye. Some of these studies further improve clinical interpretability by discovering robust and reproducible neuroimaging biomarkers.

Inspired by the data-driven scientific discovery paradigm, Diffusion with Transformers for Depression (DiT-Dep) is proposed. Specifically, DiT-Dep represents rs-fMRI data as graph structures, in which node and edge feature vectors are encoded and concatenated to form embeddings within a latent space. Subsequently, a diffusion model with a Transformer-based denoising network is employed to learn comprehensive feature representations. Ultimately, these embeddings are passed to a graph classifier to estimate the probability that the subject is diagnosed with depression. Additionally, perturbation-based post hoc explanation methods are adopted to identify brain functional networks associated with depression. Its contributions are as follows:

- The DiT has been employed for depression detection, demonstrating exceptional classification performance. When evaluated on a mixed dataset comprising three integrated datasets, DiT-Dep outperformed six competitive baselines from recent years, achieving state-of-the-art (SOTA) results.
- An entropy-based attention refinement module has been incorporated into the denoising network of DiT to further optimize the discriminative capacity of the embeddings in the latent space.
- In addition to the classification loss serving as the primary training objective, an auxiliary reconstruction loss has been introduced to constrain the relative distribution consistency between the input and output embeddings of DiT, thereby enhancing classification performance.
- By utilizing a range of perturbations in the brain functional networks, DiT-Dep quantified the rate at which HCs were misclassified as DPs and suc-

cessfully identified the default mode network as the most closely associated with depression, in addition to several potential pathological patterns of neural activity. This advancement enhances the explainability of DiT-Dep and suggests a promising future for the application of AI in scientific research.

2 Related Work

2.1 Diffusion Models and Transformers

Transformer [6] has revolutionized the landscape of deep learning by relying solely on attention mechanisms to model complex dependencies within sequential data, thereby dispensing with traditional recurrence or convolution. Its self-attention framework enabled unprecedented parallelization and rich contextual modeling, which has led to its dominance across a broad spectrum of natural language processing (NLP) tasks. Vision Transformer (ViT) [7] extended the applicability of Transformers to computer vision (CV), decomposing images into sequences of fixed-size patches and processing them analogously to token sequences in text. This architecture shift has challenged established convolutional inductive biases and has demonstrated that, when trained on sufficiently large-scale datasets, ViT outperforms convolutional neural networks (CNNs) in various vision benchmarks. Notably, the emergence of ViT also facilitated subsequent efforts to replace the traditional CNN-based U-Net backbone in diffusion models for image generation tasks with transformer-based networks.

Diffusion models formed a powerful class of generative methods, involving perturbing data with increasingly intense noise, followed by a reverse process that iteratively removes the noise to synthesize new samples [8]. Denoising Diffusion Probabilistic Models (DDPM) [9] laid the foundational framework for high-quality image synthesis by introducing a reverse chain parameterized with a U-Net. Building upon this, Latent Diffusion Models (LDM) [10] further advanced the field by introducing the concept of learning within a perceptually rich and low-dimensional latent space, thereby enabling efficient computation and scalability to high-resolution image generation without compromising fidelity. More recently, Diffusion Models with Transformers (DiT) [11] replaced the convolutional U-Net-based denoising network with pure Transformers on the latent patches, leveraging superior modeling capacity to enhance both the representation power and sampling quality. The evolution of Transformers and diffusion models has motivated the design of the DiT-Dep framework.

2.2 fMRI-Based Detection of Depression with Deep Learning

Graph Neural Networks (GNNs) have been widely applied to brain modeling, representing brain regions of interest (ROIs) as nodes and functional connectivity derived from fMRI as weighted edges [4,12–15]. Building upon the foundational GNNs architecture, variants such as Graph Convolutional Networks (GCNs) [16] and Graph Attention Networks (GATs) [17,18] have been introduced to facilitate more expressive aggregation and adaptive propagation of information across the graph. These refinements enabled the modeling of intricate relationships by dynamically weighting the influence of neighboring nodes. Furthermore, to characterize the dynamic aspects of brain activity, spatio-temporal attention mechanisms have been incorporated [19–22].

Interpretable deep learning methods have been leveraged for depression-specific neuroimaging biomarkers identification. Built-in interpretable GNNs are designed to generate explanations through their architectures. For example, CI-GNN [14] was able to identify the most influential subgraph via Granger causality, BPI-GNN [15] utilized prototype learning to produce intuitive explanations, and GNNMA [17] performed Singular Value Decomposition (SVD) on the attention adjacency matrix of the brain modules. In contrast, post hoc explanations, which are more flexible and model agnostic [23], have also been widely adopted. For instance, N2V-GAT [18] combined the classifier with the Permutation Importance method to study feature importance and DGCN [16] used class activation map (CAM) to determine the contribution of each brain area.

3 Method

3.1 Graph Construction from rs-fMRI

DiT-Dep models each participant's rs-fMRI as a graph $\mathcal{G}$ by leveraging the Brainnetome Atlas [24], which provides a parcellation of the entire brain into 246 subregions: 210 cortical and 36 subcortical. Specifically, each subregion is represented as a node, collectively forming the node set $\mathcal{V} = \{v_1, v_2, \ldots, v_N\}$, where $N = 246$. To construct node features, the BOLD time series of each subregion is first extracted according to the parcellation. For node v_i, the time series $\mathbf{x}_i \in \mathbb{R}^M$ is obtained by averaging the BOLD signal across all voxels within the i-th subregion. In practice, the initial 5 volumes of each node's time series are discarded to mitigate scanner instability, and only the remaining M volumes are used for all subsequent analyses. By stacking all such vectors, the node embedding matrix $\mathbf{X} = [\mathbf{x}_1; \mathbf{x}_2; \ldots; \mathbf{x}_N] \in \mathbb{R}^{N \times M}$ is formed, where each row reflects the temporal dynamics of a specific subregion. Subsequently, to characterize functional connectivity between subregions, the weight of each edge connecting nodes (v_i, v_j) is defined as the Pearson correlation coefficient between their respective time series $\mathbf{x}_i$ and $\mathbf{x}_j$. The set of all edges is denoted by $\mathcal{E}$, and the corresponding symmetric matrix of edge weights $\mathbf{A} \in \mathbb{R}^{N \times N}$ encapsulates the strength of interaction between subregions, serving as the edge embedding. Formally, the rs-fMRI data is represented as a graph $\mathcal{G} = (\mathcal{V}, \mathcal{E})$, with node embedding capturing intra-regional activity and edge embedding characterizing inter-regional relationships.

3.2 The Framework of DiT-Dep

The architecture of DiT-Dep, as illustrated in Fig. 1, comprises 3 main stages: (1) projection of node and edge embeddings into a latent space, (2) transformer-based diffusion model for latent representation refinement, and (3) graph-level classification for depression detection.

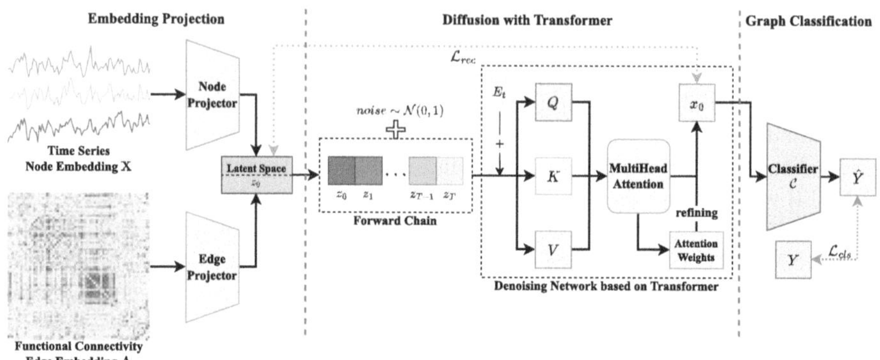

Fig. 1. The pipeline of DiT-Dep. Red vertical dashed lines delineate the 3 stages. (Color figure online)

Initially, during the projection of graph embedding into the latent space, the node projector and edge projector respectively map $\mathbf{X}$ and $\mathbf{A}$ into vectors of identical dimensionality L, which are then stacked to construct $\mathbf{z}_0 \in \mathbb{R}^{S \times L}$, with S representing the stacked dimension. The projectors, utilizing multi-layer perceptrons (MLPs) as their backbones, are designed to map high-dimensional feature representations derived from the graph $\mathcal{G}$ into a lower-dimensional latent space (i.e. $L \ll N \times N + N \times M$). This projection stage aims to preserve the original information to the greatest possible extent while facilitating efficient computations in the subsequent DiT module.

Subsequently, DiT-Dep implements the forward diffusion process as outlined in Eq. 1, which enables direct sampling of the noisy latent $\mathbf{z}_t$ at any time step t from the initial embedding $\mathbf{z}_0$ in closed form, where $\boldsymbol{\epsilon}$ follows a standard Gaussian distribution $\mathcal{N}(\mathbf{0}, \mathbf{I})$, $\sqrt{\bar{\alpha}_t}$ and $\sqrt{1-\bar{\alpha}_t}$ serve as the signal retention and noise strength coefficients, respectively, both of which depend on the time step t.

$$\mathbf{z}_t = \sqrt{\bar{\alpha}_t} \cdot \mathbf{z}_0 + \sqrt{1-\bar{\alpha}_t} \cdot \boldsymbol{\epsilon}, \ \bar{\alpha}_t = \prod_{i=1}^{t} \alpha_i, \ \alpha_i \in (0,1), \ t \in \{1, \dots, T\} \tag{1}$$

DiT-Dep leverages a Transformer-based deep neural network for denoising, drawing on the foundational architecture of the original DiT [11] while introducing targeted modifications. Consistent with DiT, the current time step t is projected onto a time embedding E_t that aligns with the shape of $\mathbf{z}_t$, followed by element-wise addition to incorporate temporal conditioning. This representation is then projected via linear transformations to the query ($\mathbf{Q}$), key ($\mathbf{K}$), and value ($\mathbf{V}$) matrices. The $\mathbf{Q}, \mathbf{K}, \mathbf{V}$ matrices are subsequently fed into a multi-head attention mechanism, which performs self-attention computations to yield an approximate fitting to the clean latent representation $\mathbf{x}_0'$, serving as an initial estimation of the underlying noise-free $\mathbf{z}_0$, alongside the corresponding attention weights $\mathbf{W} \in \mathbb{R}^{S \times S}$. The self-attention step is crucial for harnessing the whole graph-embedded information of $\mathbf{z}_0$ to distill emergent relational dynamics from noisy latent projections, empowering the denoising process to reconstruct hierarchical dependencies with unprecedented contextual fidelity. Diverging from DiT, DiT-Dep incorporates an entropy-based attention refinement module to further optimize $\mathbf{x}_0'$. Specifically, the entropy formula (Eq. 2) is utilized to quantify the uncertainty within the distribution, resulting in an entropy vector $\mathbf{e} \in \mathbb{R}^S$. During the scaling step (Eq. 3), the Sigmoid function $\sigma(\cdot)$ is employed. The entropy values are transformed through a scaling mechanism with a threshold of 0.5, a scaling amplitude of 0.5, and a bias of 0.75. This adjustment serves to intensify the model's focus on uncertain regions, producing a broadcasted scaling factor vector $\mathbf{s} \in \mathbb{R}^{S \times S}$. The computed scaling factors are then applied to the original attention weights $\mathbf{W}$ via element-wise multiplication, resulting in the scaled attention weights $\mathbf{W}' \in \mathbb{R}^{S \times S}$. The Softmax function is subsequently applied to ensure $\mathbf{W}'$ is properly normalized. Finally, as illustrated in Eq. 4, the refined representation $\mathbf{x}_0 \in \mathbb{R}^{S \times L}$ is obtained through matrix multiplication.

$$\mathbf{e} = -\sum_{j=1}^{S} \mathbf{W}_{i,j} \log \mathbf{W}_{i,j} \tag{2}$$

$$\begin{aligned} \mathbf{s} &= \sigma(\mathbf{e} - 0.5) \cdot 0.5 + 0.75 \\ \mathbf{W}' &= \text{Softmax}(\mathbf{W} \odot \mathbf{s}) \end{aligned} \tag{3}$$

$$\mathbf{x}_0 = \mathbf{W}'\mathbf{x}_0' \tag{4}$$

Ultimately, a classifier $\mathcal{C}$ conducts graph-level prediction tasks, taking the refined embedding $\mathbf{x}_0$ as input and producing probability estimates $\hat{Y}$ for HCs and DPs. $\mathcal{C}$ is constructed by stacking a series of residual networks (ResNets) and MLPs, wherein the ResNets are employed to alleviate the vanishing gradient problem, while the MLPs progressively reduce the dimensionality of the tensor.

DiT-Dep adopts a dual-objective optimization strategy, as delineated in Eq. 5. The primary objective $\mathcal{L}_{cls}$ leverages the cross-entropy loss function to quantify the divergence between the predicted class probabilities $\hat{Y}$ and the ground-truth labels Y. Complementing this, the auxiliary objective $\mathcal{L}_{rec}$ employs the mean squared error (MSE) loss, which exhibits increased sensitivity to errors and pronounced responsiveness to outliers, thereby enforcing relative consistency between the denoised reconstruction $\mathbf{x}_0$ generated by DiT and the original embedding input $\mathbf{z}_0$. In practice, the auxiliary $\mathcal{L}_{rec}$ is scaled by a modest weight $\beta = 0.4$ to balance its influence. This composite loss formulation empowers DiT-Dep to concurrently refine the projectors, DiT, and $\mathcal{C}$ throughout end-to-end training, yielding substantial improvements in the robustness of depression detection.

$$\mathcal{L} = \mathcal{L}_{cls}(\hat{Y}, Y) + \beta \mathcal{L}_{rec}(\mathbf{x}_0, \mathbf{z}_0) \tag{5}$$

3.3 Post Hoc Explanations Based on Subgraph Perturbation

Owing to the model-agnostic property, post hoc explanations represent the most prevalent methods in interpretable deep learning [23], thus enabling their seamless application to intricate black-box models such as DiT-Dep. DiT-Dep is initially trained on an unperturbed training dataset, followed by perturbing combinations of features in the test set during inference. By analyzing the changes in model performance, it becomes possible to evaluate the importance contributed by each feature combination to DiT-Dep's decision-making process.

Brain networks provide a powerful paradigm for investigating cognitive and affective dysfunctions in psychiatric disorders, including depression [25]. Based on the fine-grained functional network partitioning scheme proposed by Yeo et al. [26] and the triple network theory of psychopathology [25], DiT-Dep categorizes the entire brain, which consists of 246 subregions, into 8 distinct networks. Formally, the complete graph $\mathcal{G}$ with 246 nodes is divided into 8 subgraphs $\mathcal{G}_1, \ldots, \mathcal{G}_8$. Subsequently, perturbations are applied to the node embedding $\mathbf{X}_i$ and edge embedding $\mathbf{A}_i$ of $\mathcal{G}_i$. By observing changes in performance for classification between DPs and HCs, it is feasible to investigate the temporal signal variations within subregions of the corresponding network and the interactions between these subregions, further elucidating their association with depression.

4 Experiments

4.1 Datasets and Metrics

In this study, three datasets characterized by diverse demographic features are consolidated from two different sites for experimental purposes. There are 80 DPs and 21 HCs in datasets ds002748 [27] and ds003007 [28]. To mitigate the negative impact of class imbalance, 59 HCs are randomly selected from Cambridge-Buckner dataset of the Functional Connectomes Project [29] for data augmentation. The mixed dataset is partitioned using a 5-fold cross-validation approach, with final metrics calculated as the mean values obtained from each fold.

In this context, DPs and HCs are defined as positive and negative samples, respectively. To evaluate the performance of depression detection, several binary classification metrics are selected, including Accuracy (ACC), Precision (PRE), Sensitivity (SEN), F1 Score (F1S), and Area Under the Curve (AUC). All of them range from 0 to 1, with higher values indicating stronger classification performance of the model. Furthermore, the False Positive Rate (FPR) is selected as a vital metric for identifying neuroimaging biomarkers, as a higher FPR indicates that the model misdiagnoses an increasing number of HCs as DPs.

4.2 Quantitative Comparison on Depression Detection

Six competitive deep learning algorithms based on fMRI are selected as baselines, with the quantitative comparison results illustrated in Table 1. In the mixed depression dataset, DiT-Dep outperforms other baseline models across the majority of metrics, demonstrating optimal performance in depression detection. Although DiT-Dep exhibits a lower SEN compared to BrainGNN and N2V-GAT, the significant imbalance in SEN and PRE of these two models results in their overall F1S scores being less favorable than that of DiT-Dep. This indicates that BrainGNN and N2V-GAT may be overly sensitive to positive samples, leading to a higher misdiagnosis rate among HCs. In contrast, DiT-Dep achieves a favorable balance between PRE and SEN.

Table 1. Quantitative comparison results on the mixed depression dataset. The results marked in bold indicate the optimal performance.

Models	ACC	PRE	SEN	F1S	AUC
IBGNN [12]	0.7750	0.7555	0.8125	0.7813	0.8523
BrainGNN [13]	0.8438	0.8023	**0.9125**	0.8538	0.9250
N2V-GAT [18]	0.8250	0.8052	0.8625	0.8281	0.8844
STANet [19]	0.8063	0.8217	0.7875	0.8025	0.8914
STAGIN [20]	0.7875	0.8254	0.7375	0.7725	0.8766
DSAM [21]	0.8063	0.8006	0.8250	0.8046	0.8402
DiT-Dep	**0.8563**	**0.8689**	0.8500	**0.8551**	**0.9352**

DiT-Dep distinguishes itself by integrating a more advanced Diffusion Transformer to learn the subtle patterns embedded in the temporal features of each subregion, as well as the interaction features among them derived from fMRI.

4.3 Ablation on Key Components

This study conducts a thorough ablation analysis on the components of the input data for DiT-Dep and the key modules within the framework to explore their respective contributions. In Table 2, there are five variants of DiT-Dep. The two variants represent ablation studies on the data: "wo E" indicates the removal of the edge embedding $\mathbf{A}$, with the model trained using only the node embedding $\mathbf{X}$; while "wo N" signifies the exclusive use of $\mathbf{A}$. Additionally, three variants represent ablation studies on the modules: "wo D" indicates the absence of DiT, wherein $\mathcal{C}$ classifies directly using $\mathbf{z}_0$ instead of $\mathbf{x}_0$; "wo A" signifies the deactivation of attention-based refinement, meaning that the update calculations in Eq. 4 are not being performed; "wo M" denotes that $\mathcal{L}_{rec}$ is not utilized as an auxiliary loss, with the model relying solely on $\mathcal{L}_{cls}$ as the training objective.

In the ablation analysis of graph embedding, "wo E" variant shows a significantly lower AUC than "wo N", suggesting that its probability predictions deviate further from the ground truth. This finding potentially highlights a stronger correlation between cerebral functional connectivity and depression. The ablation experiments on the key modules also exhibit varying degrees of performance

Table 2. Ablation results on the mixed depression dataset. Bold formatting indicates the optimal performance, while underlined formatting signifies the lowest.

Variants	ACC	PRE	SEN	F1S	AUC
DiT-Dep wo E	0.8250	0.8031	0.8625	0.8300	0.8688
DiT-Dep wo N	0.8250	0.7916	**0.9000**	0.8394	0.9172
DiT-Dep wo D	<u>0.7750</u>	0.7696	<u>0.8000</u>	<u>0.7795</u>	0.8262
DiT-Dep wo A	0.8188	0.7955	0.8750	0.8283	0.8957
DiT-Dep wo M	0.7813	<u>0.7551</u>	0.8375	0.7869	<u>0.8227</u>
DiT-Dep	**0.8563**	**0.8689**	0.8500	**0.8551**	**0.9352**

degradation, indicating that each module plays a crucial role in the overall framework: (1) DiT effectively extracts more discriminative features within the graph embedding; (2) the attention-based refinement enhances the model's focus on relevant characteristics; (3) the auxiliary loss contributes to improved classification performance by providing Y supervision to DiT.

4.4 Identification of Neuroimaging Biomarkers for Depression

The eight subgraphs correspond to the following brain networks: Visual, Somatomotor, Dorsal Attention, Ventral Attention, Salience, Limbic, Control, Default. In each iteration of inference on the test set, only one subgraph $\mathcal{G}_i$ is perturbed by altering either $\mathbf{X}_i$ or $\mathbf{A}_i$. Specifically, for $\mathbf{X}_i$, the values of each row are set to an alternating sequence of minimum and maximum values normalized within the range of $[-1, 1]$, simulating the high volatility and active neurophysiological processes occurring in the subregions. The values within $\mathbf{A}_i$ are uniformly set to -1 to reflect the asynchronous activity and heterogeneity among subregions within the corresponding brain network. Fluctuations in FPR resulting from the perturbations of different subgraphs are observed to identify neuroimaging biomarkers. Networks that exhibit higher FPR are deemed more susceptible to misclassifying HCs as DPs, suggesting that the corresponding simulated pathological patterns may serve as potential markers for the diagnosis of depression.

As illustrated in the results following the perturbations presented in Fig. 2, Default (Default Mode Network, DMN) demonstrates the most pronounced effects. Building upon the aforementioned perturbation patterns, it is reasonable to infer the following three neuroimaging characteristics that may prominently represent individuals suffering from depression: (1) the time series of subregions within DMN display significant volatility; (2) there is a marked enhancement in functional connectivity between subregions of DMN; however, their respective activities tend towards disarray rather than synchronization; (3) the disruptions within Salience (Salience Network) and Control (Frontoparietal Control Network), as shown in Fig. 2 a and 2 b, serve as second most significant markers.

These findings align closely with prevailing psychological research [25,30], which indicates that DMN is involved in self-referential activities. Elevated DMN

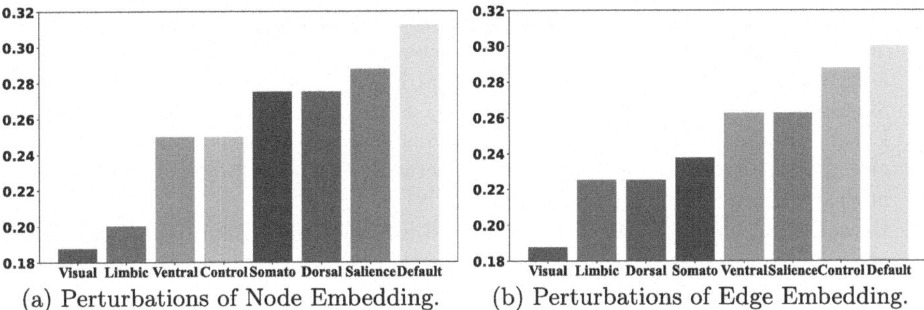

(a) Perturbations of Node Embedding. (b) Perturbations of Edge Embedding.

Fig. 2. FPR following perturbations across distinct brain networks.

activity during the resting state can exacerbate rumination, particularly regarding negative emotions, such as persistent feelings of low mood, self-doubt, and self-neglect, ultimately leading to the development of depression. Similar findings are observed in research on interpretable deep learning methods [16,18]; however, DiT-Dep advances this understanding by not only identifying significant brain networks but also revealing potential pathological neural activity patterns.

5 Conclusions

DiT-Dep not only enhances the upper limits of depression detection capabilities but also accurately identifies DMN that is highly correlated with depression, offering neural activity patterns that may serve as potential neuroimaging biomarkers. This study focuses on the activities and interrelations within brain functional networks, with plans for a more detailed examination of the connectivity between different networks in future research. Additionally, there is an intention to extend this interpretable framework to other types of mental disorders, aiming to develop broader clinical applications.

Acknowledgments. This study was funded by Noncommunicable Chronic Diseases National Science and Technology Major Project (2024ZD0529100) and National Natural Science Foundation of China (grant No. U22A2041).

Disclosure of Interests. The authors declare that they have no conflict of interest.

References

1. Haque, U.M., Kabir, E., Khanam, R.: Detection of depression and its likelihood in children and adolescents: evidence from a 15-years study. In: Health Information Science, pp. 3–16. Springer Nature Singapore, Singapore (2023)
2. Gopalakrishnan, A., Gururajan, R., Venkataraman, R., Zhou, X., Chan, K.C.: A combined attribute extraction method for detecting postpartum depression using social media. In: Health Information Science, pp. 17–29. Springer Nature Singapore, Singapore (2023)

3. Li, X., Li, S., Liu, Y.: Network analysis of relationships and change patterns in depression and multiple chronic diseases based on the china health and retirement longitudinal study. In: Health Information Science, pp. 30–39. Springer Nature Singapore, Singapore (2023)
4. Liu, S., et al.: An objective quantitative diagnosis of depression using a local-to-global multimodal fusion graph neural network. Patterns **5**(12), 101081 (2024). https://doi.org/10.1016/j.patter.2024.101081
5. Biswal, B.B., Uddin, L.Q.: The history and future of resting-state functional magnetic resonance imaging. Nature **641**(8065), 1121–1131 (2025). https://doi.org/10.1038/s41586-025-08953-9
6. Vaswani, A., et al.: Attention is all you need. In: Proceedings of the 31st International Conference on Neural Information Processing Systems, pp. 6000–6010. NIPS'17, Curran Associates Inc., Red Hook (2017)
7. Dosovitskiy, A., et al.: An image is worth 16x16 words: transformers for image recognition at scale. In: International Conference on Learning Representations (2021)
8. Yang, L., et al.: Diffusion models: a comprehensive survey of methods and applications. ACM Comput. Surv. **56**(4) (Nov 2023). https://doi.org/10.1145/3626235
9. Ho, J., Jain, A., Abbeel, P.: Denoising diffusion probabilistic models. In: Proceedings of the 34th International Conference on Neural Information Processing Systems. NIPS '20, Curran Associates Inc., Red Hook (2020)
10. Rombach, R., Blattmann, A., Lorenz, D., Esser, P., Ommer, B.: High-resolution image synthesis with latent diffusion models. In: 2022 IEEE/CVF Conference on Computer Vision and Pattern Recognition (CVPR), pp. 10674–10685 (2022). https://doi.org/10.1109/CVPR52688.2022.01042
11. Peebles, W., Xie, S.: Scalable diffusion models with transformers. In: 2023 IEEE/CVF International Conference on Computer Vision (ICCV), pp. 4172–4182 (2023). https://doi.org/10.1109/ICCV51070.2023.00387
12. Cui, H., Dai, W., Zhu, Y., Li, X., He, L., Yang, C.: Interpretable graph neural networks for connectome-based brain disorder analysis. In: Medical Image Computing and Computer Assisted Intervention – MICCAI 2022, pp. 375–385. Springer Nature Switzerland, Cham (2022)
13. Li, X., et al.: Braingnn: interpretable brain graph neural network for FMRI analysis. Med. Image Anal. **74**, 102233 (2021). https://doi.org/10.1016/j.media.2021.102233
14. Zheng, K., Yu, S., Chen, B.: CI-GNN: a granger causality-inspired graph neural network for interpretable brain network-based psychiatric diagnosis. Neural Netw. **172**, 106147 (2024). https://doi.org/10.1016/j.neunet.2024.106147
15. Zheng, K., Yu, S., Chen, L., Dang, L., Chen, B.: BPI-GNN: interpretable brain network-based psychiatric diagnosis and subtyping. Neuroimage **292**, 120594 (2024). https://doi.org/10.1016/j.neuroimage.2024.120594
16. Zhou, N., et al.: Using dynamic graph convolutional network to identify individuals with major depression disorder. J. Affective Disorders **371**, 188–195 (2025). https://doi.org/10.1016/j.jad.2024.11.035
17. Si, W., Wang, G., Liu, L., Zhang, L., Qiao, L.: Graph neural network with modular attention for identifying brain disorders. Biomed. Sign. Process. Control **102**, 107252 (2025). https://doi.org/10.1016/j.bspc.2024.107252
18. Su, S., et al.: Classification of major depressive disorder using graph attention mechanism with multi-site RS-FMRI data. Neuroinformatics **23**(2), 34 (2025). https://doi.org/10.1007/s12021-025-09731-8

19. Zhang, W., et al.: Stanet: a novel spatio-temporal aggregation network for depression classification with small and unbalanced fmri data. Tomography **10**(12), 1895–1914 (2024). https://doi.org/10.3390/tomography10120138
20. Kim, B.H., Ye, J.C., Kim, J.J.: Learning dynamic graph representation of brain connectome with spatio-temporal attention. In: Proceedings of the 35th International Conference on Neural Information Processing Systems. NIPS '21, Curran Associates Inc., Red Hook (2021)
21. Thapaliya, B., et al.: DSAM: a deep learning framework for analyzing temporal and spatial dynamics in brain networks. Med. Image Anal. **101**, 103462 (2025). https://doi.org/10.1016/j.media.2025.103462
22. Zheng, K., Ma, B., Chen, B.: Dynbraingnn: towards spatio-temporal interpretable graph neural network based on dynamic brain connectome for psychiatric diagnosis. In: Machine Learning in Medical Imaging, pp. 164–173. Springer Nature Switzerland, Cham (2024). https://doi.org/10.1007/978-3-031-45676-3_17
23. Chen, V., Yang, M., Cui, W., Kim, J.S., Talwalkar, A., Ma, J.: Applying interpretable machine learning in computational biology–pitfalls, recommendations and opportunities for new developments. Nat. Methods **21**(8), 1454–1461 (2024). https://doi.org/10.1038/s41592-024-02359-7
24. Jiang, T.: Brainnetome: a new -ome to understand the brain and its disorders. Neuroimage **80**, 263–272 (2013). https://doi.org/10.1016/j.neuroimage.2013.04.002
25. Menon, V.: Large-scale brain networks and psychopathology: a unifying triple network model. Trends Cogn. Sci. **15**(10), 483–506 (2011). https://doi.org/10.1016/j.tics.2011.08.003
26. Thomas Yeo, B.T., et al.: The organization of the human cerebral cortex estimated by intrinsic functional connectivity. J. Neurophysiol. **106**(3), 1125–1165 (2011). https://doi.org/10.1152/jn.00338.2011
27. DD, B., ME, M., AA, S., ED, P.: Resting state with closed eyes for patients with depression and healthy participants (2021). https://doi.org/10.18112/openneuro.ds002748.v1.0.5
28. DD, B., ME, M., AA, S., ED, P.: Two sessions of resting state with closed eyes for patients with depression in treatment course (NFB, CBT or no treatment groups) (2021). https://doi.org/10.18112/openneuro.ds003007.v1.0.1
29. Biswal, B.B., et al.: Toward discovery science of human brain function. Proc. Nation. Academy Sci. **107**(10), 4734–4739 (2010). https://doi.org/10.1073/pnas.0911855107
30. Bezmaternykh, D.D., et al.: Brain networks connectivity in mild to moderate depression: resting state FMRI study with implications to nonpharmacological treatment. Neural Plasticity **2021**(1) (2021). https://doi.org/10.1155/2021/8846097

Elderly Health Consultation System Implemented with Large Language Models and Multi-Agent Systems

Shaojie Wang[1], Shaofu Lin[1](✉), Zhisheng Huang[2,3,4], Haoru Su[1], Fengyuan Zuo[1], Jing Bai[1], and Kang Peng[1]

[1] College of Computer Science, Beijing University of Technology, Beijing 100124, China
linshaofu@bjut.edu.cn
[2] Department of Computer Science, Vrije University Amsterdam, Amsterdam, The Netherlands
[3] Clinical Research Center for Mental Disorders, Shanghai Pudong New Area Mental Health Center, Tongji University School of Medicine, Shanghai, China
[4] Deep Blue Technology Group, Shanghai, China

Abstract. With the accelerating aging of the population, there is growing demand among elderly individuals for personalized and proactive health management. However, current systems face multiple challenges such as fragmented health data hindering comprehensive assessment and insufficient personalization to meet the diverse needs of the elderly. To address these challenges, an intelligent elderly healthcare system integrating LLMs with a multi-agent system is proposed to achieve personalized health management. The system constructs a unified knowledge base by integrating Q&A on common geriatric diseases, drug databases, and medical literature databases on geriatric diseases. It employs voice-dominant natural language interaction to guide elderly users in actively inputting data. An LLM optimized through prompt engineering serves as the core intelligent engine, enhancing both senior-friendly adaptation and comprehensibility of health consultation services. Two specialized agents—for medication guidance and health knowledge consultation—perform tasks such as drug-drug interaction detection and elderly health Q&A under the coordination of LLM. System efficacy was validated with Sensibleness-Specificity Assessment (SSA) scores evaluating the rationality and relevance of multi-turn health consultations and Precision and Recall metrics assessing medication guidance accuracy. Experimental results demonstrate that the system delivers professional yet comprehensible health recommendations during consultations while achieving high accuracy in critical healthcare services like medication management.

Keywords: Intelligent Elderly Care · Medication Guidance · Large Language Models · Multi-Agent Systems · Natural Language Interaction

1 Introduction

Recent advances in artificial-intelligence agent systems—particularly those that combine large language models (LLMs) [1] with advanced reasoning—are opening new opportunities for geriatric medicine and elderly health management. As populations age

E. R. Kaburuan and S. Goundar (Eds.): HIS 2025, LNCS 16392, pp. 46–58, 2026.
https://doi.org/10.1007/978-981-95-6304-3_5

worldwide, the working-age share of the population is shrinking while elderly dependency ratios rise. Traditional healthcare and long-term care systems are therefore under mounting pressure from workforce shortages and rising service costs. In this context, intelligent health-management technologies capable of continuous monitoring and personalized reply have become both an urgent need and a promising approach to improving older adults' quality of life and supporting the sustainable operation of health systems.

Recent evaluation and system design efforts have not only fully demonstrated the application potential of relevant technologies in the field of elderly care but also clearly revealed the existing shortcomings in current practices. Langston et al. (2025) [2] conducted a systematic comparative study on four mainstream intelligent agents (ChatGPT-4, Bard, Alexa, and Google Assistant). The results indicated that agents based on Large Language Models (LLMs) are significantly superior to traditional intelligent tools across three core dimensions including accuracy, depth of information, and contextual adaptability. In terms of exploring specific application systems, the ColaCare system proposed by Wang et al. (2025) [3] exhibits considerable innovation. By coordinating domain expert agents and coordination agents, this system simulates the multidisciplinary clinical consultation process and provides a novel paradigm for managing complex elderly health issues. Similarly, the SAGE [4] architecture adopts a design approach of central coordination agent plus tree-structured task decomposition. The central agent parses the natural language input from elderly users and dynamically dispatches tool agents (e.g., medication reminders or emergency calls), effectively reducing the operational difficulty for users with cognitive impairments. Despite the phased breakthroughs achieved by the aforementioned studies, the implementation of key needs such as medication management in real-world elderly care scenarios still faces numerous challenges that require urgent resolution.

The practical application of current systems mainly faces three significant limitations. First, from the perspective of user interaction, the complex interactive workflows designed for the system [5] are mismatched with the operational habits and cognitive abilities of elderly users. This not only increases the probability of operational errors by users but also directly impairs the practicality of the system in daily use, preventing the technology from being truly implemented to serve the elderly population. Second, focusing on the core technical support, general-purpose Large Language Models [6] have obvious shortcomings in adaptability to clinical scenarios. Their outputs exhibit probabilistic characteristics, are prone to bias influenced by training data, and hallucinations occur from time to time. In high-risk tasks directly related to life and health, such as polypharmacy management, these technical risks are further amplified. Finally, even at the system architecture level, although multi-agent systems [7, 8] provide a sound paradigm for simulating expert collaboration and show broad application prospects, they still face enormous challenges in achieving stable and reliable coordination among agents in dynamically changing real-world environments. This is due to factors such as numerous scene interference elements and real-time changes in task requirements, which further restricts the system's ability to cope with complex geriatric care scenarios.

To address the aforementioned challenges, we have developed a geriatric health consultation system that integrates Large Language Models (LLMs) with a multi-agent collaboration framework. Leveraging domain-specific prompt engineering and a structured knowledge base, we have enhanced the reliability of LLMs in specialized clinical scenarios such as polypharmacy management, reducing probabilistic biases and factual errors. Through the adoption of multi-agent coordination mechanisms and dynamic workflow orchestration, the system, relying on natural voice-driven interaction, maintains contextual consistency in extended multi-turn conversations, enables scalable and trustworthy collaboration among professional agents, and adapts to the needs of elderly users.

The rest of this article is organized as follows. The second section describes the data sources and data process, the third section describes the research methods, the fourth section displays and analyzes the experimental results, and the fifth section draws conclusions and looks forward to the future.

2 Data Resources and Data Processing

2.1 Data Resources

The core knowledge base of this study integrates three categories of data resources including Q&A data on common diseases of the elderly, a drug database, and a medical literature repository for the elderly, covering practical health needs, drug information, and academic research content. The Q&A data on common diseases of the elderly, sourced from dxy.com and Xywy.com, contains over 100,000 valid question-answer pairs focusing on common geriatric conditions such as hypertension and diabetes, with each pair stored in JSON format as shown in Table 1. The drug database, derived from www.yaozh.com, includes 59 types of commonly used drugs for chronic diseases of the elderly and more than 100 types of drugs frequently used for respiratory, digestive, surgical, and other diseases, encompassing both basic drug information and key usage information. The medical literature repository for the elderly, collected from core academic databases such as CNKI and PubMed, comprises over 100 peer-reviewed literatures focusing on geriatric diseases and health care. These documents are stored in PDF format.

Table 1. Q&A data on common diseases of the elderly

ID	Question	Answer
1	In addition to hearing loss, what specific hearing impairment-related situations might elderly people with deafness encounter in their daily lives?	When the elderly suffer from deafness, in addition to obvious hearing loss, they may also encounter the following specific hearing impairment-related situations: 1. Diminished speech discrimination ability: Even if they can hear sounds, they may struggle to understand the content and require others to repeat what they say. 2. Auditory recruitment: Their perception of sound is non-linear—they cannot hear soft sounds, yet loud sounds feel excessively noisy. 3.Phoneme regression: Although their pure-tone hearing may still be relatively good, their ability to understand language decreases significantly…
2	I have a hypertension issue and am very worried that it might lead to lacunar infarction. What is the specific connection between them?	Hypertension is the main direct cause of lacunar infarction. It affects the small blood vessels in the brain through two mechanisms: 1. Persistent hypertension may cause damage to the vessel walls of the deep penetrating arteries and other tiny arteries in the brain, increase vascular permeability, lead to abnormal coagulation function, and result in fibrinoid necrosis, hyaline degeneration of the microvascular walls, as well as microaneurysms—all of which contribute to small artery occlusion and microembolism…
3	The elderly at home have been experiencing some abnormal heart conditions recently. I want to know what specific symptoms atrial flutter usually presents in the elderly?	Atrial flutter in the elderly may present with the following symptoms: dizziness, tachycardia, palpitations, angina pectoris, and hypotension. In some cases, it may also lead to heart block, and in severe instances, it can trigger shock. If you suspect that an elderly person has symptoms of atrial flutter, they should seek medical attention and undergo examination in a timely manner
…	…	…

2.2 Data Processing

For the Q&A dataset on common diseases in the elderly, refined cleaning was conducted under a human-led plus rule-based verification framework. This framework included three key operations: first, removing duplicate entries and redundant information to eliminate data redundancy; second, correcting non-standard content (such as inconsistent medical terminology or ambiguous descriptions) to ensure content normalization; and third, optimizing the structure of JavaScript Object Notation (JSON) format to convert unstructured data into a standardized, machine-readable structure.Regarding the pharmaceutical database, its data were first subjected to text segmentation using section identifiers, with each segment having a maximum length of 1024 characters, and underwent format regularization to unify inconsistent text layouts. Subsequently, the preprocessed text was converted into high-dimensional semantic vectors via the text-embedding-3-large model. Finally, a hybrid retrieval mechanism was adopted, integrating full-text retrieval, vector retrieval, and secondary ranking using the bce-reranker-base v1 reranking model, to enable data retrieval.For the elderly medical literature database, valid literatures were initially screened based on inclusion criteria, which required publication in journals within the past decade and a focus on the field of elderly health. Thereafter, the same workflow applied to the pharmaceutical database—including text segmentation, vectorization, and hybrid retrieval—was implemented.Through the aforementioned processes, unified processing and retrieval of the three types of data were ultimately achieved.

3 Research Methods

3.1 Modeling of Large Language Model

Large Language Models (LLMs) act as the core driver of multi-agent systems, and this study innovatively realizes the adaptation of general models to the medical field through a dual-model collaborative architecture combined with targeted prompt engineering, breaking the bottleneck of general LLMs in professional medical scenario application.

We selected DeepSeek-R1-Distill-Qwen-7B [9] and Qwen3-8B [10] as the base models and integrated them with the unified knowledge base (covering geriatric disease Q&A, drug databases, and medical literature). For DeepSeek-R1-Distill-Qwen-7B, specialized prompt templates were designed to prioritize the extraction of elderly health-related key information and intent recognition. The template structure includes fixed slots such as "User Age: ____, Chronic Diseases: ____, Current Medications (name & dosage): ____, Consultation Demand Type: [Medication Safety/Common Disease Inquiry/Daily Care]", which guides the model to parse voice-transcribed user input (e.g., "I'm 78, have high blood pressure, take nifedipine, and want to know if I can add aspirin") into structured data. This ensures the model accurately identifies user intent and diverts it to the Medication Guidance Agent, reducing misclassification caused by ambiguous natural language.

For Qwen3-8B, prompt strategies tailored to geriatric medical scenarios were adopted to enhance professional reliability and elderly-friendliness. First, medical knowledge anchoring: the prompt explicitly requires the model to reference the unified knowledge base, e.g., "When answering questions about atrial flutter symptoms in the elderly, prioritize content from the geriatric disease Q&A database and PubMed geriatric literature"; second, professional output constraint: the prompt limits the use of complex medical terms and specifies actionable guidance (e.g., "When advising on hypertension care, include 1 specific daily measure, such as 'Measure blood pressure at 7 a.m. before eating'"). Additionally, the prompt adds a hallucination suppression rule: "If the knowledge base has no clear record of a disease/drug interaction, output 'This situation requires further confirmation by a doctor' instead of speculative content", avoiding misleading information.

This design not only exerts the lightweight efficiency of DeepSeek-R1-Distill-Qwen-7B and the strong reasoning ability of Qwen3-8B [11] but also realizes the deep adaptation of general models to elderly health scenarios through prompt engineering—addressing the issues of general LLMs' probabilistic bias and poor scenario adaptability. It improves the system's professionalism (e.g., accurate DDI reasoning) and reliability (e.g., reduced factual errors) in medical health management while avoiding additional computational costs from full-model fine-tuning.

3.2 Voice Interaction

In this study, the speech interaction module employs SenseVoice-Small for automatic speech recognition. The model is optimized for low latency and multilingual support, demonstrating robust performance in Mandarin, Cantonese, and English. It further integrates language identification and paralinguistic cues such as emotion and event detection. These capabilities make it particularly suitable for elderly-oriented interaction, where continuous speech and noisy acoustic conditions often occur, providing reliable input for downstream multi-agent understanding and decision-making [12].

For speech synthesis, CosyVoice2–0.5B is adopted. It incorporates streaming generation with block-aware causal alignment, enabling real-time synthesis with reduced delay while preserving naturalness and fluency of the generated speech. The model also employs quantization strategies to improve the efficiency of speech codebooks, ensuring realistic voice output even under limited computational resources. This efficiency facilitates timely task reporting and agent feedback, which are crucial in multi-agent coordination [13].

By integrating the ASR timestamps with the block-based TTS streaming pipeline, the system establishes a seamless listening-understanding-responding loop. For elderly users, such smooth and natural voice interaction enhances accessibility and comfort, while also improving the perceived reliability and usability of multi-agent systems in real-world applications.

3.3 Multi-Agent Architecture

In the intelligent elderly healthcare management system proposed in this study, multi-agents serve as key execution modules. Under the collaborative scheduling of the Large Language Model (LLM), they implement specialized task division tailored to the healthcare management needs of the elderly population, effectively addressing the shortcomings of traditional systems in service relevance and execution accuracy.The multi-agents integrated into the system do not operate in isolation; instead, they take the LLM optimized through prompt engineering as the core coordination hub. Relying on a unified knowledge base that integrates Q&A repositories for common geriatric diseases, authoritative drug databases, and medical literature databases on geriatric diseases, they form a collaborative working mode of centralized scheduling, professional execution, and knowledge support.Among them, two types of core professional agents undertake differentiated key tasks:

- Medication Guidance Agent: Focusing on the core demand of medication safety for the elderly, this agent accurately conducts drug-drug interaction detection based on drug data (such as drug components, indications, contraindications, etc.) in the unified knowledge base. Meanwhile, it can generate medication plan recommendations adapted to the physiological characteristics of the elderly by combining users' medication history and underlying diseases, thereby avoiding health risks caused by polypharmacy.
- Health Knowledge Consultation Agent: Aimed at addressing the diverse health inquiries of elderly users, this agent retrieves authoritative medical literature and standardized Q&A resources from the knowledge base around topics such as prevention of common geriatric diseases, daily care for chronic diseases, and healthy lifestyles. It answers users' consultations in plain language, helping the elderly proactively acquire health management knowledge.

Under the overall coordination of the LLM, these two types of agents not only achieve the accurate implementation of professional tasks but also adapt to the operating habits of the elderly by connecting with the voice-dominated natural language interaction module. The structure of the system is shown in Fig. 1. The system visualisation is shown in Fig. 2.

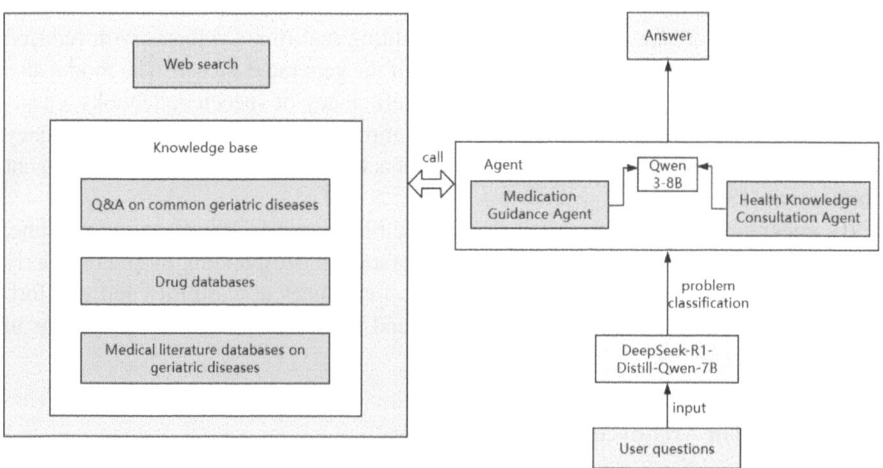

Fig. 1. System frame diagram

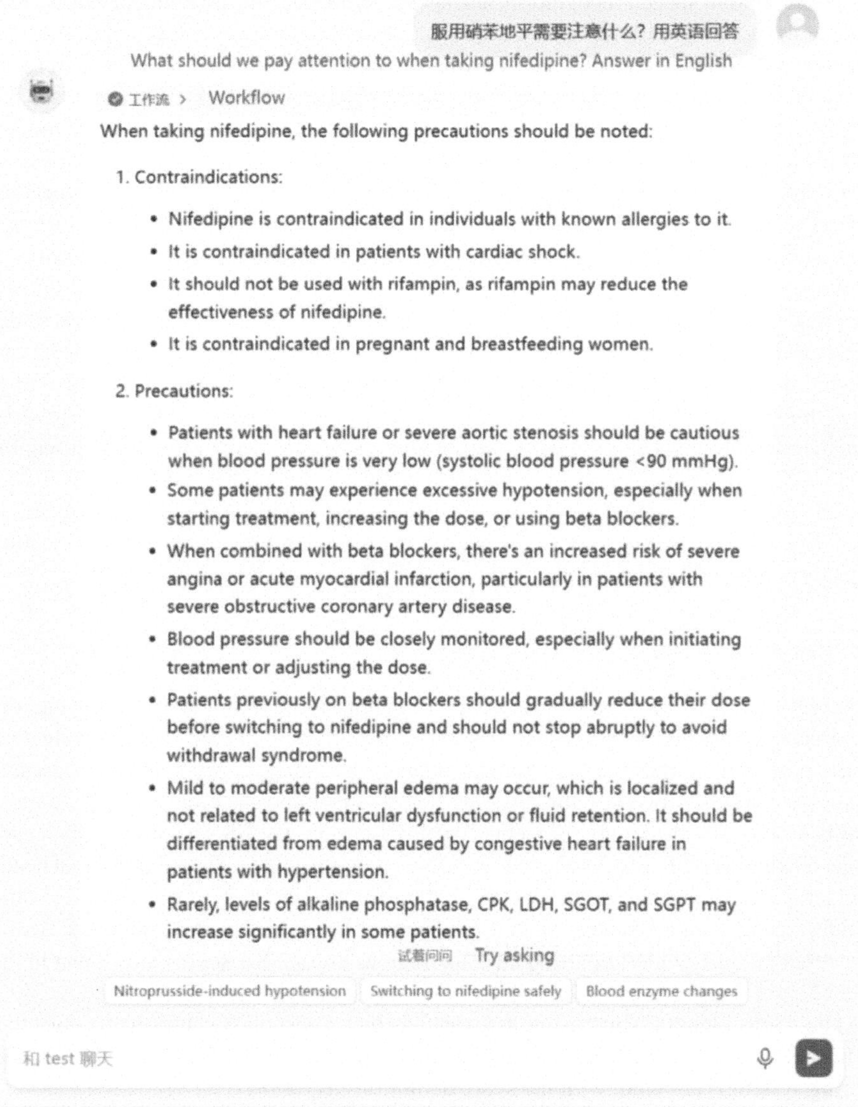

Fig. 2. System display

4 Experimental Results Display and Analysis

4.1 Experimental Setup

The underlying operating environment of this experiment is built on the Ubuntu 22.04 LTS operating system. At the hardware level, an NVIDIA A100 graphics processing unit is adopted, which provides stable computing power support for model training, inference, and the collaborative operation of multi-tasking. To cover the three core tasks of text generation, speech recognition, and speech synthesis, this experiment selects four types of models with differentiated functions. The text generation category includes the DeepSeek-R1-Distill-Qwen-7B and Qwen3-8B models, which are utilized to achieve high-quality text content generation. The speech processing category encompasses the open-source SenseVoiceSmall model and the open-source CosyVoice2–0.5B model, forming a complete speech signal processing chain.

In order to enable the autonomous decision-making capability and tool invocation capability of large language models, the experiment designs and adopts a tool-prioritized invocation strategy. This strategy explicitly grants the intelligent agent permission to invoke two types of tools: knowledge base retrieval and Tavily web search, with knowledge base retrieval configured as the preferred tool through priority settings. Meanwhile, to standardize the task execution logic of the agent, a standardized pompt template is constructed in the experiment. This template integrates rules for user requirement parsing, rules for judging tool invocation conditions, and rules for integrating tool results. In addition, the experimental results and interaction processes are visualized using the Streamlit framework. This visualization system supports multiple interactive functions, including speech input, speech output, dialogue opening remarks, suggestions for follow-up questions, and real-time monitoring of the agent's decision-making process, tool invocation trajectory, and task output results.

4.2 Sensibleness-Specificity Assessment

Proposed by the Google team during their research on the dialogue robot Meena, the Sensibleness-Specificity Assessment (SSA) Score serves as a core manual evaluation metric designed to measure the "human-likeness" of machine-generated responses. It primarily comprises two key dimensions: Sensibleness and Specificity. In the content quality evaluation of dialogue systems for elderly users, the SSA Score acts as a core subjective indicator. It effectively determines whether responses align with the real needs of elderly users in scenarios such as health consultation and daily life assistance, while avoiding generalized expressions that are "correct but useless". We conducted actual user research on 15 elderly participants and regular users, SSA scores are shown in the Table 2.

The "Sensibleness" dimension assesses whether a response conforms to objective facts, maintains logical consistency, and is free from common-sense errors. A 1–5 point scoring system is adopted, with the score definitions as follows:

- 1 point: The response completely violates objective common sense or medical standards and contains obvious misleading information.
- 2 points: The response has numerous common-sense flaws, poor logical coherence, and extremely low practicality.
- 3 points: The response generally conforms to common sense and logic but has minor flaws and moderate practicality.
- 4 points: The response aligns with objective facts and logic, has no obvious flaws, and can meet the basic needs of elderly users.
- 5 points: The response is logically rigorous, factually accurate, fully considers the characteristics of the elderly user group, and has strong practicality.

The "Specificity" dimension focuses on whether a response closely addresses the user's question, avoids deviating from the topic, and refrains from overgeneralization. It also uses a 1–5 point scoring system, with the following definitions:

- 1 point: The response completely deviates from the topic of the user's question and is irrelevant to the user's needs.
- 2 points: The response has extremely low relevance to the user's question, shows obvious topic deviation, and contains no valid information.
- 3 points: The response is partially relevant to the user's question but is generalized in expression and lacks specific details.
- 4 points: The response closely targets the core of the user's question, has no topic deviation, contains certain specific information, and can provide clear guidance for the user.
- 5 points: The response accurately matches the core of the user's question, contains sufficient detailed information, and has strong operability.

Table 2. SSA score

Evaluation sample size	Number of evaluators	Average sensibleness score	Average specificity score	Final SSA score
250	15	4.1	3.8	3.95

4.3 Evaluation Indicators

This experiment focuses on the core function of the drug guidance agent—accuracy of drug-drug interaction (DDI) detection. It quantitatively assesses the agent's ability to identify medication-related risks in common polypharmacy scenarios among the elderly population using two key metrics: Precision and Recall. Elderly individuals often suffer from multiple comorbidities such as hypertension and diabetes, requiring concurrent use of three or more medications, which elevates the risk of DDIs. High Precision helps avoid medication anxiety and waste of medical resources caused by false positives, while high Recall reduces potential medication hazards resulting from false negatives. Together, these two metrics ensure the safety and reliability of the agent's service.

To align with the actual medication needs of the elderly and ensure the rigor of annotations, a dataset was constructed using a targeted screening plus hierarchical annotation approach. Thirty-five single drugs were selected from core drug categories commonly used by the elderly. These drugs were then combined into 30 drug combinations, each containing 3 to 4 drugs, to simulate complex polypharmacy scenarios. A 3-person team was responsible for annotation, including 2 core annotators and 1 conflict verifier. The 2 core annotators performed annotations based on official drug package inserts. Annotations consistent between the two annotators were designated as Ground Truth (gold standard). For conflicting annotations, the third team member conducted a review to determine the final result. Among the 30 final drug combinations, there were 22 positive samples with confirmed drug-drug interactions (DDIs) and 8 negative samples without DDIs, forming a standardized dataset as presented in Table 3.

Table 3. Drug combinations and DDIs

ID	Drug 1	Drug 2	DDI
1	Erythromycin	Lovastatin	Yes
2	Phenobarbital Tablets	Levamlodipine	Yes
3	Dexketoprofen Tablets	Aspirin	Yes
...	...	...	...

In the experiment, the drug combinations were input into the system one by one. The intelligent agent then analyzed the combinations and output risk assessment results by leveraging its capabilities of accessing drug databases, conducting web searches, and performing large language model (LLM)-based reasoning. Using the manually annotated gold standard as the reference, the system's results were compared with the gold standard on a combination-by-combination basis.Three core statistical metrics were defined:

- True Positive (TP): Samples where the system correctly identified the presence of DDIs.
- False Positive (FP): Samples where the system incorrectly judged DDIs to be present.
- False Negative (FN): Samples where the system failed to detect the presence of actual DDIs.

Through comparison and statistics, TP in this experiment is 17 groups (17 groups of 22 groups of actual positive samples were correctly identified by the system), FP is 1 group (1 group of 8 groups of actual negative samples was misjudged as having DDI), FN is 5 groups (5 groups of 22 groups of actual positive samples were not identified by the system). Based on the above statistics, the specific calculation formula of accuracy and recall rate is defined as follows in Eqs. (1)–(2):

$$\text{Precision} = \frac{\text{TP}}{\text{TP} + \text{FP}} = \frac{17}{17 + 1} = 94.4\% \tag{1}$$

$$\text{Recall} = \frac{\text{TP}}{\text{TP} + \text{FN}} = \frac{17}{17 + 5} \approx 77.3\% \tag{2}$$

In terms of the calculation results, the drug guidance intelligent agent exhibits high precision (94.4%) in the detection of drug-drug interactions (DDIs) for commonly used drug combinations in the elderly population. Only one negative sample was misjudged as a false positive, which can minimize medication anxiety among elderly patients caused by unnecessary risk alerts and reduce resource consumption resulting from redundant medical consultations. This holds positive significance for improving medication adherence in elderly patients and the efficiency of medical services. Regarding the recall rate, it reaches approximately 77.3%, enabling effective coverage of over 70% of potential DDI risks. This provides risk early-warning support for the safety of combined medication use in the elderly population and allows for the identification of medication-related risks.

5 Conclusion and Outlook

This study develops an intelligent elderly health consultation system integrating LLMs with multi-agent systems to address challenges like fragmented elderly health data and insufficient service personalization. The main achievements of this study are:

- A unified knowledge base built from 3 core resources with standardized processing and hybrid retrieval for efficient knowledge support.
- A dual-model collaboration LLM architecture and voice interaction adapting to elderly users.
- Effective multi-agent collaboration: the system scores 3.95 in SSA and the Medication Guidance Agent achieves 94.4% Precision and 77.3% Recall in DDI detection, ensuring medication safety.

Future research will focus on expanding dataset diversity (adding rare disease medications and multilingual Q&A data) and building a dynamic knowledge update mechanism with real-time data integration; optimizing multi-agent hierarchical coordination logic and developing specialized agents (e.g., emergency response, cognitive training) for special subgroups. In summary, this study verifies the feasibility of integrating LLMs with multi-agent systems in elderly health management, contributing to improving the quality of life of the elderly and promoting the development of geriatric care systems.

Acknowledgments. This study was funded by Beijing Natural Science Foundation (grant number L222048).

References

1. Gao, S., Fang, A., Huang, Y., et al.: Empowering biomedical discovery with AI agents. Cell **187**(22), 6125–6151 (2024)
2. Langston, E.M., Hattakitjamroen, V., Hernandez, M., et al.: Exploring artificial intelligence-powered virtual assistants to understand their potential to support older adults' search needs. Human Fact. Healthcare **7**, 100092 (2025)
3. Wang, Z., Zhu, Y., Zhao, H., et al.: ColaCare: enhancing electronic health record modeling through large language model-driven multi-agent collaboration. In: Proceedings of the ACM on Web Conference 2025, pp. 2250–2261. ACM (2025)
4. Rivkin, D., Hogan, F., Feriani, A., et al.: AIoT smart home via autonomous LLM agents. IEEE Internet Things J. **12**(3), 2458–2472 (2025)
5. Mahmood, A., Cao, S., Stiber, M., et al.: Voice assistants for health self-management: designing for and with older adults. In: Proceedings of the 2025 CHI Conference on Human Factors in Computing Systems, pp. 1–22. ACM (2025)
6. Rao, A., Kim, J., Lie, W., et al.: Proactive polypharmacy management using large language models: opportunities to enhance geriatric care. J. Med. Syst. **48**(1), 41 (2024)

7. Ataei, M., Cheong, H., Grandi, D., et al.: Elicitron: a large language model agent-based simulation framework for design requirements elicitation. J. Comput. Inf. Sci. Eng. **25**(2), 021012 (2025)
8. Shao, S., Lin, S., Huang, Z., et al.: A medical consultation system for geriatric disease based on multi-agent architecture and knowledge graph. In: Health Information Science. Lecture Notes in Computer Science, pp. 313–325 (2024)
9. Guo, D., Yang, D., Zhang, H., et al.: Deepseek-r1: Incentivizing reasoning capability in llms via reinforcement learning. arXiv preprint arXiv:2501.12948 (2025)
10. Bai, J., Bai, S., Chu, Y., et al.: Qwen technical report. arXiv preprint arXiv:2309.16609 (2023)
11. Thirunavukarasu, A.J., Ting, D.S.J., Elangovan, K., et al.: Large language models in medicine. Nat. Med. **29**(8), 1930–1940 (2023)
12. An, K., Chen, Q., Deng, C., et al.: FunAudioLLM: voice understanding and generation foundation models for natural interaction between humans and LLMs. arXiv preprint arXiv:2407.04051 (2024)
13. Du, Z., Wang, Y., Chen, Q., et al.: CosyVoice 2: scalable streaming speech synthesis with large language models. arXiv preprint arXiv:2412.10117 (2024)

Interiority for Sexual Disease Rehabilitation with Positive Environment Design Approach

Vincentius Raymond and Andriano Simarmata(✉)

Interior Design Department, School of Design, Bina Nusantara University, Jakarta 11480, Indonesia
andriano.simarmata@binus.ac.id

Abstract. Sexually transmitted diseases (STDs) and other sexual disorders continue to pose significant global health challenges, with cases steadily increasing, including in Indonesia. In Bandung, the rising incidence and low public awareness underscore the need for facilities that combine medical rehabilitation with comprehensive sexual education. Current rehabilitation centers often lack psychological support and user oriented spatial design, while stigma and shame hinder individuals from seeking help. This study proposes an interior design concept for a Sexual Rehabilitation and Education Center in Bandung based on the Positive Environment Design approach. The design seeks to reduce stigma and promote emotional healing through human-centered strategies. Its conceptual framework Revival, Encourage, Sanctuary, and Privacy is manifested through zoning, materials, lighting, and circulation. Using a qualitative method involving literature reviews, field observations, interviews, and fishbone diagram analysis, the research identifies user needs that inform the spatial arrangement of medical, educational, and support areas. The resulting prototype demonstrates how interior design can integrate functionality and psychological comfort, serving as a model for future sensitive healthcare environments in Indonesia.

Keywords: Interior Design · Sexual Disease Center · Positive Environment

1 Research Background

Sexual health is an essential component of holistic well-being, encompassing physical, emotional, mental, and social dimensions. In Indonesia, discussions and services related to sexual health remain limited due to sociocultural taboos, lack of proper education, and inadequate public facilities. Bandung, a metropolitan city with a dense and diverse population, faces a growing number of sexual health cases. According to 2023 public health records, the city reported 747 HIV cases, 190 AIDS cases, and a 9.75% increase in out-of-wedlock pregnancies. These data emphasize a serious public health issue that calls not only for clinical treatment but also for educational, psychological, and spatial approaches. Current rehabilitation and health centers in Indonesia often focus primarily on medical treatments, with limited attention to patients' emotional and psychological comfort. Moreover, stigma surrounding sexually transmitted diseases (STDs) often

E. R. Kaburuan and S. Goundar (Eds.): HIS 2025, LNCS 16392, pp. 59–70, 2026.
https://doi.org/10.1007/978-981-95-6304-3_6

leads to social isolation, shame, and delayed treatment. This presents a challenge that extends beyond healthcare systems into the built environment. This project introduces the interiority for sexual disease rehabilitation Bandung, incorporating the principles of Positive Environment Design. The central objective is to develop interior environments that serve not only clinical and educational functions, but also provide psychological support, foster emotional healing, ease feelings of shame, and encourage open dialogue. The overall design approach is anchored in four foundational concepts—Revival, Encourage, Sanctuary, and Privacy—which inform decisions related to spatial organization, material choices, lighting quality, and environmental ambiance. Through this user-focused and emotionally responsive design, the project aspires to create a comprehensive and inclusive model that can serve as a reference for future healthcare spaces addressing sensitive issues across Indonesia.

2 Literature Review

2.1 Sexually Transmitted Diseases and Sexual Disorders

Sexually transmitted diseases (STDs) and sexual disorders represent interconnected yet distinct aspects of sexual health that demand holistic and empathetic care. STDs such as HIV, syphilis, gonorrhea, and chlamydia cause not only physical symptoms but also psychological and social distress, including anxiety, depression, and shame linked to moral and cultural stigma (WHO, 2023; Herek, 2014). Similarly, sexual disorders such as erectile dysfunction, premature ejaculation, vaginismus, and hypersexuality are non-infectious conditions influenced by emotional, psychological, and physiological factors (McCabe et al., 2016), often leading to low self-esteem, relationship conflict, and social withdrawal (Fisher et al., 2020). Both issues are intensified by societal taboos, lack of education, and limited access to confidential healthcare, especially in conservative contexts like Indonesia. Addressing them requires not only medical and psychological treatment but also spatial environments that foster dignity, privacy, and emotional safety. As noted by Link and Phelan (2017), the design of healing spaces can play a crucial role in reducing stigma and promoting psychological recovery. Thus, interior design interventions that emphasize comfort, empathy, and acceptance are vital in supporting holistic rehabilitation for individuals affected by sexual health issues.

2.2 Positive Environment Design

Positive Environment Design is a specific approach designed to support the client's recovery process through strategies focused on reinforcing positive behavior, empathy, and psychological well-being. Corey (2017) describes it as a strategy that promotes healing by addressing not only physical needs but also the emotional and psychological dimensions of patient care. When applied effectively, this design philosophy can create environments that foster trust, dignity, and emotional safety for its users. The aspects resulting from a positive environment are summarized in Table 1.

A positive environment is multidimensional, encompassing physical, psychological, and emotional aspects (see Table 1). Physically, it ensures cleanliness, comfort, and

Table 1. The Aspect resulting from Positive Environment Design.

The Aspect	Description
Physical Aspect	A positive environment in a sexual education and rehabilitation center can support the physical recovery of patients by creating a comfortable and safe atmosphere. Clean and well-organized facilities, along with professional medical services, can reduce patients' physical stress and facilitate the healing process. The creation of spaces free from external disturbances helps patients feel more at ease, which in turn supports the body's response to medical treatment, reduces the risk of infection, and accelerates physical recovery
Physcological Aspect	A supportive environment in a sexual education and rehabilitation center can improve the psychological well-being of patients by providing a sense of safety, comfort, and acceptance. Friendly and non-judgmental counselors or medical personnel help patients feel more open to discussing their sexual health issues. This encourages patients to be more cooperative during treatment and has a positive impact on their mental state, reducing anxiety and increasing confidence in managing their sexual health problems
Emotional Aspect	A positive environment also plays a significant role in supporting patients' emotional well-being. An empathetic and attentive atmosphere, with clear and non-judgmental communication, provides patients with the space to process feelings of shame or guilt often associated with sexual illnesses. Emotional support offered by medical staff, along with opportunities to share experiences, helps patients feel valued and accepted—an essential factor in maintaining emotional balance during the recovery process

accessibility to support the healing process. Psychologically, it cultivates a sense of acceptance and openness, encouraging users to seek treatment without fear of judgment. Emotionally, it provides a nurturing atmosphere where patients can process feelings of shame and regain self-worth through empathetic interactions and supportive spatial settings.

Recent studies reinforce this concept. Baumann (2024) found that design environments emphasizing warmth, natural elements, and privacy significantly reduce stigma and enhance patient comfort. Biophilic integration, soft textures, and human-scale lighting not only promote relaxation but also symbolize care and empathy key elements in reducing emotional tension and social anxiety. International precedents such as the 56 Dean Street Clinic in London and the Royal Melbourne Hospital Sexual Health Unit demonstrate how interior design can reshape perceptions of sexual health facilities through inclusive, non-institutional aesthetics.

In contrast, many healthcare facilities in Indonesia remain sterile, rigid, and emotionally detached, which inadvertently perpetuates stigma and discourages patients from seeking help. This project seeks to reinterpret the principles of Positive Environment

Design within Indonesia's socio-cultural context by combining rehabilitation and education into an integrated spatial system. The goal is to create an interior environment that is not only functional and hygienic but also emotionally responsive, socially inclusive, and culturally empathetic facilitating both psychological healing and destigmatization.

3 Methodology

This study adopts a qualitative descriptive approach to explore the psychological, social, and spatial needs of users within the context of a sexual rehabilitation center. The qualitative method is considered suitable as it emphasizes in-depth understanding over numerical measurement, allowing richer interpretation of users' emotional and behavioral responses. The design process follows a human-centered methodology, prioritizing users' experiences and psychological conditions in spatial decision-making. As Norman (2013) explains, human-centered design involves deeply investigating users' needs, behaviors, and limitations to formulate empathetic and effective spatial solutions aligning with the principles of Positive Environment Design that emphasize comfort, dignity, and emotional well-being.

Primary and secondary data were collected to establish a comprehensive foundation. The literature review included key references such as WHO (2006) on the global context of STDs, Sternberg (2010) on design psychology, Ulrich (1991) on environmental influences in healthcare, and Baumann (2024) on positive design and healing environments. For primary data, interviews and surveys were conducted with three participant groups patients, medical personnel, and members of the general public in Bandung. Participants were selected using purposive sampling, focusing on individuals aged 20–50 with prior experience or awareness of sexual health issues. A total of 15 respondents were involved: 5 patients, 5 medical professionals, and 5 members of the public. Interviews were semi-structured to allow open discussion on topics such as stigma, spatial privacy, emotional comfort, and perceptions of sexual health facilities. Field observations were also carried out in selected clinics and hospitals across Bandung to assess spatial configurations, user circulation, and environmental quality.

Qualitative data from interviews and observations were analyzed using thematic analysis, where responses were coded, grouped, and interpreted to identify recurring themes related to user needs and spatial experiences. These themes informed the Fishbone Diagram Analysis, which was used to trace root problems such as insufficient privacy, confusing wayfinding, and the lack of emotional warmth. The findings were then synthesized into conceptual keywords and visual frameworks (e.g., moodboards and zoning diagrams) to guide design development. The process culminated in spatial programming, schematic planning, and 3D visualization to propose a healing-oriented interior prototype. Given the sensitivity of the research topic, ethical considerations were strictly observed. All participants provided informed consent, and their identities were kept anonymous to ensure confidentiality and emotional safety. Data collection was conducted with approval from relevant institutional review procedures, maintaining respect, empathy, and non-judgmental communication throughout the process.

4 Proposed Design Implementation

The layout of this rehabilitation center is designed based on the principle of privacy, with clearly defined zones separating male and female users, as well as distinct entry and exit circulation paths to minimize patient interaction. The presence of private waiting rooms and labyrinth partitions, such as frosted glass and wooden screens, ensures a sense of safety and maintains patient confidentiality, allowing users to undergo treatment without feelings of shame or anxiety. The sanctuary aspect is reflected in the calming spatial design, particularly in therapy and inpatient areas, which utilize organic forms and spatial arrangements that avoid an institutional and rigid atmosphere. Meanwhile, encourage is embodied in the flowing curved forms used in educational spaces like the library and audiovisual room, which create a warmer and more welcoming ambiance, fostering openness and positive interaction. The revival principle is expressed through abundant natural lighting and the use of natural materials such as wood and soft textiles, supporting physical and emotional healing (Figs. 1 and 2).

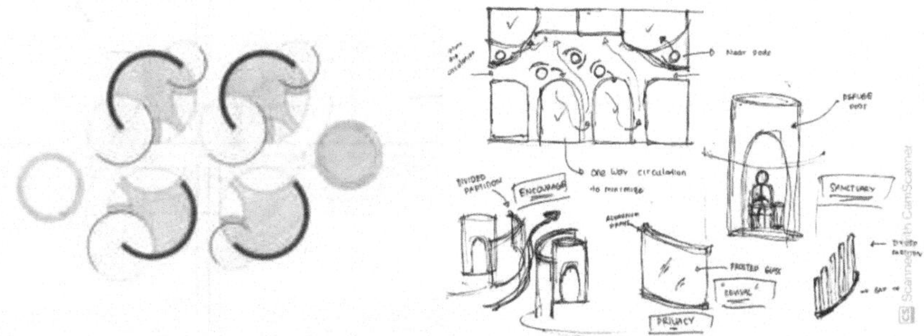

Fig. 1. Creative Concept : Initial Sketch of Circulation and Sanctuary Refuge Pods, Author (2025)

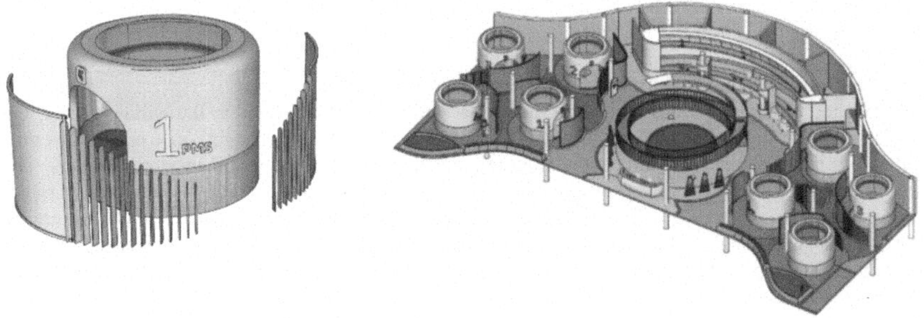

Fig. 2. Application of the Labyrinth Waiting Area and Refuge Pods. Author (2025)

The waiting area in this design is created with an organic form that follows a labyrinthine pattern, representing the keyword privacy. This labyrinth concept is implemented through a one-way circulation system to minimize direct encounters between patients, thereby enhancing psychological comfort. The organic shape of the partitions reflects the keyword encourage, aiming to create a more welcoming and less rigid atmosphere. Additionally, the waiting space is designed as individual pods to evoke a sense of sanctuary, allowing users to feel safe, comfortable, and protected while they wait. Meanwhile, the keyword revival is realized through a mirroring layout concept, intended to facilitate orientation and navigation within the space, enabling users to easily and intuitively find their desired functions.

In terms of color, the palette selection is also grounded in the four key principles. Neutral tones like beige and warm white create a calm and secure atmosphere (Sanctuary), sage green and pastel blue promote tranquility and mental recovery (Revival), while soft yellow accents are applied in educational areas to stimulate enthusiasm and user engagement (Encourage). Overall, this color composition not only reinforces a positive environment but also supports Privacy through soft, non-intimidating tones. For more information, the design implementation is presented in Table 2.

Table 2. Design Concept Implementation.

Area & Layout	Perspective
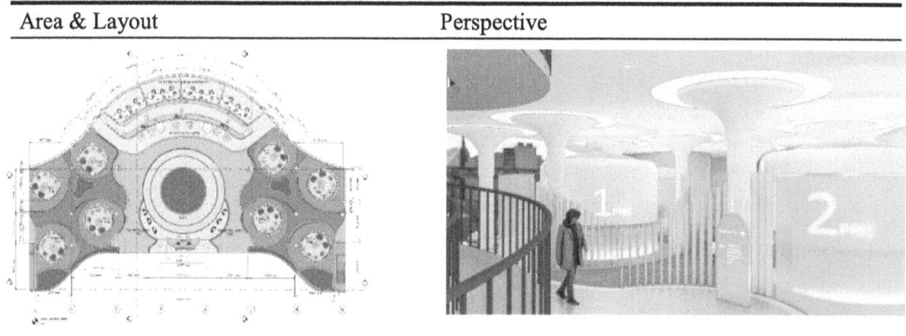	
1. Lobby	
Design Implementation Description: In the existing architectural design, which features a central spiral ramp within the building mass, the layout is arranged in a mirrored configuration to divide the waiting areas. The rationale behind this mirrored layout refers to the Revival concept, aiming to evoke a sense of calm and comfort for users. The main focus in the lobby area is the private waiting room and labyrinth-like corridor, as these spaces represent the added value offered by this rehabilitation center. The intended atmosphere for the waiting area is one of sanctuary, highlighted through the use of organic forms in every interior element. To support both privacy and safety, partitions made of frosted glass and wooden slats are used—reinforcing the Privacy concept by minimizing direct contact between patients.	

(*continued*)

Table 2. (*continued*)

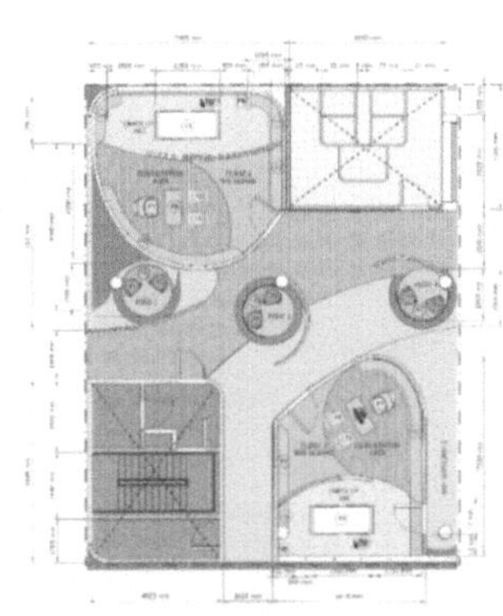

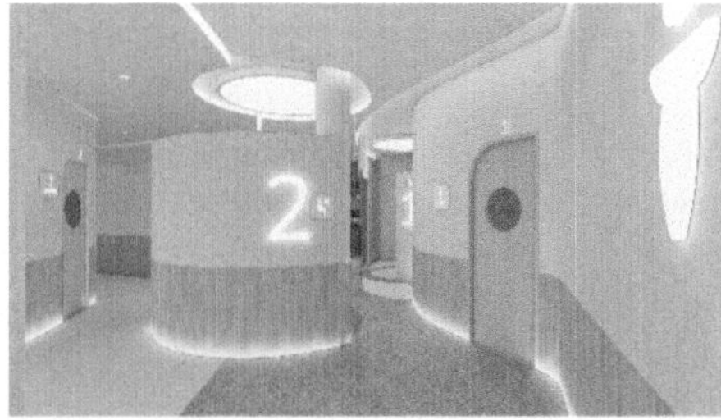

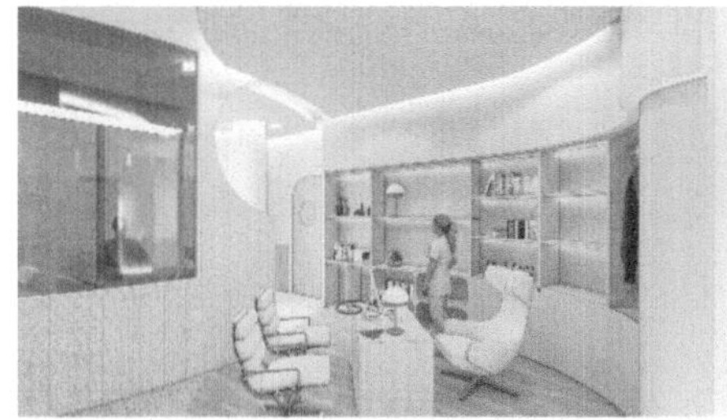

2. STD Clinics

Design Implementation Description:
The layout of this STD clinic is also designed to support the Privacy concept through the use of labyrinth partitions, private waiting areas, and separate circulation paths for entering and exiting the clinic, aiming to minimize contact between patients. On this floor, the Sexually Transmitted Disease (STD) Clinic includes 4 examination rooms, 1 medical post, and 5 private waiting pods. Inside the clinic, there are two main areas: a consultation area and an examination area, separated by frosted glass partitions to enhance privacy while also creating a modern and clean impression.

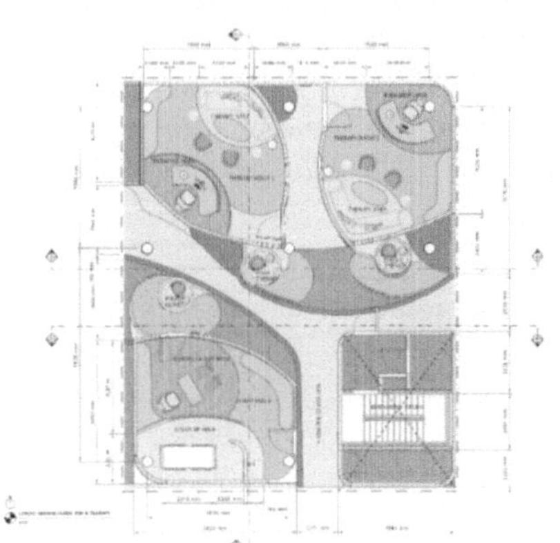

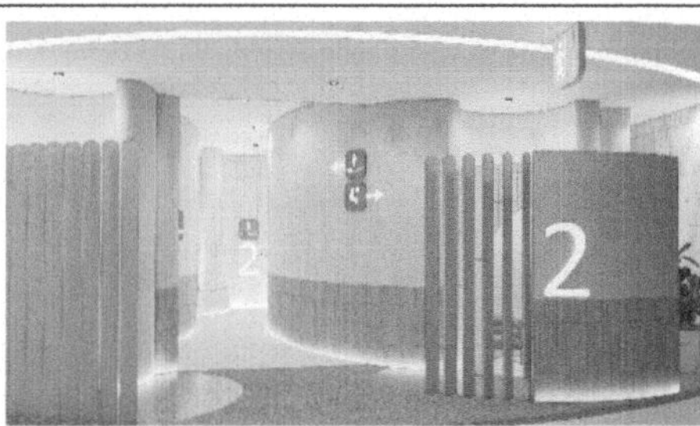

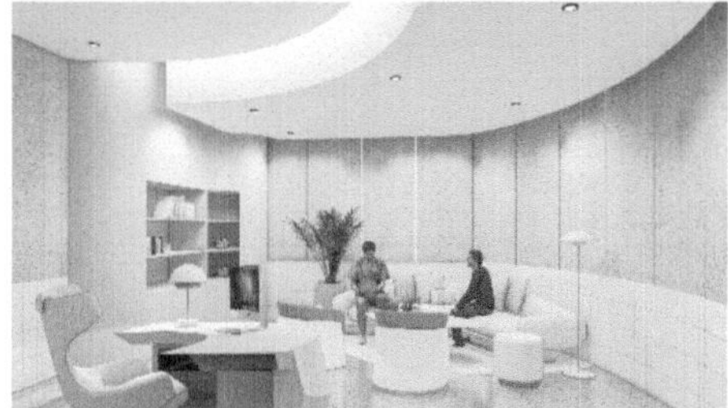

3. Sexual Disorder Clinic & Therapy

(*continued*)

Table 2. *(continued)*

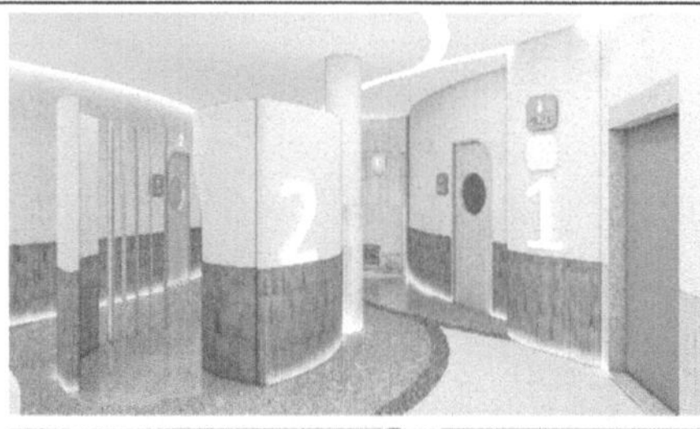

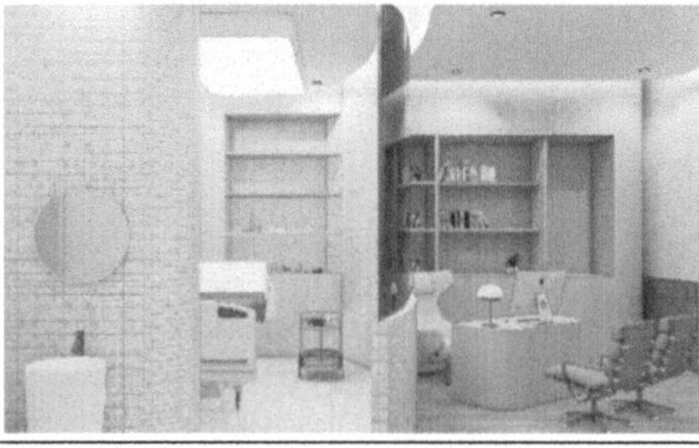

Design Implementation Description:
The layout of the Sexual Disorder and Therapy Clinic is also designed to support the Privacy concept through the use of labyrinth partitions, private waiting areas, and separate circulation paths for entering and exiting the clinic to minimize contact between patients. This clinic includes two private waiting rooms for the therapy area and one private waiting room for the clinic area. These private waiting rooms are located near both the clinic and therapy rooms to ensure ease of access for patients.
Inside the Sexual Disorder Clinic, the space is divided into two main areas: the consultation area and the examination area. These areas are separated by frosted glass partitions to enhance privacy while also creating a modern and clean impression. The therapy area is also divided into two zones: the therapist's desk area and the CBT (Cognitive Behavioral Therapy) area. This space is designed to be more flexible by using a sofa and two easy chairs, allowing patients to feel more comfortable and open during CBT sessions. All interior elements incorporate organic forms to support the Encourage concept.

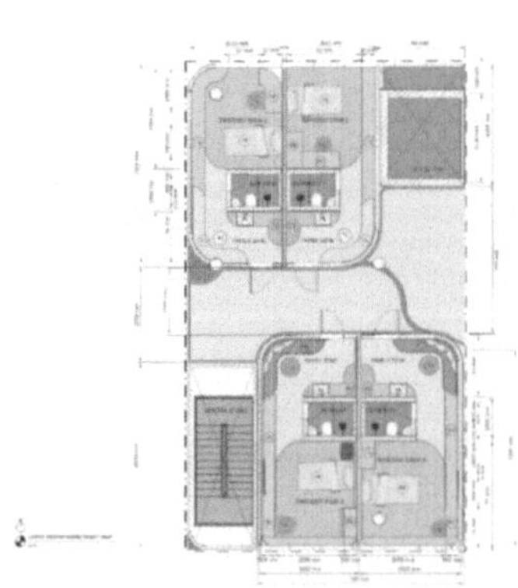

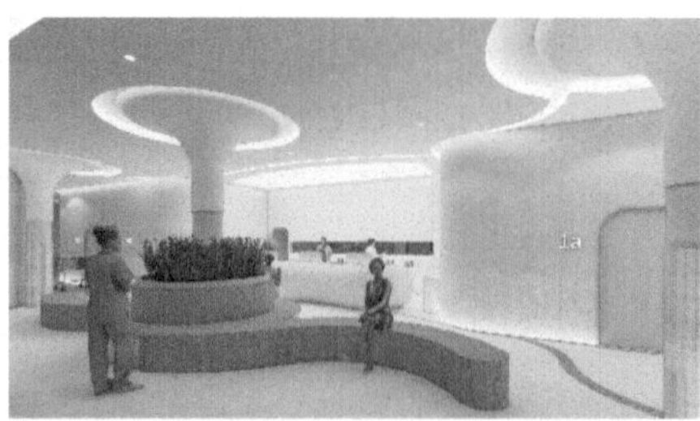

(continued)

Table 2. *(continued)*

4. Inpatients Area

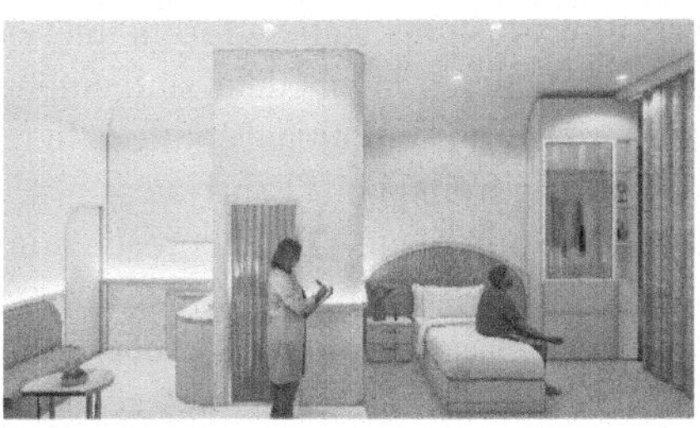

Design Implementation Description:
The inpatient room layout is designed similarly to the other rooms. Each inpatient room is equipped with facilities such as a mini pantry, a sofa for visitors, a bed, a bedside table, a desk and chair, built-in wardrobe, and a private bathroom. Outside the inpatient rooms, there is a medical post and office, as well as benches for visitors. The layout features organic forms while still prioritizing functionality and user comfort. In the bedroom area, the lighting design is intended to reduce negative impacts on health by maximizing daylight and integrating natural elements within both shared and private spaces. Effective healing environments require careful regulation of sensory input. Designers should minimize glare, reduce noise, and balance light quality to support user orientation and a sense of familiarity.

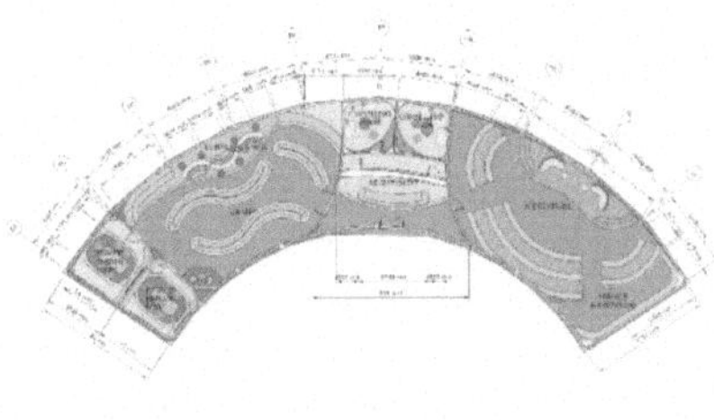

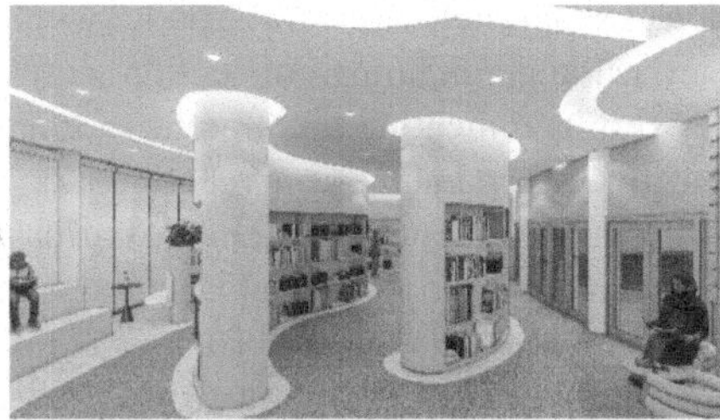

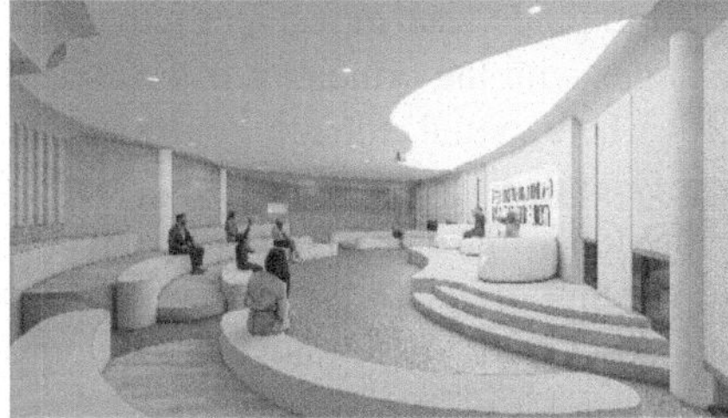

5. Education Area (Education Floor)

Design Implementation Description:
The Education Area is designed to prioritize privacy, sanctuary, and revival.
The private reading room offers a quiet, secluded space for focused study, while the library features individual study booths for personal reflection. The counseling area ensures confidentiality with high partitions and soft lighting, creating a secure environment for sensitive conversations.
The audiovisual room is designed for both group learning and personal reflection, with flexible seating for comfort.
Overall, the space fosters emotional healing by balancing privacy and comfort, encouraging social empowerment and growth.

5 Result and Discussion

The resulting spatial configuration of the Sexual Rehabilitation and Education Center reflects direct insights gathered from interviews, surveys, and field observations. Users particularly patients and medical staff emphasized the need for clear spatial hierarchy to support privacy and emotional comfort. In response, the design establishes a gradient of spaces ranging from public to private zones, each addressing distinct functional and psychological requirements. This approach minimizes social discomfort, especially among users who reported feeling vulnerable due to the stigma surrounding sexual health issues. Interview feedback revealed that gender sensitivity was crucial in creating a safe environment; therefore, the design applies gender-based segregation for clinical and inpatient areas. These are located on separate floors, ensuring both cultural appropriateness and emotional security, as several respondents expressed unease when treatment areas lacked gender separation.

Emotional comfort was another recurring theme in user interviews and observations, where participants highlighted the importance of warm, quiet, and non-judgmental spaces. To address this, therapy and counseling rooms incorporate curved layouts, acoustic treatment, and soft materials to reduce anxiety and foster psychological well-being. Field data showed that patients often felt tense in open waiting areas, leading to the integration of semi-enclosed "refuge pods" within transitional zones spaces that offer partial privacy while maintaining connection with staff visibility. Educational areas, based on survey results indicating a preference for approachable and stigma-free environments, are positioned separately from rehabilitation zones and designed with organic forms and playful visual elements to encourage curiosity and reduce resistance to learning.

Observations across several Bandung clinics indicated that lighting quality and spatial flow significantly influenced user comfort and willingness to participate in therapy. Accordingly, warm lighting, tactile finishes, and single-direction circulation were adopted to guide user movement intuitively and promote a calm, trusting atmosphere. This aligns with the principles of Positive Environment Design, as noted by Baumann (2024), where spatial empathy contributes to behavioral engagement and recovery motivation. Overall, the integration of user-derived data within spatial strategies demonstrates how interior design can bridge clinical functionality with emotional safety. The proposed prototype thus offers a replicable model for designing sensitive healthcare environments in Indonesia where psychological support and social inclusion are as vital as medical treatment.

6 Conclusion

This project presents a comprehensive interior design strategy for a Sexual Rehabilitation and Education Center in Bandung that holistically responds to both clinical and emotional user needs. By employing the Positive Environment Design framework, the project introduces spatial solutions that actively reduce stigma, encourage psychological healing, and create a culturally sensitive environment. The four conceptual pillarRevival, Encourage, Sanctuary, and Privacy form the foundation of spatial organization, material selection, and lighting strategies. These principles translate into clear zoning, natural daylighting, and the application of soft, ergonomic materials that enhance user comfort and safety.

In comparison with existing rehabilitation centers in Indonesia most of which focus primarily on medical functionality and lack spaces dedicated to psychological recovery this design provides a significant advancement. Observations from clinics and rehabilitation facilities in Bandung revealed that current facilities often have minimal privacy, generic layouts, and limited emotional consideration in their interiors. The proposed design directly addresses these limitations by offering gender-segregated treatment areas, emotionally adaptive waiting zones, and therapy rooms designed for psychological safety. This contrast highlights how an empathetic spatial framework can transform the rehabilitation experience from purely clinical to holistically healing.

Beyond this specific project, the design model carries broader implications for healthcare design in Indonesia. It presents a prototype for facilities that manage socially sensitive health issues, such as mental health, reproductive health, and addiction recovery. Its emphasis on empathy, cultural appropriateness, and user dignity aligns with emerging global trends toward trauma-informed and inclusive healthcare environments. The approach can be adapted across regions, though challenges such as cost, staff training, and societal stigma remain key factors in implementation.

Finally, this research acknowledges its limitations. The study's findings are grounded primarily in qualitative data obtained from a limited sample of participants and field sites, and the design remains at a prototypical stage without post-occupancy evaluation. Future studies should expand on quantitative validation, cross-site comparison, and longitudinal assessment to measure the effectiveness of Positive Environment Design in real rehabilitation contexts. Despite these limitations, the project provides a solid foundation for reimagining interior environments that balance clinical effectiveness with emotional and social healing.

Authorship Statement. Vincentius Raymond (Interior Design, BINUS University, Bandung Campus) served as the student member and corresponding author, responsible for conceptualization, data curation, drafting the manuscript, and creating de-sign illustrations. Andriano Simarmata, S.Ds., M.Ds. (Lecturer, Interior De-sign, BINUS Bandung) acted as the research leader, guiding the methodology, supervising students, data curation, methodology development, ergonomic theory analysis, refinement of the literature review and reviewing and editing the manuscript. All authors actively discussed, provided critical feedback, and approved the final manuscript.

Data Availability. This research used qualitative methods by combining literature review and observation with design-based approaches to study visual impairment experiences. The datasets generated are qualitative in nature and contain sensitive information from participants. Therefore, the data is not publicly available due to privacy and ethical considerations. However, anonymized excerpts may be made available from the corresponding author upon reasonable re-quest.

References

1. Baumann, M.: The role of positive environment in healing architecture. J. Environ. Psychol. **48**(1), 55–68 (2024)
2. Corey, S.: Positive environment design: a strategy for psychological healing. Healthc. Archit. J. **12**(1), 45–58 (2017)

3. Day, C.: Spirit and Place: Healing our Environment, Healing Environment. Architectural Press, Oxford (2002)
4. Devlin, A.S., Arneill, A.B.: Health care environments and patient outcomes: a review of the literature. Environ. Behav. **35**(5), 665–694 (2003)
5. Dilani, A.: Psychosocially supportive design: a salutogenic approach to the design of the physical environment. Des. Health Sci. Rev. **1**(1), 59–65 (2001)
6. Hamilton, D.K., Watkins, D.H.: Evidence-Based Design for Multiple Building Types. Wiley, Hoboken (2009)
7. Herek, G.: [Lengkapi judul artikel/perujukannya jika tersedia] (2014)
8. McCabe, M.P., et al.: Risk factors for sexual dysfunction in men and women: a consensus statement. J. Sex. Med. **13**(2), 153–167 (2016)
9. McCormack, B., McCance, T.: Person-Centred Practice in Nursing and Health Care: Theory and Practice, 2nd edn. Wiley-Blackwell, Oxford (2017)
10. Ministry of Health RI. Regulation No. 9 of 2014 on Clinics. Jakarta (2014)
11. Ministry of Health RI. Regulation No. 24 of 2016 on Technical Standards of Health Services. Jakarta (2016)
12. Norman, D.A.: The design of everyday things (Revised ed.). New York: Basic Books (2013)
13. Pallasmaa, J.: The Eyes of the Skin: Architecture and the Senses. Wiley, Chichester (2005)
14. Setiawati, N.: Sex education in Indonesian society. Jurnal Pendidikan dan Kebudayaan **16**(2), 135–142 (2010)
15. Sui, T.Y., McDermott, S., Harris, B., Hsin, H.H.: The impact of physical environments on outpatient mental health recovery. PLoS ONE **18**(4), e0283962 (2023)
16. Sternberg, E.M.: Place Advantage: Applied Psychology for Interior Architecture. Wiley, Hoboken (2010)
17. Stichler, J.F.: Creating healing environments in critical care units. Crit. Care Nurs. Q. **46**(1), 19–30 (2023)
18. Ulrich, R.: Effects of healthcare environmental design on medical outcomes. Environ. Behav. **23**(3), 395–413 (1991)
19. Zainuddin.: Learning resource centers in modern education. Jakarta: Ministry of Education and Culture (1984)
20. Zakiyah, N., Fadilah, L.N., Nurhayati, R.: Sexual violence and social responsibility in children. Jurnal Sosialita **8**(1), 22–29 (2016)

Epilepsy Detection from EEG Signals Using an SXTD-Weighted Visibility Graph and a Novel Transitive Amplification Index Features

Supriya Supriya[1,2(✉)], Nandini Sidnal[1,2], and Tony Jan[2]

[1] Torrens University, Melbourne, VIC 3000, Australia
{supriya.supriya,nandini.sidnal}@torrens.edu.au
[2] Centre for Artificial Intelligence Research and Optimisation (AIRO), Torrens University, Adelaide, Australia
tony.jan@torrens.edu.au

Abstract. Electroencephalogram (EEG) signal analysis plays a significant role in recognizing brain function and supporting the diagnosis of Epilepsy. Existing graph approaches are binary or use endpoint-only (slope/correlation) weights that do not capture the interior fluctuations and trend departures, which limit robustness for epilepsy detection. Many rely heavily on preprocessing and lack shift/scale robustness, which compromises generalization and reliability across subjects and recording conditions. The research aims to propose a novel SXTD-Weighted Visibility Graph framework with an information-rich edge weighting scheme to enhance interpretability and diagnostic accuracy in epilepsy EEG analysis. In addition, new EEG graph features such as Transitive Amplification Index (TAI), MedianWeightEps are developed that capturing the interior fluctuations and trend deviations, remaining shift-invariant and scale-equivariant, providing tunable noise–structure control, and requiring no additional assumptions. The proposed framework achieved 100% accuracy, precision, recall, and specificity across all binary test cases (A–E vs. E) when investigated using multiple classifiers on the Bonn University epileptic EEG dataset. Short, quick EEG changes (spikes, sharp waves) are regularly amplified by the framework, providing a clear difference between ictal and non-ictal segments.

Keywords: Weighted Graph · Topological · Statistical or Graphical Features · EEG signals · Classification of EEG · Visibility graph · Time Series analysis · Complex Network · Epilepsy · fluctuations

1 Introduction

Over 70 million people worldwide suffer from epilepsy, a common neurological condition characterized by frequent, unprovoked seizures [1]. Electroencephalography (EEG) continues to be the most promising noninvasive biomarker to understand the brain electrophysiology [2]. EEG is frequently used for seizure monitoring and diagnosis [3]. However, seizure identification is still mostly done by hand in standard clinical workflows, which is manual, time-consuming, and expert-dependent [4, 5]. These drawbacks

E. R. Kaburuan and S. Goundar (Eds.): HIS 2025, LNCS 16392, pp. 71–81, 2026.
https://doi.org/10.1007/978-981-95-6304-3_7

highlight the necessity for real-time, scalable computer aided systems that can function continuously and almost instantly for automated seizure identification from EEG [6]. Accurate and timely automation can speed up intervention, lessen the workload for clinicians, and significantly enhance the health and well-being of individuals with epilepsy [7]. Therefore, artificial intelligence automation systems capable of accelerating diagnosis and optimizing treatment are extensively desired and continue to be the subject of substantial research investment.

Graph technique has emerged as a powerful approach in the analysis of EEG time series data by advancing a structural and dynamic perspective of brain activity that goes beyond traditional signal processing [8–10]. By modeling the EEG signal as graph/network, exclusively via visibility graph techniques, the temporal structure of the signal is preserved that are enabling the extraction of topological features that plays a critical role in reflecting the underlying neurological state [11–13]. For epilepsy detection, graph-based methods are particularly promising, especially for single-channel EEG signals as they can capture the abrupt transitions, nonlinear dynamics, and especially the chaotic nature of seizure events that conventional features like entropy, variance, or power often not able to capture efficiently [14].

However, most existing graph models either treat edges as binary (i.e., unweighted) or apply simplistic weighting schemes that fail to account for rich intra-segment signal dynamics [15]. This limits the graph's ability to reflect both magnitude and structural variability, which are critical in distinguishing seizure from non-seizure activity. To address these challenges, we propose a novel SXTD-Weighted Visibility Graph framework, that extracts novel graphical features. These features allow for more expressive graph representations, capturing both amplitude-driven and topology-driven characteristics of epileptic seizures, thus significantly improving classification performance on the Bonn University dataset with 100% classification performance with different classifiers such as KNN, SVM (linear, rbf, poly, sigmoid), decision tree, Random Forest and Gradient Boosting.

The key contributions of this research are:

- Introduction of a novel edge weight SXTD (Slope × eXcess Total variation × Trend Deviation) that captures slope, fluctuation, and temporal distortion between EEG points.
- A novel feature: Transitive Amplification Index (TAI), a multi-scale feature that quantifies closure-based amplification within the graph.
- A new adaptive normalization factor named MedianWeightEps, that ensures scale robustness and numerical stability.

Overall, this research study offers a computationally effective and technically sound method for EEG-based seizure detection. More scalable and interpretable clinical support systems will be made possible by the suggested framework's easy extension to real-time applications and adaptation to multi-channel or cross-subject studies.

The organization of the paper comprises the methodological framework in Sect. 2 that describes the epilepsy detection approach in detail. Section 3 includes discussion of the experimental evaluation. Section 4 concluded the research study.

2 Methodological Framework

This section discusses in more detail the proposed framework of EEG signals analysis using the SXTD-Weighted Visibility Graph (SXTD-WVG). Initially, the time series EEG data (Bonn University epileptic EEG data) is converted into an SXTD-Weighted Visibility Graph, which is directional in nature. To characterize the structural connectivity and weight-based dynamics, Transitive Amplification Index Feature and MedianWeightEps are extracted as discriminative novel features from the SXTD-WVG. Using these features, the automated classification is performed on the classifiers: k-Nearest Neighbors (KNN), Random Forest, Support Vector Machine (SVM), and Decision Tree. Finally, to evaluate the performance of the framework, the standard performance metrics (Accuracy, sensitivity and specificity) are systemically deployed to validate its efficiency in distinguishing pathological patterns in EEG such as epilepsy (Fig. 1).

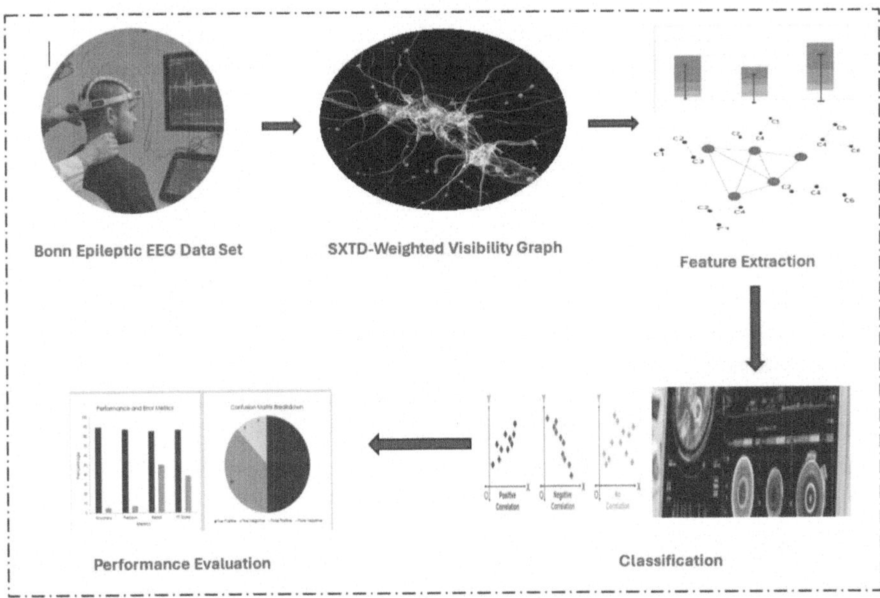

Fig. 1. The systematical representation of the framework, which outlines the major phases of the methodology, including SXTD-Weighted Visibility Graph construction from EEG signals, feature extraction, classification, and performance evaluation.

2.1 SXTD (Slope × eXcess Total Variation × Trend Deviation) Weighted Visibility Graph Construction

Let an EEG time series (of single channel) be represented (possibly non-uniformly) as

$$X = \left(t_{k,} x_{k,}\right)_{k=1}^{N}, \quad t_{k+1} > t_k, \, x_k \in \mathbb{R} \tag{1}$$

For a graph $G = (V, E)$ a vertex for each sample is defined as $V = \{1, \ldots\ldots, N\}$. For any pair $i < j$, , create a directed graph edge (link)$i \rightarrow j$ if all intermediate points are "visible" under the Lucas–Lucasa (natural visibility) condition [16]:

$$x_k < x_i + \frac{x_j - x_i}{t_j - t_i}(t_k - t_i), \quad \forall k \in \{i+1, \ldots, j-1\} \tag{2}$$

The resulting directed graph is $G^{\rightarrow} = (V, E^{\rightarrow})$, with

$$E^{\rightarrow} = \{(i, j) : i < j \text{and } (1) \text{ holds}\} \tag{3}$$

The (binary) directed adjacency is:

$$A_{ij} = \begin{cases} 1, (i, j) \in E^{\rightarrow}, \\ 0, \textit{otherwise}. \end{cases} \tag{4}$$

Edge Weight SXTD (Slope × eXcess Total Variation × Trend × Deviation)
For every visible pair that is directed $(i, j) \in E^{\rightarrow}$, the SXTD weigh is calculated as:

$$w_{ij}^{SXTD} = \frac{|x_j - x_i|}{(t_j - t_i)}(1 + \alpha V_{ij})^{\mu}(1 + \lambda D_{ij})^{\nu} \tag{5}$$

where, α, λ, μ and $\nu > 0$. $\varepsilon \approx 10^{-6}$ for stability.

- The slope term describes the signals gradient connecting two points.
- V_{ij} represents the excess of total variation that quantifies the accumulated fluctuations among two nodes i and j, beyond the direct slope.
- D_{ij} denotes the trend deviation that measures how much the intermediate signal deviates from the expected linear interpolation.
- Hyperparameters α, $\lambda > 0$ and exponents μ,$\nu \geq 0$, regulate how strongly these fluctuations and deviations influence the weight.

The fluctuation terms are:

$$V_{ij} = \frac{\sum_{k=i}^{j-1} |x_{k+1} - x_k| - |x_j - x_i|}{|x_j - x_i| + \varepsilon}, \tag{6}$$

$$D_{ij} = \frac{1}{j - i - 1} \sum_{k=i+1}^{j-1} \frac{|x_k - \hat{x}_k|}{|x_j - x_i| + \varepsilon}, \hat{x}_k = x_i + \frac{x_j - x_i}{t_j - t_i}(t_k - t_i), \tag{7}$$

- V_{ij} is excess total variation
- D_{ij} is the mean deviation from trend
- α, λ control how strongly fluctuations amplify the weight
- Exponents μ, ν ϵ[0.5,1.5] shape the sensitivity (we use in experiment $\alpha = \lambda = 1, \mu = \nu = 1$).
- $\varepsilon > 0$ ensures numerical stability.

The weighted directed edge (weighted adjacency matrix) is then:

$$W_{ij} = \begin{cases} w_{ij}^{SXTD}, (i,j) \in E^{\rightarrow}, \\ 0, otherwise. \end{cases} \tag{8}$$

This W_{ij} is the major input for feature extraction (e.g., TAI Index, MedianWeightEps) and classification.

2.2 Feature Extraction

The quality of the features improves the classification performance, boost robust-ness, enhances accuracy and generalization of a model. Given a SXTD-Weighted Visibility Graph directed, $G^{\rightarrow}$=(V, $E^{\rightarrow}$, , W) built from the Epileptic EEG time series data, the feature extraction is a mapping:

$$\Phi : G^{\rightarrow} \rightarrow \mathbb{R}^d, \tag{9}$$

that represents the structure of $G^{\rightarrow}$ into low-dimensional, discriminative features for classification.

Triplet Set

Let's consider all forward triplets that form a 2-step chain:

$$T = \{(i, j, k) : i < j < k, (i, j) \in E, (j, k) \in E\} \tag{10}$$

Define the chain strength and closure for a triplet (i, j, k) :

$$C_{ijk} = \sqrt{w_{ij} w_{jk}}, K_{ijk} = \begin{cases} w_{ik}, (i, k) \in E, \\ 0, otherwise. \end{cases} \tag{11}$$

A small data-adaptive stability constant has been used:

$$\varepsilon_w = \tau median\{w_{ij} : (i, j) \in E\}, \tau \in (0,1)(\text{we use } \tau = 10^{-2}) \tag{12}$$

Once the SXTD-Weighted Visibility Graph is constructed, we compute the following novel features:

1. **Transitive Amplification Index (TAI)**

   The log-gain per triplet is:

$$g_{ijk} = \log\left(\frac{K_{ijk} + \epsilon_w}{C_{ijk} + \epsilon_w}\right) \tag{13}$$

   The global TAI is the average of these gains:

$$TAI = \frac{1}{|T|} \sum_{(i,j,k) \in T} g_{ijk} \tag{14}$$

2. **TAIIndex (Multi-Scale Summary)**
   Bin triplets by their span Δ_{ik} (uniform sampling: $\Delta_{ik} = k - i$; non-uniform: $\Delta_{ik} = t_k - \Delta_i$ into bins $\{\mathcal{B}_m\}(e.g., dyadic[1,2], [2,4], [4,8], \ldots.)$.
   Per bin,

$$TAI_m = \frac{1}{|T_m|} \sum_{(i,j,k)\in T_m} g_{ijk}, T_m = \{(i,j,k), \in T : \Delta_{ik} \in \mathcal{B}_m\} \tag{15}$$

   Aggregate with a short-scale-biased average:

$$TAIIndex = \frac{\sum_m w_m (TAI_m)^q}{\sum_m w_m}, w_m = 2^{\beta(m-1)}, \beta < 0 \text{ emphasizes short spans}, q \in \{1,2\} \tag{16}$$

3. **NumTriples**

$$NumTriples = |T| = \sum_{i<j<k} 1\{(i,j) \in E\} 1\{(j,k) \in E\} \tag{17}$$

   (Equivalently, with adjacency indicator $A_{ij} = 1\{(i,j) \in E\}$: $NumTriples = \sum_{i<j<k} A_{ij} A_{jk}$
4. **MedianWeightEps**
   The stability constant used in all gains:

$$MedianWeightEps = \epsilon_w = \tau median\big\{w_{ij} : (i,j) \in E\big\}, \tag{18}$$

Notes for reproducibility:

- If any $K_{ijk} = 0$ (no closure edge), the log-gain remains well-defined due to $\varepsilon_w > 0$.
- All logs are natural logs
- These definitions are scale-free with respect to a global scaling of ω (TAI and TAI Index are unchanged if all weights are multiplied by a constant).

2.3 Classification

During classification process, the feature vectors are mapped to discrete labels by learning a decision function from labeled data (training data). In this study, the above extracted features used as input to different classifiers (Decision Tree, SVM, Random Forest, KNN and Gradient Boosting) to check how informative they are to differentiate between healthy and epileptic seizure activity [17, 18]. Decision tree is used for interpretability and fast non-parametric splits. SVM has margin maximization and flexible kernelized boundaries. Random Forest is excellent for variance reduction and robustness to noisy/high information variables. KNN for leveraging local geometry without distributional assumptions. KNN has an advantage of leveraging local geometry without distributional assumptions and Gradient Boosting for sequentially improving errors to obtain subtle interactions.

2.4 Performance Evaluation

The classification performance of the extracted novel features is evaluated using the following metrics [19, 20]:

$$\text{Precision} = \frac{\text{TP}}{\text{TP} + \text{FP}} \tag{19}$$

$$\text{Recall} = \frac{\text{TP}}{\text{TP+FN}} \tag{20}$$

$$\text{Accuracy} = \frac{\text{TP+TN}}{\text{TP+FN+TN+FP}} \tag{21}$$

$$\text{Specificity} = \frac{\text{TN}}{\text{TN+FP}} \tag{22}$$

where, positive class is the epileptic seizure and negative class is the non-epileptic (healthy control):

- TP (True Positive): Positive class EEG correctly predicted as epileptic.
- FP (False Positive): Healthy control class EEG incorrectly predicted as epileptic.
- TN (True Negative): Healthy control class EEG correctly predicted as non-epileptic.
- FN (False Negative):Positive class EEG incorrectly predicted as non-epileptic.

2.5 EEG Epileptic Dataset

In this study, the publicly available Bonn University Epileptic EEG data set is used to evaluate the performance of the proposed framework. The data set includes five different categories (Set A to E) of EEG brain activities. Every single set includes 100 segments of single channel EEG with a sampling rate of data is 173.61 Hz, duration of 23.6 s with 4096 samples. Set A and Set B are the data of healthy control EEG during an awake state with their eyes open and eyes closed. Set C (hippocampal formation of the opposite hemisphere) and Set D (epileptogenic zone) data recordings are of seizure free duration. Set E contains epileptic seizure data. The additional information regarding the dataset is available at [21].

3 Results and Discussion

The proposed framework was evaluated on the Bonn University Epileptic EEG data set (Sets A–E). Each single-channel EEG was converted to a directed SXTD-Weighted Visibility Graph. Initially, these features were extracted: MedianWeightEps TAI _[1, 2], TAI_[2, 4],TAI_[4, 8],TAI_[8, 16],TAI_[16,32],TAI_[32,64],TAI_[64,128],TAI _[128,256],TAI_[256,512], TAI_[512,1024], TAI_[1024,2048],TAI_[2048,4096], were extracted using multi-scale TAI to capture typical edge strength and transitive amplification across ranges. However, among all tested combinations of features, these six features achieved the highest classification performances: MedianWeightEps, TAI_[2, 4], TAI_[4, 8], TAI_[64,128], TAI_[128,256], TAI_[256,512]. Single stratified with 80% training and 20% testing split were deployed (RANDOM_STATE = 42). There was no cross-validation or tuning implemented. Standard Scaler applied to SVM and KNN only (inside pipelines) to prevent leakage.

Table 1 represents the classification performance of the test-case: E vs. A and E vs. C. For the test-case, E vs. C, all classifiers attained 100% classification performance in terms of accuracy, precision, recall and specificity. For the test-case E vs. A, the classification accuracy for different classifiers is broadly consistent across metrics. However, SVM (with kernel: linear, rbf) and KNN (k = 3,5,7,11) achieved the 100% classification performance among all metrices.

Table 1. The classification performance of different test-cases using different classifiers

Classifiers	E vs. C				E vs. A			
	Accuracy (%)	Precision (%)	Recall (%)	Specificity (%)	Accuracy (%)	Precision (%)	Recall (%)	Specificity (%)
DecisionTree	100.0	100.0	100.0	100.0	97.5	95.24	100.0	95.0
SVM (linear, rbf)	100.0	100.0	100.0	100.0	100.0	100.0	100.0	100.0
SVM_poly	100.0	100.0	100.0	100.0	95.0	100.0	90.0	100.0
SVM_sigmoid	100.0	100.0	100.0	100.0	95.0	99.01	100.0	90.0
Random Forest_50	100.0	100.0	100.0	100.0	95.0	90.91	100.0	90.0
Random Forest (100, 200)	100.0	100.0	100.0	100.0	97.5	95.24	100.0	95.0
KNN (k = 3,5,7,11)	100.0	100.0	100.0	100.0	100.0	100.0	100.0	100.0
Gradient Boosting	100.0	100.0	100.0	100.0	97.5	95.24	100.0	95.0

Table 2 illustrates the classification performance of the test-case: E vs. D and E vs. B. For test-case, E vs. D, decision tree, SVM_poly, Random Forest (50, 100, 200) and KNN (k = 3, 5) attained 100% accuracy, precision, recall and specificity. Whereas, for the test-case, E vs. B, Random Forest (50, 100, 200), KNN (k = 3), SVM_linear and Gradient Boosting classifiers achieved 100% classification performance. Overall, across all of the four test cases, KNN (k = 3) and SVM with linear-kernel, consistently achieved the highest classification performance.

Table 3 presents a comparative analysis of the classification performance of our directed, SXTD-weighted visibility-graph framework with MedianWeightEps and multi-scale TAI feature sets. The performance was evaluated on the Bonn University EEG dataset, with A–D as non-seizure and E as seizure, and consider pairwise test cases (e.g., E vs. A). The table clearly depicts our proposed novel weight mechanism and novel extracted features of a weighted graph that yield competitive-to-superior seizure identification compared with current techniques while remaining compact and interpretable.

In summary, the proposed SXTD-weighted visibility-graph framework is more informative in comparison to other weighted visibility graph because it presents fluctuation sensitivity. As two edges can have the same endpoint slope but very different interior

Table 2. The classification performance of different test-cases using different classifiers

Classifiers	E vs. D				E vs. B			
	Accuracy (%)	Precision (%)	Recall (%)	Specificity (%)	Accuracy (%)	Precision (%)	Recall (%)	Specificity (%)
DecisionTree	100.0	100.0	100.0	100.0	92.5	94.8	90.0	95.0
SVM_poly	100.0	100.0	100.0	100.0	85.0	100.0	70.0	100.0
Random Forest (50, 100, 200)	100.0	100.0	100.0	100.0	100.0	100.0	100.0	100.0
KNN (k = 3)	100.0	100.0	100.0	100.0	100.0	100.0	100.0	100.0
KNN_k5	100.0	100.0	100.0	100.0	97.5	100.0	95.0	100.0
KNN_k7	97.5	95.24	100.0	95.0	95.0	100.0	90.0	100.0
SVM_linear	95.0	99.01	90.0	100.0	100.0	100.0	100.0	100.0
SVM_rbf	95.0	99.01	90.0	100.0	97.5	100.0	95.0	100.0
SVM_sigmoid	95.0	99.01	100.0	90.0	80.0	73.08	95.0	65.0
KNN_k11	95.0	99.01	90.0	100.0	97.5	100.0	95.0	100.0
Gradient Boosting	95.0	99.01	100.0	90.0	100.0	100.0	100.0	100.0

Table 3. Comparative analysis of the proposed framework with current techniques using same dataset

Authors	Year	Method	Accuracy (%)
Wang, J. et al. [22]	2023	Weighted Neighbour Graph	99.9
Shyu, K. et al. [23]	2023	LBPMAD-LR	96.4
Cao, X. et al. [24]	2025	CNN-BiLSTM	97.30
Silpa, B. et al. [25]	2025	DSLWNet	99.5
Proposed		SXTD-Weighted Visibility Graph	100

volatility. The weight based on simple slope cannot distinguish them whereas, w_{ij}^{SXTD} increases via V_{ab} (oscillation/roughness) and D_{ab} (departure from linear trends. In addition, it exhibits the trend awareness information such as D_{ab} penalizes/boost according to how far the path strays from straight line, capturing transient excursions that are very important in EEG/physiological signals. In addition, each feature has a clear physical meaning such as edge strength, closure gain, and clustering that is creating the clinical narratives easier. This method can be used for both offline analysis and possibly real-time deployment.

4 Conclusion

In this research, we introduced a novel weighted complex network-based framework for the automatic detection of epilepsy utilizing single-channel EEG recordings. The main emphasis is the SXTD-Weighted Visibility Graph, which uses a new edge-weighting method that considers slope, local variation, and temporal distortion. This gives a more detailed picture of EEG dynamics than typical binary or simple weights. We also introduce the Transitive Amplification Index (TAI), which is a multi-scale characteristic that measures how signal patterns get stronger along closure paths in the graph. This, along with MedianWeightEps for steady normalization, gives you strong and easy-to-understand characteristics even when the signal strength changes. The proposed framework, when examined on the Bonn University dataset, showed 100% classification accuracy in all binary class test cases and successfully separating seizure from non-seizure segments. The combination of advanced edge weighting and transitive topological features makes for a scalable, understandable, and effective way to detect seizures in EEG data.

References

1. Kuhlmann, L., Lehnertz, K., Richardson, M.P., Schelter, B., Zaveri, H.P.: Seizure prediction—ready for a new era. Nat. Rev. Neurol. **14**(10), 618–630 (2018)
2. Supriya, S., Jan, T., Sidnal, N., Thompson-Whiteside, S.: Alcoholic EEG data classification using weighted graph-based technique. In: Traina, A., Wang, H., Zhang, Y., Siuly, S., Zhou, R., Chen, L. (eds.) Health Information Science. HIS 2022. Lecture Notes in Computer Science, vol. 13705, pp 266–276 . Springer, Cham (2022)
3. Tawhid, M.N.A., Siuly, S., Wang, K., Wang, H.: GENet: A generic neural network for detecting various neurological disorders from EEG. IEEE Trans. Cogn. Dev. Syst. **16**(5), 1829–1842 (2024)
4. Busia, P., Leone, G., Matticola, A., Raffo, L., Meloni, P.: Wearable epilepsy seizure detection on FPGA with spiking neural networks. IEEE Trans. Biomed. Circ. Syst. (2025)
5. Supriya, S., Siuly, S., Wang, H., Zhang, Y.: New feature extraction for automated detection of epileptic seizure using complex network framework. Appl. Acoust. **180**, 108098 (2021)
6. Zhang, X., Zhang, X., Huang, Q., Chen, F.: A review of epilepsy detection and prediction methods based on EEG signal processing and deep learning. Front. Neurosci. **18**, 1468967 (2024)
7. Tawhid, M.N.A., Siuly, S., Wang, K., Wang, H.: Automatic and efficient framework for identifying multiple neurological disorders from EEG signals. IEEE Trans. Technol. Soc. **4**(1), 76–86 (2023)
8. Alke, D., et al.: The importance of graph databases and graph learning for clinical applications. Database (Oxford), 2023, baad045 (2023)
9. Supriya, S., Siuly, S., Wang, H., Zhang, Y.: EEG sleep stages analysis and classification based on weighted complex network features. IEEE Trans. Emerg. Top. Comput. Intell. **5**(2), 236–246 (2021)
10. Awais, M., Belhaouari, S.B., Kassoul, K.: Graphical insight: revolutionizing seizure detection with EEG representation. Biomedicines **12**(6), 1283 (2024)
11. Supriya, S., Siuly, S., Wang, H., Zhang, Y.: Weighted complex network based framework for epilepsy detection from EEG signals. In: Modelling and Analysis of Active Biopotential Signals in Healthcare, vol. 1, chap. 3, pp. 3–1–3–22. IOP Publishing, Bristol (2020)

12. Díaz-Montiel, A.A., Zhang, R., Lankarany, M.: Optimal graph representations and neural networks for multichannel time series data in seizure phase classification. Sci. Rep. **15**(1), 19552 (2025)
13. Supriya, S., Siuly, S., Wang, H., Cao, J., Zhang, Y.: Weighted visibility graph with complex network features in the detection of epilepsy. IEEE Access **4**, 6554–6566 (2016)
14. Supriya, S., Sidnal, N., Jan, T., Thompson-Whiteside, S.: Epilepsy detection from weighted EEG graph (WEG) using novel feature-normalized weighted forgotten topological index (NWFT-index). In: Siuly, S., Xing, C., Li, X., Zhou, R. (eds.) Health Information Science. HIS 2024. Lecture Notes in Computer Science, vol. 15336, pp. 234–244. Springer, Singapore (2025)
15. Supriya, S., Siuly, S., Wang, H., Zhang, Y.: Epilepsy detection from EEG using complex network techniques: a review. IEEE Rev. Biomed. Eng. **16**, 292–306 (2023)
16. Lacasa, L., Luque, B., Ballesteros, F., Luque, J., Nuño, J.C.: From time series to complex networks: the visibility graph. Proc. Natl. Acad. Sci. U.S.A. **105**(13), 4972–4975 (2008)
17. Untoro, M.C., Aziz, M.H., Wardoyo, R., Jumadi, J., Ramdhani, M.A.: Evaluation of decision tree, K-NN, naive Bayes and SVM with MWMOTE on UCI dataset. J. Phys. Conf. Ser. **1477**(3), 032025 (2020)
18. Simarmata, N., et al.: Comparison of random forest, gradient tree boosting, and classification and regression trees for mangrove cover change monitoring using landsat imagery. Egypt. J. Remote Sens. Space Sci. **28**(1), 138–150 (2025)
19. Supriya, S., Siuly, S., Wang, H., Zhang, Y.: An efficient framework for the analysis of big brain signals data. In: Wang, J., Cong, G., Chen, J., Qi, J. (eds.) Databases Theory and Applications. ADC 2018. Lecture Notes in Computer Science, vol. 10837, pp. 199–207. Springer, Cham (2018)
20. Oksuz, K., Cam, B.C., Akbas, E., Kalkan, S.: Localization recall precision (LRP): a new performance metric for object detection. IEEE Trans. Pattern Anal. Mach. Intell. **42**(8), 1884–1897 (2020)
21. Andrzejak, R.G., Lehnertz, K., Rieke, C., Mormann, F., David, P., Elger, C.E.: Indications of nonlinear deterministic and finite-dimensional structures in time series of brain electrical activity: dependence on recording region and brain state. Phys. Rev. E **64**(6), 061907 (2001)
22. Wang, J., et al.: EEG signal epilepsy detection with a weighted neighbor graph representation and two-stream graph-based framework. IEEE Trans. Neural Syst. Rehabil. Eng. **31**, 3174–3187 (2023)
23. Shyu, K.K., Huang, S.C., Lee, L.H., Lee, P.L.: A low complexity estimation method of entropy for real-time seizure detection. IEEE Access **11**, 5990–5999 (2023)
24. Cao, X., Zheng, S., Zhang, J., Chen, W., Du, G.: A hybrid CNN-Bi-LSTM model with feature fusion for accurate epilepsy seizure detection. BMC Med. Inform. Decis. Mak. **25**(1), 6 (2025)
25. Silpa, B., Hota, M.K.: DSLWNet: a dual-stream lightweight deep learning network for the detection of epileptic seizures using EEG signals. In: Connection Science, vol. 37, no. 1, p. 2518985 (2025)

Reassessing Digital Care: Sociotechnological Drivers of Telemedicine Disengagement Among Filipino Physicians

Michelle Bernabe[1,2](✉) and Ryan Ebardo[2]

[1] University of St. La Salle, Bacolod City 6100, Philippines
m.bernabe@usls.edu.ph
[2] De La Salle University, 1004 Manila, Philippines
ryan_ebardo@usls.edu.ph

Abstract. Physician disengagement from telemedicine remains a critical yet underexplored challenge to the long-term viability of digital health systems. While adoption has been widely promoted, the reasons clinicians reduce or discontinue its use after initial uptake are less understood. This study explores the sociotechnological factors influencing Filipino physicians' decisions to scale back telemedicine use in post-adoption settings. Using a qualitative design, in-depth interviews were conducted with physicians across various specialties and practice locations. Thematic analysis revealed that discontinuance is shaped by a combination of diagnostic limitations, poor system usability, lack of interoperability, medico-legal concerns, emotional exhaustion, and financial burden. Physicians reported that virtual consultations often hindered accurate assessments, strained communication, and disrupted professional boundaries. This research offers a novel contribution by reframing telemedicine disengagement as a professional and clinical recalibration rather than a mere reaction to technical issues. It extends discontinuance models by integrating clinical judgment, ethical accountability, and work-life balance considerations. The study provides practical insights for designing telemedicine systems that are not only technologically reliable but also aligned with physicians' workflow realities and care standards. These findings are particularly relevant for health systems in low- and middle-income countries seeking sustainable digital health integration.

Keywords: Telemedicine · Discontinuance · Health Information · Sociotechnological Barriers

1 Introduction

Physician disengagement from telemedicine has become a critical concern in the digital transformation of healthcare. During the COVID-19 pandemic, virtual care was rapidly scaled to maintain continuity of services and protect both patients and providers. While this expansion demonstrated the potential of telemedicine, many physicians who initially adopted it are now reducing or abandoning its use in routine practice [1–3]. This trend

E. R. Kaburuan and S. Goundar (Eds.): HIS 2025, LNCS 16392, pp. 82–93, 2026.
https://doi.org/10.1007/978-981-95-6304-3_8

suggests that disengagement is not driven solely by technical dissatisfaction, but also by deeper professional, clinical, and organizational concerns, raising questions about the long-term sustainability of telemedicine as a mainstream care model [4–7].

Previous research has focused largely on barriers to adoption, such as infrastructure limitations, reimbursement and regulatory gaps, and variable digital literacy among providers and patients [8–10]. However, fewer studies examine what happens after adoption, specifically, why physicians disengage even after incorporating telemedicine into their workflows. This is a critical gap because discontinuance can limit the health system's resilience and reduce patient access, particularly in low- and middle-income countries (LMICs), such as the Philippines, where infrastructural instability, limited policy support, and ethical or legal ambiguities may amplify the risks of disengagement [6, 11, 12]. Studying discontinuance is important because it ensures that telemedicine is not only implemented during crises but also sustained in ways that are safe, trusted, and equitable.

This study addresses that gap by examining the sociotechnological factors influencing physicians' disengagement from telemedicine in the Philippine context. Using a qualitative design, semi-structured interviews were conducted and analyzed thematically to uncover the lived experiences of physicians who have scaled back or abandoned virtual consultations. The strength of this approach lies in capturing how clinical judgment, workflow demands, ethical obligations, and technological limitations interact in shaping professional decisions, an area often overlooked in quantitative surveys or policy reports [13–16].

This study explains telemedicine disengagement not as simple dissatisfaction but as a professional response shaped by clinical limitations, fragmented systems, disrupted workflows, and clinical-technical risks. In the Philippine setting as a low- and middle-income country, these issues are intensified by unstable infrastructure, poor interoperability, limited training, and weak regulatory support, which collectively push physicians to reduce or discontinue telemedicine use [4–6, 12]. The findings contribute by highlighting the importance of hybrid care models, user-centered platforms, stronger privacy and legal safeguards, comprehensive training for both providers and patients, and institutional policies that reduce workload and restore physician confidence in sustaining telemedicine [15, 17–20].

2 Related Literature

The sustainability of telemedicine depends on both its technological infrastructure and its ability to meet clinical demands. A major challenge is the inadequacy of virtual consultations, where the absence of physical examinations, reliance on patient self-reports, and poor visual quality reduce diagnostic accuracy, especially among elderly and multilingual patients facing communication barriers [7, 21, 22]. These clinical limitations are compounded by infrastructural deficiencies such as unstable internet, power interruptions, and poor platform usability, which disrupt session continuity and frustrate physicians, particularly in rural settings [10, 23, 24]. In addition, insufficient training, technical glitches, and lack of interoperability create fragmented workflows, redundant documentation, and inefficiency, further discouraging long-term engagement [15, 16].

Collectively, these sociotechnological barriers undermine both diagnostic reliability and workflow sustainability, contributing to declining physician confidence and reduced telemedicine use in the post-pandemic period.

Beyond technical issues, institutional factors play a critical role in physicians' decisions to continue or discontinue telemedicine. A key concern is legal and ethical accountability, as the lack of standardized consent forms, clear documentation protocols, and well-defined liabilities heightens physicians' fear of legal disputes [6]. In the Philippines, these challenges are worsened by economic and operational barriers, including costly platform subscriptions, limited institutional support, and the absence of reimbursement, which often force physicians to shoulder expenses themselves [12, 25, 26]. Physicians also face a dilemma between using formal platforms that meet compliance requirements but are complex and time-consuming, and informal tools like Messenger or Viber that are easier to use but raise serious concerns about data privacy and professionalism [20, 21]. Without stronger institutional policies and leadership to address these issues, physicians are more likely to withdraw from telemedicine, reinforcing the view that it is not yet viable as a sustainable model of care.

At the individual level, physicians' personal experiences and emotional responses played a major role in their decision to disengage from telemedicine. Virtual care disrupted established workflows and added administrative tasks such as uploading results, managing pre-consultation requirements, and documenting across non-integrated systems, which often extended beyond clinic hours and led to fatigue and burnout [15, 22, 27]. The constant intrusion into personal time, compounded by blurred work-life boundaries and occasional ethical discomfort from inappropriate patient behaviors, further eroded physicians' willingness to continue telemedicine [17, 28].

In response, many restricted its use to follow-ups or familiar patients, while others returned entirely to face-to-face care for greater diagnostic control, ethical clarity, and emotional stability. Patient-side limitations, including caregiver dependency and the unsuitability of telemedicine for chronic disease management, reinforced this shift back to traditional consultations [24, 29]. Together, these experiences highlight how the intersection of technological burdens, professional fatigue, and patient-side constraints makes telemedicine difficult to sustain as a long-term model of care.

3 Methodology

This study used a qualitative descriptive design to examine how sociotechnological factors influenced physicians' decisions to discontinue telemedicine after the pandemic. This approach was chosen to capture participants' experiences in their own words [30–32]. Sixteen (16) licensed physicians from Eastern Visayas, Western Visayas, and Metro Manila participated, all with at least two years of telemedicine experience and who reported reduced or discontinued use post-pandemic. The sample included 11 female and 5 male physicians across both public and private practice, representing general practice, internal medicine, pulmonology, EENT, pediatrics, family medicine, and OB-Gyn.

Data were collected through semi-structured interviews conducted between March and July 2025, either online (Zoom) or face-to-face, lasting 15–30 min. Informed consent was secured, and all sessions were audio-recorded. Transcripts were analyzed using Braun & Clarke (2019)[34]six-phase thematic analysis framework, supported by Dedoose software. Codes were generated inductively, refined into coherent themes, and supported with illustrative excerpts. Data saturation was reached by the 14th interview.

To ensure rigor, iterative data review and cross-validation of codes were conducted with an interrater who received training and immersion to ensure familiarity with the dataset, followed by an interrater validity test to confirm coding reliability (Ahmed, 2023; Nowell et al., 2017). Participants were assured confidentiality, voluntary participation, and the right to withdraw, with anonymized transcripts securely stored throughout the research process.

4 Results and Discussions

This study sought to address the research question: How do sociotechnological factors affect physicians' decisions to discontinue the use of telemedicine in the post-pandemic period? Thematic analysis uncovered four major themes that illustrate these dynamics: (1) Clinical Limitations in Virtual Consultations, (2) System Fragmentation in Physician Workload, (3) Workflow Disruption in Medical Practice, and (4) Clinical-Technical Risk in Telemedicine. Each theme represents a cluster of sociotechnological factors that highlight how the challenges of diagnostic adequacy, system integration, professional workflow, and risk perception intersect to shape physician decisions regarding telemedicine use. Thematic patterns were developed based on code occurrences and relationships generated from the Dedoose analysis, ensuring that each theme was grounded in systematic data co-occurrence rather than isolated narratives. The following sections will discuss these themes in detail, supported by participant excerpts and existing literature, to explain how these interconnected factors contributed to the decline of telemedicine adoption after the height of the COVID-19 pandemic.

4.1 Clinical Limitations in Virtual Consultations

This theme highlights how diagnostic, and communication challenges influenced physicians' decision to discontinue telemedicine after the pandemic. Physicians emphasized that the absence of physical examinations weakened their diagnostic confidence, creating blind spots and raising safety concerns: "Unable to perform physical examinations on my patients online" (P11). Poor video quality, such as pixelated or blurry calls, further limited visual assessment and increased fears of missed diagnoses or poor outcomes (P3, P5) [21, 36].

Beyond technical issues, physicians reported heavy reliance on patient self-reports, often inaccurate or incomplete: "It relies on what the patient tells you. Sometimes inaccurate" (P7). This discouraged them from using telemedicine with new patients, reserving it mainly for follow-ups (P4) [19, 37]. Communication barriers, including difficulties in explaining medications and language differences, further reduced clarity of care (P1, P2). These findings show how technological deficits (unstable connections, poor video) combined with social realities (communication gaps, inaccurate testimony, language barriers) eroded physician confidence in telemedicine. Unless these gaps are addressed with better tools, training, and multilingual support, telemedicine is likely to remain limited to follow-ups rather than being sustained as a mainstream model of care [19, 23]. Refer to Table 1 for the summary of themes.

Table 1. Thematic Narrative with Sub-Themes

Theme	Sub-theme	Codes	Description
1. Clinical Limitations in Virtual Consultations	1.1 Diagnostic Blind Spots	Physical check-up needed, Visual assessment, Poor prognosis, Blurry calls	Physicians faced limitations in visual assessment and feared inaccurate diagnoses due to absence of physical exam
	1.2 Incomplete Patient Histories	Reliant on patient's health testimony, Patient history preference	Heavy reliance on vague or inaccurate self-reported symptoms from patients
	1.3 Communication Difficulties	Difficulty in explaining the medication, Language barriers	Challenges in communication, especially with elderly or multilingual patients, reduced clarity of care instructions

4.2 System Fragmentation in Physician Workload

This theme shows how infrastructural, technical, and organizational shortcomings combined to create stress for physicians, ultimately leading to discontinuance of telemedicine. Physicians cited connectivity and power instability as a major challenge: *"Sometimes there are frequent disconnections, especially when power interruptions happen"* (P8). These disruptions hindered continuity of care and undermined trust in telemedicine, consistent with evidence that poor connectivity remains a persistent barrier in low- and middle-income settings [4]. Beyond infrastructure, platform usability and training gaps also emerged. As one physician stated, *"We were not trained well, so it caused delays in consultation"* (P10). Insufficient digital literacy and lack of structured training have been shown to impair integration of telemedicine and cause clinicians to revert to face-to-face care [5, 38].

Another key barrier was tool misalignment and inappropriateness, with physicians struggling between informal yet convenient tools and formal but cumbersome systems: *"Patients prefer Messenger, but we are required to use the official platform which is costly and tedious"* (P14). This reflects broader challenges of platforms poorly aligned with user needs, which reduce efficiency and patient access [39]. Fragmentation also extended to lack of interoperability, as physicians described duplicate tasks: *"I still had to manually encode patient information because the systems were not connected"* (P6). Interoperability gaps are well-documented in digital health literature, contributing to inefficiency and dissatisfaction [37, 40].

Finally, blurred boundaries and burnout emerged as telemedicine intruded into personal time. One physician admitted, *"There were constant messages from patients even after clinic hours, which was exhausting"* (P2). This shows how technological design (always-on communication channels) intersects with social expectations of continuous physician availability, leading to stress and eventual withdrawal [14, 41]. This theme highlights that discontinuance is driven not only by weak infrastructure or glitches but by the compounded sociotechnological strain of poor connectivity, usability challenges, system misalignment, interoperability gaps, and boundary violations. Addressing these issues requires reliable infrastructure, interoperable platforms, training, and institutional safeguards for physician well-being. Refer to Table 2 for the summary of themes.

Table 2. Thematic Narrative with Sub-Themes

Theme	Sub-theme	Codes	Description
2. System Fragmentation in Physician Work Strain	2.1. Connectivity and Power Instability	Unstable internet connection, Power interruptions	Frequent disconnections and blackouts impeded session continuity, especially in rural settings
	2.2. Platform Usability and Training Gaps	System quality, Poor technological training, Technical glitches, Unfamiliarity with the system	Lack of training and usability issues led to delays and frustration for both patients and physicians
	2.3. Tool Misalignment and Inappropriateness	Platform inappropriateness, Access to technology, Formal Platform, Informal Platform	Mismatch between platform functions and clinical requirements; poor patient access to technology
	2.4. Lack of Interoperability	Poor interoperability	Manual data handling and lack of integration across platforms hindered efficiency
	2.5. Blurred Boundaries and Burnout	Disruption to personal time	Unregulated after-hours communication led to physician burnout and dissatisfaction

4.3 Workflow Disruption in Medical Practice

This theme shows how the mismatch between telemedicine technologies and clinical routines disrupted physicians' roles and contributed to discontinuance. Physicians described increased administrative burden from pre-consultation requirements, uploading results, and manual workarounds, which extended tasks beyond usual workflows: "I still had to prepare documents before every consult and upload them after, which took more time than in-person" (P9). Such inefficiencies reflect how digital platforms often add parallel documentation instead of integrating smoothly, increasing workload and reducing efficiency [5].

Temporal frustration also emerged, as extended consultation times and frequent delays slowed clinical flow and caused fatigue: "Consultations took longer, and sometimes I had to wait because of platform delays" (P12). These interruptions mirror findings that prolonged consults and technical issues reduce productivity and contribute to telemedicine fatigue [18, 42]. Finally, physicians reported diminished confidence due to inaccurate information, misuse of telemedicine, and fears of poor prognosis: "Without examining the patient physically, I am worried I might miss something serious" (P5). This erosion of trust aligns with studies showing that diagnostic uncertainty reduces physician confidence and predicts discontinuance [4, 14, 43]. Together, these findings highlight that administrative inefficiencies, prolonged consults, and diagnostic risks create unsustainable workloads and distrust, ultimately driving physicians to disengage. Addressing these challenges requires systems that streamline documentation, improve efficiency, and support accurate diagnosis. Refer to Table 3 for the summary of themes.

Table 3. Thematic Narrative with Sub-Themes

Theme	Sub-theme	Codes	Description
3. Workflow Disruption in Medical Practice	3.1 Increased Administrative Burden	Pre-consultation requirement, Uploading of results to the platform, Manual workaround	Additional preparation and documentation efforts increased workload beyond typical workflows
	3.2 Temporal Frustration and Work Impediment	Delay in consultation, Long consultation hours, Contact outside clinic hours, Frustrations, Perceived Work Impediment	Extended consult durations, unscheduled contacts, and constant availability caused fatigue
	3.3 Erosion of Professional Confidence	Misusage of telemedicine, Inaccurate information, Poor prognosis	Inaccurate or misused information and tools led to poor clinical outcomes and eroded physician trust

4.4 Clinical-Technical Risk in Telemedicine

This theme shows how concerns about liability, caregiver competence, and diagnostic limitations influenced physicians' decisions to discontinue telemedicine after the pandemic. Legal and ethical vulnerabilities were a major issue, as physicians felt pressured by the constant need for consent forms: "I always needed to secure a consent form to protect myself, but it added pressure every time" (P6). While these forms safeguarded data privacy and ethical standards, they also reinforced perceptions of telemedicine as legally uncertain, echoing concerns about data breaches and unclear liability [5, 6, 44].

Caregiver and patient competence also affected reliability. Physicians noted that caregivers often struggled to describe symptoms, while patients failed to provide complete histories: "First-time patients rarely gave the full history I needed" (P8). Such gaps created diagnostic uncertainty, consistent with studies showing that dependence on non-professional caregivers and patient self-reports weakens clinical accuracy [16, 29].

Finally, diagnostic and safety concerns led many physicians to restrict telemedicine to follow-ups or referrals, since physical exams remained essential: "If I cannot do a physical check-up, I might miss something serious" (P3). Evidence confirms that while telemedicine works for monitoring and follow-ups, it falls short for complex or first-time cases [9, 37, 45]. Altogether, legal uncertainties, limited caregiver competence, and safety risks eroded physician trust and contributed to disengagement. Sustainable adoption will require stronger privacy protections, clearer legal frameworks, caregiver and patient training, and hybrid models that integrate digital consultations with in-person diagnostics. Refer to Table 4 for the summary of themes.

Table 4. Thematic Narrative with Sub-Themes

Theme	Sub-theme	Codes	Description
4. Clinical-Technical Risk in Telemedicine	4.1 Legal and Ethical Vulnerabilities	Perceived Risk, Consent form agreement	Telemedicine raises liability concerns, with consent forms serving as safeguards but adding pressure on physicians
	4.2 Caregiver and Patient Competence Limitations	Incapable caregivers, Patient history preference	Inadequate caregiver support and incomplete patient histories reduce reliability of remote consultations
	4.3 Diagnostic and Safety Constraints	Patient referral, Physical check-up needed	Doctors accept only referred or previously engaged patients, since a physical check-up is needed for accurate diagnosis

In summary, this study found that sociotechnological factors strongly influenced why physicians stopped using telemedicine after the pandemic. Major challenges included clinical limitations, such as the lack of physical examinations, poor video quality, and overreliance on patient self-reports, which reduced diagnostic [36, 46, 47]. System fragmentation, including unstable internet connections, weak interoperability, and limited training, increased workload and reduced efficiency [28]. Workflow disruptions, such as extra administrative tasks, longer consultations, and inaccurate information, also contributed to physician fatigue and loss of confidence in the medium [18, 19]. Finally, clinical-technical risks tied to consent forms, data privacy, caregiver inexperience, and safety concerns reinforced the perception of telemedicine as unreliable [6, 29]. Taken together, these results show that discontinuance is not caused by technology alone but by the interaction of technical shortcomings with social and professional demands. This means that sustaining telemedicine in the long term requires not only better infrastructure and platform design but also clear legal and privacy safeguards, comprehensive training for both physicians and patients, and hybrid models that integrate digital consultations with essential face-to-face care to ensure safety, efficiency, and trust [15].

5 Conclusion

Physicians' voices remind us again that digital health cannot succeed on technology alone; it must integrate with clinical judgment, workflow realities, and professional responsibilities. This study found that Filipino physicians' disengagement from telemedicine in the post-pandemic period is not merely due to technical issues but reflects a broader professional response shaped by clinical limitations, fragmented systems, workflow disruptions, and clinical-technical risks. The findings demonstrate how the absence of physical examination, poor video quality, reliance on patient testimony, unstable connectivity, and medico-legal uncertainty collectively eroded diagnostic confidence, strained workflows, and reinforced perceptions of telemedicine as unsustainable [36, 46].

The findings suggest that improving telemedicine requires more than just fixing technology. Healthcare leaders should listen to physicians' feedback and develop systems that support clinical needs. This includes better-designed platforms that are easier to use, allow smooth data sharing, and provide support for communication during consultations. Policies should also protect physicians' time and help manage patient expectations about online consultations. Training should include not only how to use the system, but also how to handle legal, ethical, and communication issues in virtual settings. Helping patients and caregivers improve their digital skills is also crucial for making telemedicine more effective and equitable.

Future work may adopt mixed-methods or longitudinal designs to extend these qualitative insights. Employing a meta-inference approach can make subsequent investigations more empirically grounded by linking statistical patterns with physicians' lived experiences, thereby clarifying how system quality, work impediment, and institutional factors shape sustained or discontinued telemedicine use.

This study focused on physicians in the Philippines who already had experience with telemedicine, which may limit the applicability of the results to other countries or health systems. Also, because the data were based on interviews, there may be some recall bias or socially desirable responses. Despite these limitations, the study offers useful insights into the challenges physicians face in digital care and helps explain why some choose to step back from telemedicine.

While this study offers valuable insights within the Philippine context, its findings may not be fully generalizable to high-income countries or health systems with more advanced digital infrastructures and policy frameworks. Differences in regulatory environments, resource allocation, and physician-patient dynamics may shape telemedicine use in distinct ways. Nevertheless, the themes identified, such as diagnostic constraints, workflow strain, and medico-legal uncertainty, may resonate in other low- and middle-income settings where systemic and sociotechnological challenges similarly influence digital care practices. Future comparative studies across diverse healthcare contexts could further clarify which disengagement factors are context-specific and which reflect universal concerns among physicians.

Strengthening the implementation of the Department of Health's Universal Health Care Act is essential to institutionalizing telemedicine in the Philippines [48]. Thailand serves as an example where coherent policy and government support have enabled digital health to thrive under its Universal Coverage Scheme [49]. Likewise, telemedicine in the Philippines should be positioned not as a replacement for traditional care but as a complementary approach that ensures continuity and equitable access to quality healthcare for all.

Disclosure of Interests. The authors declare that there are no conflicts of interest regarding the conduct or publication of this study.

References

1. Kaundinya, T., Agrawal, R.: Unpacking a telemedical takeover: recommendations for improving the sustainability and usage of telemedicine post-COVID-19. Qual. Manag. Health Care **31**, 68–73 (2022)
2. Shaver, J.: The state of telehealth before and After the COVID-19 pandemic. Primary Care – Clin. Off. Pract. **49**, 517–530 (2022)
3. Wosik, J., Fudim, M., Cameron, B., et al.: Telehealth transformation: COVID-19 and the rise of virtual care. J. Am. Med. Inform. Assoc. **27**, 957–962 (2020)
4. Anthony Jnr, B.: Implications of telehealth and digital care solutions during COVID-19 pandemic: a qualitative literature review. Inform. Health Soc. Care **46**, 68–83 (2021)
5. Bokolo, A.J.: Exploring the adoption of telemedicine and virtual software for care of outpatients during and after COVID-19 pandemic (2020). https://doi.org/10.1007/s11845-020-02299-z/Published
6. Solimini, R., Busardò, F.P., Gibelli, F., et al.: Ethical and legal challenges of telemedicine in the era of the covid-19 pandemic. Medicina (Lithuania) **57** (2021)
7. Schürmann, F., Westmattelmann, D., Schewe, G.: factors influencing telemedicine adoption among health care professionals: Qual. Interview Study. JMIR Form Res. **9** (2025)
8. Soontae, A., Yujin, L., Soondool, C.: The effects of digital literacy and health empowerment on elders' communication with doctors: focusing on moderating effect of health beliefs. J. Korean Acad. Community Health Nurs. **33**, 53–62 (2022)
9. Haleem, A., Javaid, M., Singh, R.P., Suman, R.: Telemedicine for healthcare: Capabilities, features, barriers, and applications. Sens. Int. **2**, 100117 (2021)

10. Boriani, G., Maisano, A., Bonini, N., et al.: Digital literacy as a potential barrier to implementation of cardiology tele-visits after COVID-19 pandemic: the INFO-COVID survey. J. Geriatr. Cardiol. **18**, 739–747 (2021)
11. Dela Cruz, L.A., Tolentino, L.K.S.: Telemedicine implementation challenges in underserved areas of the philippines. Int. J. Emerg. Technol. Adv. Eng. **11**, 60–70 (2021)
12. Ong, A.K.S., Kurata, Y.B., Castro, S.A.D.G., et al.: Factors influencing the acceptance of telemedicine in the Philippines. Technol. Soc. **70**, 102040 (2022)
13. Chunara, R., Zhao, Y., Chen, J., et al.: Telemedicine and healthcare disparities: a cohort study in a large healthcare system in New York City during COVID-19. J. Am. Med. Inform. Assoc. **28**, 33–41 (2021). https://doi.org/10.1093/jamia/ocaa217
14. Orrange, S., Patel, A., Mack, W.J., Cassetta, J.: Patient satisfaction and trust in telemedicine during the COVID-19 pandemic: retrospective observational study. JMIR Hum. Factors **8**, e28589 (2021)
15. Bhat, K.S., Kumar, N., Shamanna, K., et al.: Towards intermediated workflows for hybrid telemedicine. In: Conference on Human Factors in Computing Systems - Proceedings. Association for Computing Machinery (2023)
16. Jacob, C., Sanchez-Vazquez, A., Ivory, C.: Factors impacting clinicians' adoption of a clinical photo documentation app and its implications for clinical workflows and quality of care: qualitative case study. JMIR Mhealth Uhealth **8**, e20203 (2020)
17. Glock, H., Nymberg, V.M., Bolmsjö, B.B., et al.: Attitudes, barriers, and concerns regarding telemedicine among swedish primary care physicians: a qualitative study (2021)
18. Sharma, R., Nachum, S., Davidson, K.W., Nochomovitz, M.: It's not just facetime: core competencies for the medical virtualist. Int. J. Emerg. Med. **12**, 8 (2019)
19. Garfan, S., Alamoodi, A.H., Zaidan, B.B., et al.: Telehealth utilization during the Covid-19 pandemic: a systematic review. Comput. Biol. Med. **138**, 104878 (2021)
20. Shachar, C., Engel, J., Elwyn, G.: Implications for telehealth in a postpandemic future: regulatory and privacy issues. JAMA – J. Am. Med. Assoc. (2020)
21. Almathami, H.K.Y., Than Win, K., Vlahu-Gjorgievska, E.: Barriers and facilitators that influence telemedicine-based, real-time, online consultation at patients' homes: systematic literature review. J. Med. Internet Res. **22**, e16407 (2020)
22. Boksa, V., Pennathur, P.: Assessing contributing and mediating factors of telemedicine on healthcare provider burnout. Health Policy Technol. **13**, 100942 (2024)
23. Greenhalgh, T., Wherton, J., Shaw, S., Morrison, C.: Video consultations for covid-19. BMJ **368** (2020)
24. Vista, F.E.S., Tamondong-Lachica, D.R.: A comparison of the characteristics of adult medicine patients seeking telemedicine consultations versus in-person consultations in a Philippine public hospital. Baylor Univ. Med. Center Proc. **37**, 80–88 (2024)
25. Aban, Y.K.C., Abunto, J.V., Aliorde, J.V.E.P., et al.: The rise of telemedicine in the Philippines during COVID-19: a systematic review of utilization trends and patient outcomes. Philippine Soc. Sci. J. **6**, 9–18 (2024)
26. Jacob, J., Wan, F., Jin, A.: Is telemedicine worth the effort? A study on the impact of effort cost on healthcare platform with heterogeneous preferences. Comput. Ind. Eng. **188**, 109854 (2024)
27. Muller, E., Huysmans, M.A., van Rijssen, H.J., Anema, J.R.: Needs, expectations, facilitators, and barriers among insurance physicians related to the use of eHealth in their work: results of a survey. Disabil. Rehabil. **46**, 2374–2384 (2024)
28. Tan, S.H., Wong, C.K., Yap, Y.Y., Tan, S.K.: Factors influencing telemedicine adoption among physicians in the Malaysian healthcare system: a revisit. Digit Health **10**, 20552076241257050 (2024)

29. Panotes, A., Jocson, J., Andigan, C.M., Sy, M.P.: Lived experiences of caregivers upon receiving occupational therapy through telehealth amidst the pandemic. Braz. J. Occup. Therapy **3** (2024)
30. Creswell, J.: Research Design Qualitative, Quantitative and Mixed Methods Approaches (2009)
31. Khanassov, V., Ilali, M., Ruiz, A.S., et al.: Telemedicine in primary care of older adults: a qualitative study. BMC Primary Care **25**, 259 (2024)
32. Sandelowski, M.: Focus on research methods: whatever happened to qualitative description? Res. Nurs. Health **23**, 334–340 (2000)
33. Braun, V., Clarke, V.: Reflecting on reflexive thematic analysis. Qual Res Sport Exerc Health **11**, 589–597 (2019)
34. Ahmed, S.K.: The Pillars of Trustworthiness in Qualitative Research (2023)
35. Nowell, L.S., Norris, J.M., White, D.E., Moules, N.J.: Thematic analysis: striving to meet the trustworthiness criteria. Int J Qual Methods **16**, 1609406917733847 (2017)
36. Monaghesh, E., Hajizadeh, A.: The role of telehealth during COVID-19 outbreak: a systematic review based on current evidence. BMC Public Health **20**, 1193 (2020)
37. Scott Kruse, C., Karem, P., Shifflett, K., et al.: Evaluating barriers to adopting telemedicine worldwide: a systematic review. J. Telemed. Telecare **24**, 4–12 (2018)
38. Gajarawala, S.N., Pelkowski, J.N.: Telehealth benefits and barriers. J. Nurse Pract. **17**, 218–221 (2021)
39. Ye, J.: Transforming and facilitating health care delivery through social networking platforms: evidences and implications from WeChat. JAMIA Open **7**, ooae047 (2024)
40. Rodrigues, D.A., Roque, M., Mateos-Campos, R., et al.: Barriers and facilitators of health professionals in adopting digital health-related tools for medication appropriateness: a systematic review. Digit Health **10**, 20552076231225132 (2024)
41. Su, Z., Cheshmehzangi, A., Bentley, B.L., et al.: Technology-based interventions for health challenges older women face amid COVID-19: a systematic review protocol. Syst. Rev. **11**, 271 (2022)
42. Delemere, E., Gitonga, I., Maguire, R.: Utility, barriers and facilitators to the use of connected health to support families impacted by paediatric cancer: a qualitative analysis. Support. Care Cancer **30**, 6755–6766 (2022)
43. Ramachandran, M., Brinton, C., Wiljer, D., et al.: The impact of eHealth on relationships and trust in primary care: a review of reviews. BMC Primary Care **24**, 228 (2023)
44. El Kheir, D.Y.M., Alnufaili, S.S., Alsaffar, R.M., et al.: Physicians' perspective of telemedicine regulating guidelines and ethical aspects: a saudi experience. Int. J. Telemed. Appl. **2022**, 5068998 (2022)
45. Leochico, C.F.D., Valera, M.J.S.: Follow-up consultations through telerehabilitation for wheelchair recipients with paraplegia in a developing country: a case report. Spinal Cord Ser. Cases **6**, 58 (2020)
46. Kichloo, A., Albosta, M., Dettloff, K., et al.: Telemedicine, the current COVID-19 pandemic and the future: a narrative review and perspectives moving forward in the USA. Fam. Med. Commun. Health **8**, e000530 (2020)
47. Park, H.S., et al.: Use of video-based telehealth services using a mobile app for workers in underserved areas during the COVID-19 pandemic: a prospective observational study. Int. J. Med. Inform. **166**, 104844 (2022)
48. Tan, I.T.I.: Philippines Telemedicine-for-Health-Professionals (2020)
49. Zayar, N.N., Kittiratchakool, N., Saeraneesopon, T., et al.: Telemedicine utilization patterns and implications Amidst COVID-19 outbreaks in thailand under public universal coverage scheme. Inquiry (United States) **61** (2024)

A Deep-Learning Approach Based on BERT Model for Depression Severity Prediction

Ngonidzashe Mathew Kanyangarara(✉), Madhu Chetty, and Jiangang Ma

Institute of Innovation, Science and Sustainability, Federation University Australia, Ballarat, Australia
nkanyangarara@students.federation.edu.au,
{madhu.chetty,j.ma}@federation.edu.au

Abstract. Deep learning and large language models (LLMs) are being investigated to detect depression from social media data. However, traditional deep learning methods such as Long Short-Term Memory (LSTM) are limited by their reliance on feature engineering, resulting in time consuming and hard to capture complex patterns arising from media data. To address this issue, we propose a novel deep-learning approach that is based on Bidirectional Encoder Representations from Transformers (BERT) framework with Transformer Regression (called BERT-TR) for depression severity prediction from media data. In addition, we employ different techniques such as under sampling, oversampling and weighted loss function to ensure robust and generalizable predictions for depression. The data from X, derived from clinical assessments aligned with the fifth edition of the (DSM-5-TR) criteria, is used for investigations. We theoretically and empirically show that BERT-TR can predict depression severity from media data effectively and efficiently.

1 Introduction

Depression, a mental disorder, is a common mental health condition which can present different symptoms, such as emotional, cognitive, physical, or behavioural. For example, a person exhibiting feelings of guilt, worthlessness, or helplessness for an extended period, say, two consecutive weeks, can be suffering from emotional depressive disorder. Depression can affect a person's life, feelings, thoughts, and behaviour. For example, depression can affect one's sleeping cycle, leading to insomnia and excessive sleeping, which worsens preexisting health issues [1]. If not properly treated, depression can become chronic, resulting in recurring episodes and long-term effects [2]. A person suffering from depression may experience a lack of interest in activities, persistent sadness, and feelings of hopelessness. Such social disengagement can result in loneliness and damaged relationships. When combined with anger and mood fluctuations, this disengagement can further harm relationships in both professional and personal spheres [3]. What is more, severe depression usually can result in suicide or self-harm.

E. R. Kaburuan and S. Goundar (Eds.): HIS 2025, LNCS 16392, pp. 94–106, 2026.
https://doi.org/10.1007/978-981-95-6304-3_9

According to World Health Organization's (WHO) 2021 report [4], depression is one of the most common mental health conditions, affecting around two hundred and eighty million people.

Traditional methods of diagnosing depression often use structured interviews and self-report questionnaires. However, the drawbacks of these methods are that they are often slow, prone to bias, and resource intensive [1]. Machine learning methods like Support Vector Machines (SVM) and Random Forests and deep learning models such as LSTM are used in earlier research projects for depression detection on social media datasets like Twitter. However, LSTMs are limited by their reliance on feature engineering and failing to take advantage of transformer-based architectures for the problem, resulting in time consuming and hard capturing complex patterns. In recent times, natural language processing (NLP) has shown promise to effectively and accurately analyse social media data including recognising distressed individuals. Significant efforts are being made to apply deep learning, and LLMs to detect depression from social media data. An important underlying feature of this method is that patients with depression often use words (e.g., sad) to express their thoughts because LLM can understand, interpret, and analyse large amounts of complex and nuanced human language. This ability of LLM makes it possible to detect the mental state of an individual and the underlying deep learning methods.

BERT is a popular transformer-based model known for its success in natural language processing, such as text classification, sentiment analysis and question answering [5]. While the application of pretrained models like BERT on mental health tasks has been on the rise, available research [6] indicates that majority of earlier studies have primarily used BERT for simple classification of depression and severity.

Existing approaches like ensemble voting [7], semantic retrieval pipelines [8], LLM-based BDI questionnaire answering [9] and FastText-based classification [10] are aimed at categorising classes rather than regression on continuous severity scores. Although BERT-based LLMs can be effective for depression detection and have achieved competitive results, very limited work has been done on regression-based classification tasks in mental health sector. This paper proposes a novel LLM framework for depression severity prediction using a transformer-based approach with BERT regression. Comparisons carried out with LSTM, our methods and evaluations are performed using two well-known metrics: Mean Squared Error (MSE) and Coefficient of Determination (R^2) and real-world datasets, demonstrating the effectiveness of the proposed approach. The contributions of this research are as follows.

- We propose a novel BERT-TR system based on Transformer model to predict depression severity from social media data.
- We develop a concise BERT regression architecture comprising the Transformer encoder and the regression head to effectively predict depression severity. In addition, we develop related BERT-based regression algorithms to improve the accuracy of prediction.

- We conduct an extensive experimental evaluation over a set of real world datasets. Our experimental results show that BERT-TR can achieve a high accuracy of predicting depression severity from social media data.

The rest of the paper is arranged as follows. The related work is reviewed in Sect. 2 The proposed methodology including the description of the dataset, model architecture and training procedures, is described in Sect. 3. The experiment, results and discussion are presented in Sect. 4. Finally, Sect. 5 concludes the paper.

2 Related Work

Traditional machine learning models and deep learning approaches, such as SVM, Random Forests and LSTM, have been the primary tools applied in early depression detection studies. With the advances in NLP and the development of LLMs, there has also been focused on investigations of Transformer-Based Models and application of Social Media data for Mental Health research.

Using twitter data, Kavitha et al. [11] applied SVM to detect sadness with moderate accuracy and limitations in extrapolating to other datasets. Similarly, Pennebaker et al. [12], using Linguistic Inquiry and Word Count (LIWC) characteristics, demonstrated the importance of linguistic patterns in evaluating mental health. Nickson D. et al. [13], in a systematic review for predicting depression, summarize the machine learning methods and Electronic Health Records (EHR) identified challenges and difficulties in categorizing predictors and the demographic limitations due to these being largely based on Western Educated Industrialized Rich Democratic (WEIRD) populations.

Using Twitter data, Ghosh and Anwar [14] apply supervised learning method using an LSTM network with Swish activation to predict and measure depression levels and analyze various features like emotional and behavioral data. Prama et al. [15] combine emotional features, topical events, and behavioral-biometric signals to train LSTM-based models. Glen Coppersmith et al. [16] created a dataset for studying language patterns associated with different mental health conditions. Aldkheel and Zhou [17] developed a multidimensional framework, analyzing input features, social media platforms, disorder symptomatology, ground truth, and techniques and high-lighting the challenges in validation, generalizability, cause identification, and ethical considerations. Tahir et al. [18] provides a comprehensive review of ML and DL techniques for depression detection in social media emphasizing the need for multi-modal approaches and improved model interpretability.

Xin and Zakaria [19] address the challenges in early depression detection using advanced natural language processing techniques by leveraging social media data. Comparison of the performance of three models: fine-tuned BERT, BERT-BiLSTM, and BERT-CNN, MentalBERT is carried out using datasets from Reddit, Twitter, and the Mental Health Corpus, the study emphasizes the importance of explainability in AI models to build confidence and improve clinical decision-making in mental health care.

3 Proposed Method

To address the challenges posed above for predicting depression severity, we develop a novel method of BERT-TR for prediction of depression severity.

3.1 BERT-TR Architecture

The schematic representation of the proposed BERT-TR is illustrated in Fig. 1. Module-1 performs text preparation, including expanding contractions, replacing mentions and URLs, removing extra spaces, and then using the BERT tokenizer to convert the text data into standardized tokens suitable for transformer-based input. In Module-2, the pre-processed tokens are inputted into Transformer-Based BERT Model where token encoding and positional embeddingsthe are incorporated into BERT architecture, and transformer encoder stacks to generate context-rich hidden state representations. From this, BERT's in-built regression head then predicts continuous depression intensity scores. The Module-3 calculates the Mean Squared Error (MSE) between the model's predicted depression intensity scores and the true labels. The computed MSE guides the optimization and evaluation of the model's predictive performance. The Module-4 is a Model Training and Optimization unit, which manages the training loop, tracking performance metrics and employs a termination stopping strategy to prevent overfitting. In addition, it continuously monitors validation loss, updates the best loss achieved, and resets or increments the patience counter accordingly. Finally, Module-5 categorizes predicted continuous depression intensity scores into relevant severity labels: **non-depressed, mid, depressed**, enabling straightforward interpretation and potential applicability.

3.2 Data Preprocessing

The benchmark twitter data set under consideration is already annotated with depression intensity scores in the continuous range [0, 1] with 0 representing no signs of depression and 1 representing high depression. To prepare the tweets for processing, we applied a multi-step text normalization process, depicted by Algorithm 1. It comprises of contraction expansion, content anonymization, and tokenization. First, common contractions are expanded into their full forms (e.g., "I'm" → "I am"). Next, all user identity is anonymized by replacing occurrences of "@username" with a generic token "at_user", and any URLs are replaced with the token "url". This not only ensures privacy but also prevents the model from overfitting to a specific user or a link pattern. Next, irrelevant whitespace is removed, converting multiple spaces to a single space and the leading/trailing spaces is trimmed. The resulting text after cleaning contains only the standard vocabulary terms ready for tokenization.

3.3 BERT Tokenisation

After text cleaning, tokenization is performed using the BERT base-uncased Word Piece tokenizer shown in Algorithm 2. This tokenizer splits the input text

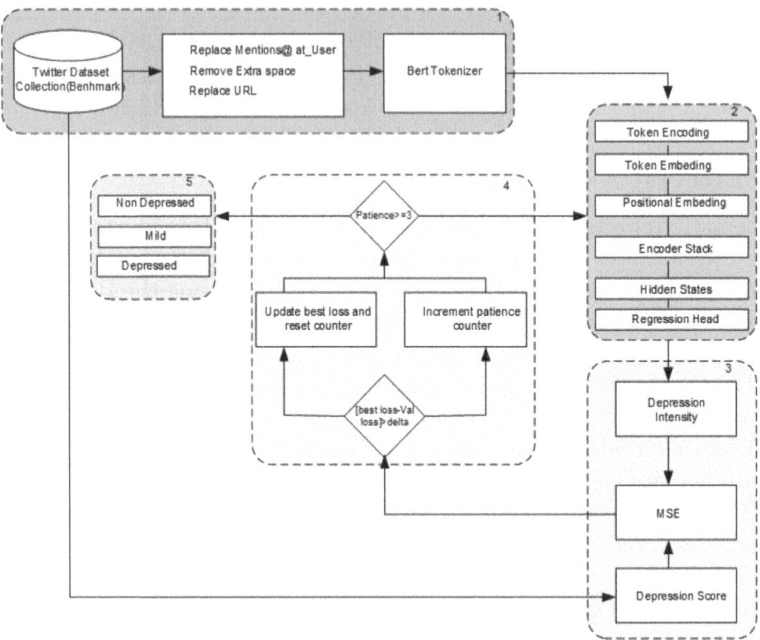

Fig. 1. Schematic of the proposed BERT-TR approach. It has five modules, namely, Module-1: text processing and Tokenization, Module-2: BERT model, Module-3: Scoring, Module-4: Termination, Module-5: Categorizing scores into severity labels.

into subword tokens from BERT's 30,000-word vocabulary [17], yield-ing consistent integer indices for each token. To ensure computational efficiency and sufficient context coverage, the sequence length is capped at 128 tokens, truncating longer tweets and zero-padding shorter ones as necessary. The special classification token [CLS] gets automatically inserted at the beginning of each sequence, along with a separator token [SEP] at the end. This produces the final model input: a padded sequence of token IDs and an attention mask indicating real tokens versus padding.

3.4 BERT Regression Process

In this section, we fine-tuned a pretrained BERT-based model for regression of depression severity. We utilize BERT as a feature extractor by leveraging the final hidden state of the [CLS] token as a compact representation of the entire tweet. On top of this, we attach a simple regression head where a single linear layer maps this 768-dimensional vector to a scalar depression severity score. This process is shown in Algorithm 3. Given the tokenized input, BERT produces a sequence of hidden embeddings for the [CLS] token and each of the N tokens in the tweet as shown by Eq. (1).

Algorithm 1. Text Prer-processing

Input: Raw tweet T_{raw}
Output: Pre-processed text T_{clean}.
Procedure TextPreprocessing (T_raw)

1. T_expanded ⟵ contraction.fix(T_raw) (e.g.,"I'm" ⟶"I am")
2. T_temp ⟵ re.(sub(r'@\w+','at_user',T_expanded)
3. T_temp ⟵ re.(sub(r'http\S+','url',T_temp)
4. T_clean ⟵ re.(sub(r'\s+',' ',T_temp).strip()
5. **return** T_clean

end procedure

Algorithm 2. BERT Tokenization

Input: Pre-processed text T_{clean}
Output: Tokenized input $X_{tokenized}$.
Procedure BERTTokenization (T_clean,max_length = 128)

1. tokenizer ⟵ BertTokenization.from_pretrained('bert-base-uncased')
2. tokens ⟵ tokenizer (
3. T_clean,
4. truncation = True,
5. padding = 'max_length',
6. max_length = max_length)
7. **return** tokens

end procedure

$$H = [h_{[CLS]}, h_1, h_2, \ldots, h_N] \tag{1}$$

The final hidden state corresponding to the [CLS] token is taken as an aggregate representation of the entire tweet [17]. This vector $h_{[CLS]} \in R^{768}$ for BERT-base(where 768 is the dimensionality of BERT-base's hidden layer) is then passed through a dropout layer for regularization, mitigating overfitting by randomly zeroing a subset of its components during training. Finally, as shown by Eq. (2), a fully connected linear layer (the regression head) maps the dropout-output vector to a single scalar, which represents the predicted depression severity.

$$\hat{y} = W_r h_{dropout} + b_r \tag{2}$$

Here, $W_r \in R^{1\times768}$ is the learnable weight matrix that transforms the 768-dimensional [CLS] representation into a single output, and $b_r \in R$ is the learnable bias term added to this linear transformation. Then $\hat{y}$ is the scalar regression output (predicted depression intensity). This formulation is a standard linear

Algorithm 3. BERT Regression Model

Input: Tokenized input $X_{tokenized}$.
Output: Depression intensity score $\hat{y}$.
Procedure BERTRegression($X_{tokenized}$)

1. H ⟵ BERT($X_{tokenized}$)
2. h_cls ⟵ H[0]
3. h_dropout ⟵ Dropout(h_cls, rate = 0.3)
4. $\hat{y}$ ⟵ Linear(h_dropout, weights = W_r, bias = b_r)
5. **return** $\hat{y}$

end procedure

regression layer on top of BERT's pooled representation [17]. The entire processing by the BERT regression architecture, comprising the Transformer encoder and the regression head, is depicted in Algorithm 3. By leveraging BERT's deep bidirectional attention mechanisms and a simple regression layer, our model can directly predict a continuous depression intensity value for each tweet.

4 Experiments

All model training and experiments were conducted using Google Colaboratory (Colab), a cloud-based Jupyter notebook environment. We utilized an NVIDIA Tesla T4 GPU as the hardware accelerator in Colab's Python 3 runtime. This GPU (16 GB VRAM) provided substantial computational power for fine-tuning the BERT-based model. For context, Colab's free tier can also allocate other GPUs such as A100 GPU or occasionally L4 GPU, though the T4 was consistently used in our case. The devel-opment and initial testing of code were done on a local machine with an Intel Core i5 CPU, 16 GB RAM, running 64-bit Windows 11, to ensure reproducibility in a standard desktop environment. We trained our models using the PyTorch framework and HuggingFace's transformer libraries. Code and configs can be accessed here.[1]

4.1 Dataset

The dataset investigated consists of 10,000 depression-related tweets, a subset of the approximately 95,000+ tweets studied by Prama et al. [15] where each tweet is annotated with a depression severity label in four classes: non-depressed, mild, moderate, or severe. Note that this results in the class distribution being highly imbalanced, with the severe class extremely underrepresented (only 61 samples out of 10000). Table 1 presents the resulting class distribution. It can be noted that the process addresses the class imbalance issue.

[1] https://github.com/ngoniematt/BERT-Model-for-Depression-Severity-Prediction.

Table 1. Class distribution before and after merging

Class Label	Original Dataset (4 classes)	After Merging (3 classes)
Non-depressed	971	971
Mild	6,838	6,838
Moderate	2,130	*merged into "depressed"*
Severe	61	*merged into "depressed"*
Depressed	–	2,191

Our corpus comprises ≈10k public tweets, and we scope claims to this setting and note dataset expansion as future work. All tweets were pre-processed in the same manner as the procedures described by Prama et al. [15] by applying the standard text cleansing steps, such as normalization, tokenization, stopwords removal and lemmatization. For experiments, we evaluate its impact on model performance. All tweets were then tokenised using the BERT WordPiece tokenizer [5] with a fixed sequence length of 128 tokens, as in the original setup.

4.2 BERT-TR and LSTM Model

We first evaluate the performance of our proposed BERT-TR model with the LSTM-model [19], which is a 4 -layer LSTM network trained to predict depression severity classes. For the dataset under investigation Table 2 presents a comparison of three metrics Mean Squared Error, R^2, and accuracy. Three training batch sizes (16, 32, 64) help examine the effect of batch size. Even with identical preprocessing, BERT dramatically outperforms the LSTM across all batch sizes. For example, with batch size of 32, the R^2 metric for BERT is 0.60, which is a +15-percentage point improvement over the LSTM value of 0.45. This is due to the BERT's transformer-based architecture which captures the linguistic context and subtle cues of depression in text far more effectively than the recurrent LSTM approach. The BERT regressor's MSE is also considerably lower (e.g. 0.0046 vs. 0.0051 for batch 32), indicating better fidelity in predicting the continuous severity score. In terms of classification accuracy, BERT achieves around 76–78% accuracy on severity categories, surpassing the LSTM baseline.

4.3 Customised Preprocessing

We now assess the impact of the new text preprocessing pipeline on BERT's performance. For this, we ignore the preprocessing steps of Prama et al. [15] and apply a customised data cleaning procedure to the tweet. We compare the BERT regressor's results with and without this custom text cleaning. The lower part of Table 2 (rows "BERT + Custom Preprocessing") shows the outcomes after applying our customized preprocessing enhancements, under the same training conditions as before. Positively, the custom preprocessing yields a significant improvement in performance. With cleaned text, BERT's MSE drops by more than half (e.g. from 0.0046 to 0.0020 at batch 32), and R^2 increases substantially (from 0.60 to 0.79 at batch 32). The accuracy on the discrete classes also rises to 84–85% (versus 78% without cus-tom cleaning). These gains suggest that noisy or inconsistent text features are hindering the model. The improvement is most pronounced at the smallest batch size (16), where R^2 reaches 0.8058, indicating that with less mini-batch noise, the benefits of cleaner input data are fully realised. Overall, across all batch sizes tested, the BERT + Custom Preprocessing configuration outperforms the original BERT results, demonstrating that accurate text cleaning can enhance model accuracy while using social media for mental health applications.

Table 2. Performance comparison of different models

Model	16			32			64		
	MSE	R^2	Acc	MSE	R^2	Acc	MSE	R^2	Acc
LSTM	0.0092	0.01	0.6	0.0051	0.45	0.72	0.0072	0.233	0.69
BERT	0.0047	0.59	0.97	0.0060	0.55	0.72	0.0040	0.598	0.78
BERT + Custom Preprocessing	0.0010	0.80	0.80	0.0020	0.78	0.84	0.0020	0.756	0.82
BERT + 3 classes	0.0018	0.80	0.85	0.0020	0.80	0.85	0.0020	0.773	0.85

4.4 Class Imbalance

Very few severe samples (61) in the severe class compared to other classes (e.g., moderate with 4161 samples) causes class imbalance in the original dataset. To address this, we merged the moderate and severe categories into a single depressed class. We trained the BERT regressor with the modified labels (non-depressed, mild, depressed). The results of this class merger (with base preprocessing) are included in Table 2 under the row "BERT+ 3 classes." We observe that simply combining the classes improves classification performance. For example, at batch size 32, the merged 3-class model reaches $R^2 = 0.8001$ and 85% accuracy, compared to 78% accuracy for the 4-class BERT under the same conditions. This indicates that the model finds it easier to regress and classify when not forced to distinguish the scarce severe cases as a separate category. The confusion matrix of the 3-class predictions on a batch size of 16 is shown in Fig. 2.

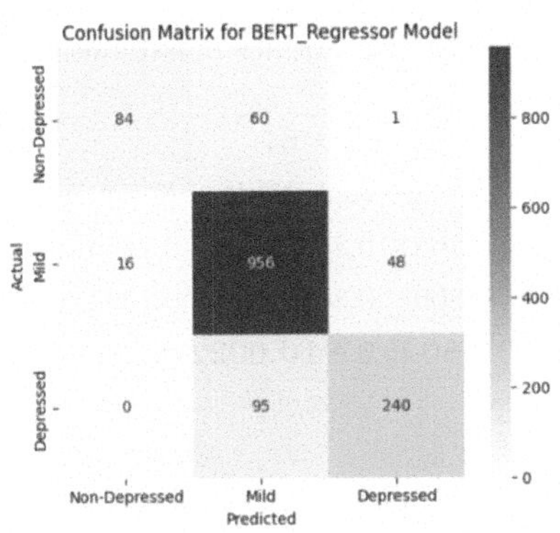

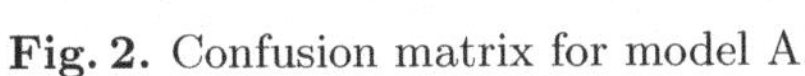
Fig. 2. Confusion matrix for model A.

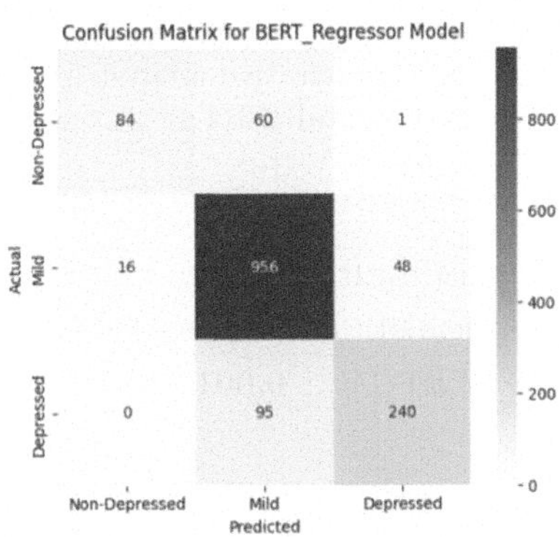

Fig. 3. Confusion matrix for model B.

Table 3. Class imbalance - Handling class imbalance in all four classes of BERT-TR.

Imbalance Technique	16			32			64		
	MSE	R^2	Acc	MSE	R^2	Acc	MSE	R^2	Acc
Under-sampling	0.0091	0.0995	0.65	0.0105	0.0480	0.62	0.0106	0.0551	0.65
Over-sampling	0.0022	0.7835	0.85	0.0023	0.7749	0.85	0.0029	0.7075	0.81
Weighted Loss	0.0026	0.7446	0.83	0.0025	0.7536	0.83	0.0033	0.6692	0.79

Table 4. Class imbalance - BERT-TR model with class imbalance handled for 3 classes.

Imbalance Technique	1			63			26		4
	MSE	R^2	Acc	MSE	R^2	Acc	MSE	R^2	Acc
Under-sampling	0.0032	0.6707	0.79	0.0036	0.6263	0.78	0.0038	0.6063	0.77
Over-sampling	0.0021	0.7820	0.86	0.0023	0.7612	0.84	0.0034	0.6513	0.80
Weighted Loss	0.0017	0.8265	0.86	0.0019	0.8046	0.85	0.0022	0.7717	0.85

4.5 Skewed Data Distribution and Class Imbalance

In the 3-class scenario, even after merging moderate and severe, the distribution remained skewed (especially with mild cases being dominant). We investigated several standard approaches to address the class imbalance in both the 4-class and 3-class settings. Tables 3 and 4 report the performance metrics for these experiments. For the four-class classification task (Table 3), our results show that oversampling and weighted loss strategies yield significantly better outcomes

Table 5. Comparative analysis of BERT-TR with transformer-based variant DistilBERT and MentalBERT.

Model	16			32			64		
	MSE	R^2	Acc	MSE	R^2	Acc	MSE	R^2	Acc
DistilBERT	0.0019	0.7970	0.85	0.0018	0.8031	0.85	0.0020	0.7869	0.85
MentalBERT	0.0019	0.7967	0.86	0.0018	0.8065	0.86	0.0020	0.7903	0.85
BERT-TR	**0.0017**	**0.8265**	**0.86**	**0.0019**	**0.8046**	**0.84**	**0.0022**	**0.7717**	**0.83**

than naive under sampling. The under-sampling approach, which discards a large portion of the abundant mild cases, leads to a drastic drop in performance with R^2 falling below 0.1 and accuracy to 65%. Table 4 shows the results of applying under-sampling, over-sampling, and weighted loss techniques to address the class imbalance in the three-class setup (non depressed, mild and depressed) dataset.

In the three-class scenario, class imbalance techniques proved more beneficial, especially when combined with the threshold optimisation approach. Here, with moderate and severe already merged, the dataset is more balanced and thus all methods performed better overall than in the 4-class case. Under-sampling still underperformed (R^2 0.67 max, and 0.79 accuracy), confirming that throwing away data is detrimental. Both oversampling and weighted loss achieved high results, with the weighted loss strategy emerging as the top performer. Training with loss weighting yielded an MSE = 0.0017, R^2 = 0.8265 and 86% accuracy (batch size 16), Fig. 3 shows classification report and confusion matrix which is the best result observed among all experiments carried out. Finally, we compare our BERT-based model with two transformer variants to evaluate generalisation and efficiency of tradeoffs: DistilBERT and MentalBERT. We fine-tuned both DistilBERT and MentalBERT on our regression task (with the custom preprocessing and 3-class threshold setup) under the same hyperparameter settings as the full BERT. Table 5 presents the results for these transformer variants in comparison to our BERT-TR. All models in this table were trained with the optimal imbalance handling (weighted loss) and moderate+severe class merge, as determined from prior experiments.

From Table 5, we see that the BERT-TR model still achieves the best overall performance. At the optimal batch size (=16), BERT-TR attains R^2 = 0.8265, edging out both DistilBERT and MentalBERT (which reach 0.80 R^2). In terms of accuracy, all three models are very close (85–86% for most settings). Our BERT-TR model remains the top performer overall, underscoring that a carefully fine-tuned standard BERT is a very strong baseline in this domain.

5 Conclusion

This study investigates the application of Transformer-based large language models for predicting depression from social media data. The proposed approach performed better than the LSTM baseline, which is currently the de facto method commonly used. BERT-TR, the proposed method achieved high accuracy (85–86%), a low MSE (0.0017), and an R^2 of around 83, even though the dataset was relatively small. Trained on Twitter, the method is platform-agnostic and expected to extend to similar short-form social platforms.

References

1. Aricioglu, F., Cetin, M.: Exploring the complex relationship between sleep, depression and the immune system. Psychiatry Clin. Psychopharmacol. **30**(4), 449–457 (2020)
2. Al-Harbi, K.S.: Treatment-resistant depression: therapeutic trends, challenges, and future directions. Patient Prefer. Adherence (6), 369–388 (2012)
3. Cacioppo, J.T., Hawkley, L.C.: Social isolation and health, with an emphasis on underlying mechanisms. Perspect. Biol. Med. **46**(3), 539–552 (2003)
4. Depression. Technical Report, World Health Organization (WHO) (2021)
5. Devlin, J., Chang, M.W., Lee, K., Toutanova, K.: Bert: pre-training of deep bidirectional transformers for language understanding. In: Proceedings of the 2019 Conference of the North American Chapter of the Association for Computational Linguistics: Human Language Technologies (NAACL-HLT), pp. 4171–4186 (2019)
6. Qasim, A., Mehak, G., Hussain, N., Gelbukh, A., Sidorov, G.: Detection of depression severity in social media text using transformer-based models. Infor **16**(2), 114 (2025)
7. Ahmed, T., Ivan, S., Munir, A., Ahmed, S.: Decoding depression: analyzing social network insights for depression severity assessment with transformers and explainable ai. Nat. Lang. Process. J. **7**, 100079 (2024)
8. Pérez, A., Warikoo, N., Wang, K., Parapar, J., Gurevych, I.: Semantic similarity models for depression severity estimation. Technical Report, http://arxiv.org/abs/2211.07624, arXiv:2211.07624 (2023)
9. Devlin, J., Chang, M.W., Lee, K., Toutanova, K.: Delving into the depths: evaluating depression severity through bdi-biased summaries. In: Proceedings of the 9th Workshop on Computational Linguistics and Clinical Psychology (2024)
10. Rizwan, M., et al.: Depression intensity classification from tweets using fasttext based weighted soft voting ensemble. CMC-Comput. Mater. Continua **78**(2), 2047–2066 (2024)
11. Chakravarthy, V.V.S.S.S., Bhateja, V., Flores Fuentes, W., Anguera, J., Vasavi, K.P.E.: Advances in signal processing, embedded systems and iot. In: Proceedings of the Seventh ICMEET-2022 (2022)
12. McCarthy, P.M., Boonthum-Denecke, C.E.: Applied natural language processing: identification, investigation and resolution. IGI Global (2012)
13. Nickson, D., Meyer, C., Walasek, L., Toro, C.: Prediction and diagnosis of depression using machine learning with electronic health records data: a systematic review. BMC Med. Inform. Decis. Mak. **23**(1), 271 (2023)
14. Ghosh, S., Anwar, T.: Depression intensity estimation via social media: a deep learning approach. IEEE Trans. Comput. Soc. Sys. **8**(6), 1465–1474 (2021)
15. Prama, T.T., Islam, M.S., Anwar, M.M., Jahan, I.: Ai-enabled deep depression detection and evaluation informed by dsm-5-tr. IEEE Trans. Comput. Soc. Sys. **11**(5), 6453–6465 (2024)

16. Coppersmith, G., Dredze, M., Harman, C., Hollingshead, K.: From adhd to sad: analyzing the language of mental health on twitter through self-reported diagnoses. In: Proceedings of From ADHD to SAD: Analyzing the Language of Mental Health on Twitter Through Self-Reported Diagnoses, pp. 1–10 (2015)
17. Aldkheel, A., Zhou, L.: Depression detection on social media: a classification framework and research challenges and opportunities. J. Healthcare Inf. Res. **8**(1), 88–120 (2023)
18. Tahir, W.B., Khalid, S., Almutairi, S., Abohashrh, M., Memon, S.A., Khan, J.: Depression detection in social media: a comprehensive review of machine learning and deep learning techniques. IEEE Access **13**, 12789–12818 (2025)
19. Xin, C., Zakaria, L.Q.: Integrating bert with cnn and bilstm for explainable detection of depression in social media contents. IEEE Access **12**, 161203–161212 (2024)

Optimal Privacy Budget Allocation Framework for Medical Data Publishing

Samsad Jahan[1], Wei Hong[1], Yong-Feng Ge[1(✉)], Hua Wang[1], Enamul Kabir[2], and Frank Whittaker[3]

[1] Institute for Sustainable Industries and Liveable Cities Victoria University, Melbourne, Australia
{samsad.jahan,wei.hong2}@live.vu.edu.au, {yongfeng.ge,hua.wang}@vu.edu.au
[2] School of Mathematics, Physics and Computing, University of Southern Queensland, Toowoomba, Australia
enamul.kabir@usq.edu.au
[3] Nexus eCare, Adelaide, Australia
frank@nexusonline.com.au

Abstract. The issue of preserving sensitive information in medical datasets while maintaining their utility is a significant concern in the implementation of Differential Privacy (DP). This paper presents a framework for allocating privacy budgets, designed to optimize the total budget for medical datasets and thereby enhance data utility. Previous strategies for allocating privacy budgets have primarily relied on fixed mathematical rules, and excessive or insufficient noise addition can impact data utility. Therefore, we propose a Genetic Algorithm (GA)-based framework that generates a privacy budget sequence through selection, crossover, and mutation operations to arrive at an attribute-wise optimal privacy budget. After that, the same individual optimal budget is utilized for each record in publishing, ensuring individual privacy guarantees. Experimental findings on two medical datasets reveal enhanced data utility when compared to heuristic budget allocation methods. This framework presents a straightforward and efficacious strategy for allocating privacy budgets within the context of privacy-preserving medical data publication. The source code used in this study is publicly available at https://github.com/Wayne-on-the-road/OPBA-MDP.

Keywords: Medical data publishing · Differential privacy · Genetic algorithm · Budget allocation

1 Introduction

The anticipated growth in health information, alongside the escalating demand for the exchange of medical data, has fostered progress in healthcare research, policy development, and clinical practice. Medical data may encompass drug research and disease surveillance, wherein personal attributes such as name, age, gender, postal code, occupation, medical condition, and health history are

E. R. Kaburuan and S. Goundar (Eds.): HIS 2025, LNCS 16392, pp. 107–118, 2026.
https://doi.org/10.1007/978-981-95-6304-3_10

collected, disseminated, and employed by third-party devices or authorities. The scrutiny and application of medical data have thus become a significant topic in recent years [16]. However, the distribution of medical information raises substantial privacy concerns and is vulnerable to inference and re-identification attacks [1].

Classical anonymization models such as k-anonymity [20], l-diversity [17], and t-closeness [14] aim to mitigate these risks. Specifically, k-anonymity protects against linkage attacks but remains vulnerable to homogeneity and background knowledge attacks. l-diversity extends k-anonymity by ensuring diversity of sensitive attributes, yet it suffers from skewness and similarity attacks. t-closeness improves resilience by restricting the distributional distance of sensitive attributes, thereby mitigating skewness and similarity attacks. Nevertheless, these models remain limited in defending against adversaries with extensive background knowledge, as their underlying threat models assume simplified attacker capabilities.

In contrast, Differential Privacy (DP) has emerged as a more rigorous privacy framework, offering strong mathematical guarantees by ensuring that the inclusion or exclusion of any individual record has a negligible effect on query outputs. This property provides resilience against a wide range of inference attacks while enabling controlled data sharing [2]. Consequently, DP has been widely applied in healthcare to facilitate the regulated dissemination of health information, reducing the risk of disclosing sensitive personal data [19,21,22]. However, the efficiency of DP critically depends on how the privacy budget is allocated among sensitive attributes. For medical datasets, attributes such as age, gender, and disease status may vary significantly in their importance to utility and sensitivity to privacy risk.

To address this challenge, recent studies have explored the use of Genetic Algorithms (GAs) for optimizing the trade-off between privacy and utility [5,8,10,11,13]. GAs are particularly well-suited for handling complex optimization problems [6,7,23]. For instance, Li et al. proposed a GA-based privacy budget allocation technique that balances privacy and utility in DP by efficiently distributing budgets among cluster centroids [15]. Similarly, Ge et al. [9] investigated an information-driven distributed GA, demonstrating the role of attribute generalization in optimal anonymization for distributed data. Furthermore, Dynamic Parameter Genetic Algorithm (DPGA) and Adaptive Parameter Memetic Algorithm (APMA) have been introduced to support multi-objective optimization in trajectory data publishing, enabling dynamic parameter adjustments that improve the privacy-utility balance [12,13]. These works highlight the adaptability of GAs and their effectiveness in enhancing privacy preservation while maintaining data usability.

Motivated by these insights, we propose a framework that leverages a GA to find near-optimal privacy budget allocation sequences for protecting medical data under DP. Specifically, a GA is employed to allocate the privacy budget among sensitive attributes in an optimal manner, and the result is then applied to each record. This GA-based allocation strategy is designed to maximize data utility while providing rigorous privacy guarantees for sensitive medical attributes. The main contributions of this work are as follows:

- We introduce a privacy-protected health data publishing framework powered by GA. It distributes the budget optimally across sensitive attributes to ensure a maximized utility under certain budget constraint.
- We design a GA-based privacy budget allocation method with an early stopping strategy to facilitate optimal and efficient allocation. A carefully crafted fitness function based test accuracy is also designed.
- Extensive experiments on real-world datasets verify the superiority of our approach in terms of utility over the traditional budget allocation approaches.

The subsequent sections of this paper are structured as follows. Section 2 describes our proposed framework. Section 3 presents the experimental results and the setup. Finally, Sect. 4 provides the conclusion.

2 Methodology

2.1 The Proposed GA-Based Framework

In this section, we propose a GA-based framework for allocating privacy budgets. The GA is employed to determine the optimal sequence of privacy budget allocation for each sensitive attribute, which is subsequently applied to individual records. The whole privacy-preserving framework is given in Fig. 1. According to this framework, the initial step involves inputting the raw dataset. Subsequently, the sensitive attributes within the data are identified. Following the identification of these sensitive attributes, it is necessary to select the total privacy budget for the dataset. We will then employ the GA to determine the optimal privacy budget sequence for each sensitive attribute. In the proposed GA, each individual represents a candidate solution for distributing the total privacy budget among the identified sensitive attributes. As represented in Fig. 1, the genes within a chromosome correspond to the per-attribute budget allocation (e.g., a portion of the total budget is allocated to age, another to gender, etc.). An individual budget vector thus encodes one possible allocation strategy. The GA starts by randomly initializing such individuals, each encoding a separate allocation sequence. Through evaluation (fitness function based on accuracy), selection, crossover, and mutation, these individuals progress toward near optimal solutions that maximize utility while maintaining total budget constraints. Once the GA achieves the near optimal accuracy for each sensitive attribute, the termination conditions are met, and the resulting privacy budget vector are selected. This optimal sequence is then applied to the corresponding sensitive attributes to generate the differentially private anonymized dataset.

2.2 DP Applications in Our Framework

A privacy mechanism M satisfies ϵ-DP if for any two neighbouring datasets D and D' differing by a single record, and for all measurable sets $S \subseteq \text{Range}(M)$,

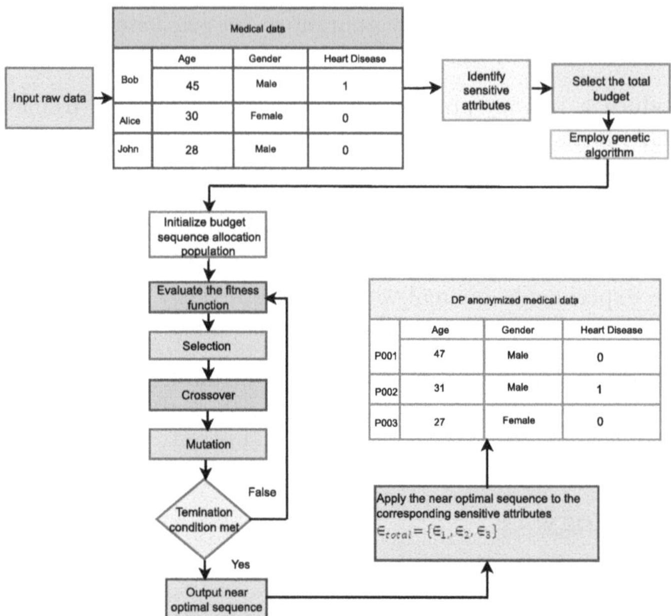

Fig. 1. GA-based privacy budget allocation framework for medical data publishing.

the probability of any output differs by at most a multiplicative factor of e^{ϵ}. The privacy budget $\epsilon > 0$ controls the amount of perturbation noise added to the data—smaller ϵ provides stronger privacy at the cost of reduced data utility [18]. DP mechanisms, such as the Laplace and Exponential mechanisms, are applied within our framework depending on the data type (numerical or categorical). The following process describes how DP is applied in detail in the GA process (when generating fitness value) and also in the final publishing stage:

$$\text{Let } D = \{x_i\}_{i=1}^{n} \text{ be the original medical dataset, with } x_i \in \mathbb{R}^d \text{ (mixed types).}$$

Each record x_i is a vector with d attributes, where some attributes are mixed, i.e. some are numerical (age), some are categorical (gender). We focus on allocating the privacy budget among these sensitive attributes in an optimal manner.

$$A = \{A_1, \ldots, A_d\}, \qquad S \subseteq A, \quad |S| = m.$$

Here, A is the set of sensitive attributes and S is the subset of sensitive attributes of size m. Only these sensitive attributes will get the privacy protection. Now the total privacy budget is as follows:

$$\epsilon > 0 \quad \text{(total privacy budget chosen by the data owner).}$$

Our focus is to distribute the total budget across the sensitive attributes, where each attribute A_j will get its own budget ϵ_j and the constraint is that the total privacy budget cannot exceed.

$$\epsilon = (\epsilon_j)_{j \in S}, \qquad \epsilon_j \geq 0, \ \sum_{j \in S} \epsilon_j \leq \epsilon. \tag{1}$$

We adopt a local DP view at the cell level: each sensitive attribute value $x_i^{(j)}$ is randomized on the client side with budget ϵ_j. For a given record x_i, the per-record total budget is $\epsilon = \sum_{j \in S} \epsilon_j$, obtained by sequential composition across attributes.

Numeric Sensitive Attribute (A_j). Let the global sensitivity, which determines the maximum possible change in attribute A_j, be

$$\Delta_j = \max_i x_i^{(j)} - \min_i x_i^{(j)}.$$

We then release

$$tildex_i^{(j)} = x_i^{(j)} + \eta_i^{(j)}, \qquad \eta_i^{(j)} \sim \text{Laplace}\left(0, \frac{\Delta_j}{\epsilon_j}\right). \tag{2}$$

Mechanism (2) is ϵ_j-DP for A_j. To preserve the privacy of categorical attributes, we employ the Exponential mechanism. *Categorical sensitive attribute* (A_j). Using the Exponential Mechanism with score function $u_j(D, r)$ and sensitivity Δu_j:

$$\Pr\left[\tilde{x}_i^{(j)} = r\right] \propto \exp\left(\frac{\epsilon_j \, u_j(D, r)}{2 \, \Delta u_j}\right). \tag{3}$$

2.3 Algorithm Process in Detail

Algorithm 1 illustrates the process of obtaining an optimal privacy budget allocation for the sensitive attributes. The algorithm begins by initializing a population of candidate budget vectors, each representing a potential split of the total privacy budget ϵ across the sensitive attributes. These vectors are sampled from a Dirichlet distribution to ensure feasibility and proportionality. Each vector is subsequently normalized so that its elements sum exactly to ϵ. In each generation, the algorithm evaluates the quality of every candidate vector by applying it to anonymize the sensitive attributes of the dataset. A classifier is then trained on the anonymized training data and evaluated against the clean test data. The resulting test accuracy is used as the fitness score of the candidate, reflecting how well the budget allocation maintains downstream utility while still enforcing privacy. Based on these fitness values, the algorithm performs tournament selection to choose parent solutions, applies blend crossover to exchange budget proportions between parents, and introduces diversity through Gaussian mutation. This evolutionary process is iterated across generations to progressively improve the population.

To enhance efficiency and avoid unnecessary iterations, an early stopping strategy is employed. Specifically, the algorithm tracks the best fitness value across generations. If the improvement in the best fitness does not exceed a small tolerance δ for K consecutive generations, the search is terminated prematurely. This prevents over-computation when the population has converged and the likelihood of further improvements is low.

Finally, the algorithm outputs the budget vector with the highest fitness value encountered during the search. This vector represents the allocation sequence that achieves the most favorable trade-off between privacy preservation and utility retention.

Algorithm 1 GA for per-attribute privacy budget allocation

Input: Dataset D with sensitive attributes S; Total privacy budget ϵ; Population size N, number of generations G; Crossover probability p_c, mutation probability p_m; Early stopping parameters: tolerance δ, patience K
Output: Optimal budget vector $\mathbf{b}^*$
Initialize population P_0 of N budget vectors sampled from a Dirichlet distribution of dimension $|S|$
Set $best\_fitness \leftarrow -\infty$, $no\_improvement\_count \leftarrow 0$
for generation $t = 1$ to G **do**
  for each individual budget vector $\mathbf{b}_i \in P_t$ **do**
    Normalize $\mathbf{b}_i$ so that $\sum_j b_{i,j} = \epsilon$
    Apply anonymization to D using $\mathbf{b}_i$ for attributes S
    Train classifier on noised data, evaluate on clean test data
    Compute utility u_i (classification accuracy)
    Assign fitness $f(\mathbf{b}_i) \leftarrow u_i$
  end for
  Select parents using tournament selection
  Apply blend crossover with probability p_c
  Apply Gaussian mutation with probability p_m
  Form next generation P_{t+1}
  Let $gen\_best \leftarrow \max_{\mathbf{b}_i \in P_t} f(\mathbf{b}_i)$
  if $gen\_best > best\_fitness + \delta$ **then**
    $best\_fitness \leftarrow gen\_best$, $no\_improvement\_count \leftarrow 0$
  else
    $no\_improvement\_count \leftarrow no\_improvement\_count + 1$
  end if
  if $no\_improvement\_count \geq K$ **then**
    break {Early stopping}
  end if
end for
Return: $\mathbf{b}^* = \arg\max_{\mathbf{b}_i \in P} f(\mathbf{b}_i)$

3 Experiment

3.1 Dataset and Experimental Settings

We evaluated our framework in two medical datasets: i) Diabetes[1], and ii) Heart disease data[2]. The diabetes dataset contains 5132 samples, 9 dimensions, and 2 clusters, and the heart disease dataset contains 1025 samples with 13 dimensions and 2 clusters. For the experiment, we pick "age", "sex", "cp" as sensitive attributes for the heart disease dataset and "age', "gender", "BMI" for the diabetes dataset. Furthermore, we have compared our GA-based optimal allocation framework with the Dichotomous Allocation Strategy (DAS) and Series Sum of Allocation Strategy (SSAS). Descriptions of these two strategies are given below:

- **DAS:** This method was originally introduced by Dwork as a privacy budget allocation strategy utilizing a dichotomy allocation technique. DAS assigns a privacy budget $\epsilon_i = \frac{\epsilon}{2i}$ throughout each attribute [3,4,15].
- **SSAS:** This strategy is based on $\epsilon = \sum_{i=1}^{\infty} \frac{\epsilon}{i(i+1)}$ with a privacy budget of $\epsilon_i = \frac{\epsilon}{i(i+1)}$. It permits an unlimited allocation of the privacy budget [15].

The GA method was configured with a population size of 40 and a maximum of 50 generations. Tournament selection (size = 3), blend crossover ($p_c = 0.7$), and Gaussian mutation ($p_m = 0.3$) were applied in each generation. All experiments were repeated across 30 random seeds for robustness concerns.

3.2 Experimental Result

In our DP design, we employed test accuracy on a clean dataset (without noise injection) as the fitness value and experimented with total budget values ranging from 1 to 10. We used information loss to show how the data is distorted after anonymization, which is measured by comparing original and noised sensitive attributes: for numerical attributes, normalized mean absolute error (scaled by the attribute's range); for categorical attributes, the fraction of altered values; and the final score was the average of these components. Other commonly used metrics, such as precision and F1 score, are also adopted to offer a comprehensive view.

Table 1 shows the accuracy comparison of the GA-based framework with DAS and SSAS on the diabetes dataset. From this table, it is observed that the accuracy improves for all methods as the privacy budget increases from 1 to 10, representing the expected privacy-utility trade-off, which indicates that weaker privacy yields better accuracy. The GA-based allocation strategy consistently outperforms the DAS and SSAS at every budget level in terms of accuracy. At a lower budget ($\epsilon = 1$), GA achieves 0.7232, compared to 0.7202 (DAS) and 0.7208 (SSAS). However, as the budget increases, the improvement margin widens. For instance, for $\epsilon = 10$, the accuracy of GA is 0.7641, which is (1.5-1.6)% higher than DAS (0.7484) and SSAS (0.7487).

[1] https://www.kaggle.com/datasets/simaanjali/diabetes-classification-dataset.

[2] https://archive.ics.uci.edu/dataset/45/heart+disease.

Figure 2 shows that for the diabetes dataset, the accuracy, F1 score, and precision improve steadily for GA as the privacy budget increases. It shows a better outcome in all aspects compared to DAS and SSAS, including the information loss, as higher information loss indicates better privacy preservation.

Table 1. Accuracy of GA, DAS, and SSAS on the diabetes dataset with Wilcoxon significance tests.

Budget	GA	DAS	SSAS	GA vs. DAS	GA vs. SSAS
1	**0.7232** (0.0075)	0.7207 (0.0077)	0.7208 (0.0078)	**	**
2	**0.7275** (0.0077)	0.7233 (0.0075)	0.7236 (0.0076)	**	**
3	**0.7316** (0.0078)	0.7258 (0.0078)	0.7261 (0.0077)	**	**
4	**0.7375** (0.0079)	0.7278 (0.0078)	0.7280 (0.0076)	**	**
5	**0.7431** (0.0085)	0.7303 (0.0077)	0.7307 (0.0077)	**	**
6	**0.7483** (0.0080)	0.7344 (0.0079)	0.7347 (0.0077)	**	**
7	**0.7520** (0.0082)	0.7381 (0.0080)	0.7384 (0.0078)	**	**
8	**0.7564** (0.0076)	0.7417 (0.0079)	0.7420 (0.0077)	**	**
9	**0.7602** (0.0072)	0.7452 (0.0076)	0.7454 (0.0073)	**	**
10	**0.7641** (0.0072)	0.7484 (0.0076)	0.7487 (0.0072)	**	**

Note: Wilcoxon signed-rank test significance levels are indicated as * ($p < 0.05$), ** ($p < 0.01$).

Table 2 shows a similar trend for the heart disease dataset as it is shown for the diabetes dataset. For example, at $\epsilon = 1$, the accuracy of GA is 0.8420, whereas DAS and SSAS both show similar accuracy, 0.8359. At $\epsilon = 10$, GA exhibits higher accuracy 0.8743 compared to DAS (0.8704) and SSAS(0.8705). Moreover, for each privacy budget level, the Wilcoxon signed-rank test shows that GA's improvement over DAS and SSAS is statistically significant at the 1% level of significance.

On the other hand, Fig. 3 also shows a similar pattern; GA exhibits higher accuracy, precision, and F1 from $\epsilon = 1$ to $\epsilon = 10$. In terms of information loss, GA-based framework preserves better privacy than DAS and SSAS. Overall our GA-based framework exhibits better outcomes for all metrics compared to DAS and SSAS.

Across both datasets, information loss decreases as ϵ increases for all methods, reflecting the standard privacy–utility trade-off. However, GA's information loss often remains *higher* than DAS/SSAS at the same ϵ, even as GA achieves higher accuracy. This pattern is consistent with GA allocating more budget to predictive attributes (lowering their noise) and less to weak attributes (raising their noise), which improves downstream utility while keeping the per-record total budget fixed. In contrast, DAS/SSAS spread budget more evenly, yielding lower average distortion but lower accuracy.

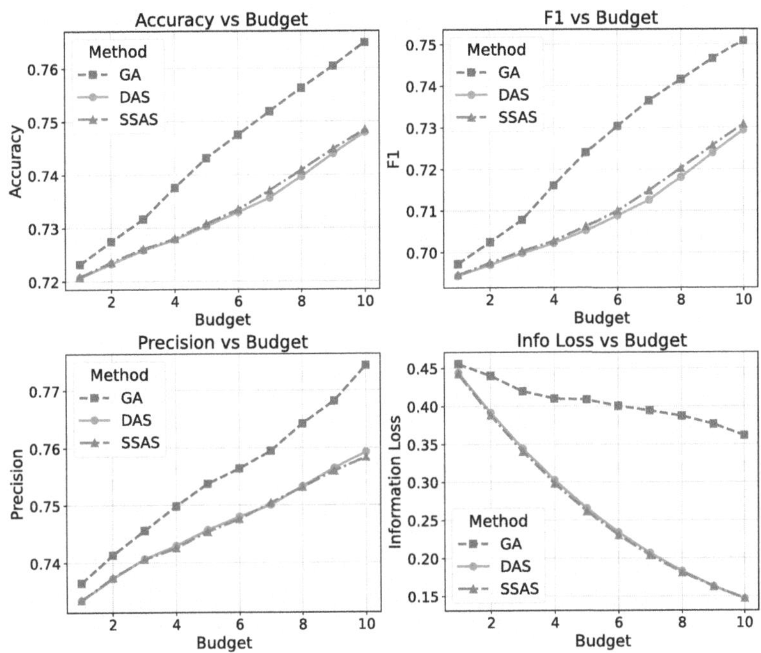

Fig. 2. Comparison for diabetes data.

Table 2. Accuracy of GA, DAS, and SSAS on the heart dataset with Wilcoxon significance tests.

Budget	GA	DAS	SSAS	GA vs. DAS	GA vs. SSAS
1	**0.8420** (0.0148)	0.8359 (0.0155)	0.8359 (0.0155)	**	**
2	**0.8461** (0.0137)	0.8415 (0.0149)	0.8416 (0.0150)	**	**
3	**0.8512** (0.0140)	0.8468 (0.0155)	0.8469 (0.0155)	**	**
4	**0.8547** (0.0129)	0.8506 (0.0146)	0.8507 (0.0146)	**	**
5	**0.8583** (0.0130)	0.8542 (0.0146)	0.8543 (0.0146)	**	**
6	**0.8610** (0.0132)	0.8571 (0.0147)	0.8572 (0.0147)	**	**
7	**0.8649** (0.0135)	0.8610 (0.0150)	0.8611 (0.0150)	**	**
8	**0.8681** (0.0132)	0.8642 (0.0148)	0.8643 (0.0148)	**	**
9	**0.8712** (0.0126)	0.8673 (0.0142)	0.8674 (0.0142)	**	**
10	**0.8743** (0.0125)	0.8704 (0.0141)	0.8705 (0.0141)	**	**

Note: Wilcoxon signed-rank test significance levels are indicated as * ($p < 0.05$), ** ($p < 0.01$).

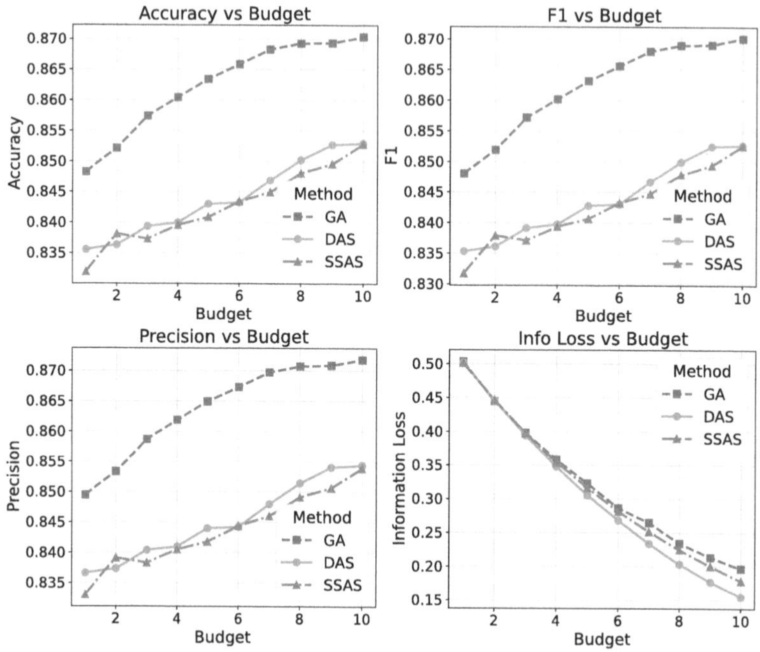

Fig. 3. Comparison for heart disease data.

4 Conclusion

In this work, we introduced a GA-based privacy budget allocation framework for medical data publishing under DP. Unlike fixed allocation strategies such as DAS and SSAS, our approach adaptively distributes the total privacy budget across sensitive attributes to maximize data utility. By applying Laplace and Exponential mechanisms to numeric and categorical attributes respectively, the framework ensures rigorous privacy guarantees while producing privatized datasets that remain useful for predictive modeling. Experimental results on two standard medical datasets demonstrate that GA consistently achieves higher accuracy than heuristic methods across a range of privacy budgets. These findings highlight the value of data-driven allocation strategies in balancing privacy and utility. Future work may extend this framework to multi-objective optimization, larger and more diverse health datasets, and other privacy models, further enhancing the practicality of privacy-preserving medical data publishing.

References

1. Anjum, A., et al.: An efficient privacy mechanism for electronic health records. Comput. Secur. **72**, 196–211 (2018)
2. Dwork, C.: Differential privacy. In: Bugliesi, M., Preneel, B., Sassone, V., Wegener, I. (eds.), In: International Colloquium on Automata, Languages, and Programming, vol. 4052, pp. 1–12. Springer, Berlin, Heidelberg (2006). https://doi.org/10.1007/11787006_1
3. Dwork, C., McSherry, F., Nissim, K., Smith, A.: Calibrating noise to sensitivity in private data analysis. In: Halevi, S., Rabin, T. (eds.), Theory of Cryptography, vol. 3876, pp. 265–284. Springer Berlin Heidelberg (2006). https://doi.org/10.1007/11681878_14
4. Fan, Z., Xu, X.: APDPK-Means: a new differential privacy clustering algorithm based on arithmetic progression privacy budget allocation. In: 2019 IEEE 21st International Conference on High Performance Computing and Communications; IEEE 17th International Conference on Smart City; IEEE 5th International Conference on Data Science and Systems (HPCC/SmartCity/DSS), pp. 1737–1742. IEEE (2019)
5. Ge, Y.F., Bertino, E., Wang, H., Cao, J., Zhang, Y.: Distributed cooperative coevolution of data publishing privacy and transparency. ACM Trans. Knowl. Discov. Data **18**(1), 1–23 (2023)
6. Ge, Y.-F., Orlowska, M., Cao, J., Wang, H., Zhang, Y.: MDDE: multitasking distributed differential evolution for privacy-preserving database fragmentation. VLDB J. , 1–19 (2021). https://doi.org/10.1007/s00778-021-00718-w
7. Ge, Y.F., Wang, H., Bertino, E., Cao, J., Zhang, Y.: Multiobjective privacy-preserving task assignment in spatial crowdsourcing. IEEE Tran. Cybern. **55**(8), 3584–3597 (2025)
8. Ge, Y.F., et al.: Evolutionary dynamic database partitioning optimization for privacy and utility. IEEE Trans. Dependable Secure Comput. **21**(4), 2296–2311 (2023)
9. Ge, Y.F., Wang, H., Cao, J., Zhang, Y., Jiang, X.: Privacy-preserving data publishing: an information-driven distributed genetic algorithm. World Wide Web **27**(1), 1 (2024)
10. Ge, Y.F., Wang, H., Cao, J., Zhang, Y., Kambourakis, G.: Federated genetic algorithm: two-layer privacy-preserving trajectory data publishing. In: Proceedings of the Genetic and Evolutionary Computation Conference, pp. 749–758 (2024)
11. Jahan, S., Ge, Y.F., Kabir, E., Wang, H.: Analysis and protection of public medical dataset: From privacy perspective. In: International Conference on Health Information Science, pp. 79–90. Springer, Heidelberg (2023). https://doi.org/10.1007/978-981-99-7108-4_7
12. Jahan, S., Ge, Y.F., Wang, H., Kabir, E.: Dynamic-parameter genetic algorithm for multi-objective privacy-preserving trajectory data publishing. In: International Conference on Web Information Systems Engineering, pp. 46–57. Springer, Heidelberg (2024). https://doi.org/10.1007/978-981-96-0576-7_4
13. Jahan, S., Ge, Y.F., Wang, H., Kabir, E.: Adaptive-parameter memetic algorithm for privacy-preserving trajectory data publishing: a multi-objective optimization approach. Computing **107**(7), 151 (2025)
14. Li, N., Li, T., Venkatasubramanian, S.: T-Closeness: privacy beyond k-anonymity and l-diversity. In: 2007 IEEE 23rd International Conference on Data Engineering, pp. 106–115. IEEE (2006)

15. Li, Y., Song, X., Tu, Y., Liu, M.: Gapbas: genetic algorithm-based privacy budget allocation strategy in differential privacy k-means clustering algorithm. Comput. Secur. **139**, 103697 (2024)
16. Liu, W., Zhang, Y., Yang, H., Meng, Q.: A survey on differential privacy for medical data analysis. Ann. Data Sci. **11**(2), 733–747 (2024)
17. Machanavajjhala, A., Kifer, D., Gehrke, J., Venkitasubramaniam, M.: l-diversity: privacy beyond k-anonymity. ACM Trans. Knowl. Disc. Data (TKDD) **1**(1), 3–es (2007)
18. Pang, X., Wang, Z., Liu, D., Lui, J.C., Wang, Q., Ren, J.: Towards personalized privacy-preserving truth discovery over crowdsourced data streams. IEEE/ACM Trans. Network. **30**(1), 327–340 (2021)
19. Sun, Z., Wang, Y., Shu, M., Liu, R., Zhao, H.: Differential privacy for data and model publishing of medical data. IEEE Access **7**, 152103–152114 (2019)
20. Sweeney, L.: k-anonymity: a model for protecting privacy. Int. J. Uncertain. Fuzziness Knowl.-Based Syst. **10**(05), 557–570 (2002)
21. Yin, J., Hong, W., Wang, H., Cao, J., Miao, Y., Zhang, Y.: A compact vulnerability knowledge graph for risk assessment. ACM Trans. Knowl. Discov. Data **18**(8), 1–17 (2024)
22. Yin, J., Tang, M., Cao, J., You, M., Wang, H., Alazab, M.: Knowledge-driven cybersecurity intelligence: software vulnerability Coexploitation behavior discovery. IEEE Trans. Ind. Inf. **19**(4), 5593–5601 (2022)
23. You, M., Ge, Y.F., Wang, K., Wang, H., Cao, J., Kambourakis, G.: Hierarchical adaptive evolution framework for privacy-preserving data publishing. World Wide Web **27**(4), 49 (2024)

Towards AI-Assisted Doctors: Exploring Factors Affecting the Use and Acceptance of ChatGPT by Medical Doctors in the Philippines using Integrated TTF-UTAUT

Francis Marlon Cabredo(✉) and Ryan Ebardo

De La Salle University, Manila, Philippines
{francis_cabredo,ryan.ebardo}@dlsu.edu.ph

Abstract. Artificial Intelligence in the healthcare sector has been highlighted as a key technology to tackle the major challenges facing healthcare systems today. ChatGPT, a large language model developed by OpenAI, shows promise as a support tool for healthcare workers. This study investigates the adoption and usage of ChatGPT among medical doctors in the Philippines by utilizing an integrated theoretical framework combining Task-Technology Fit (TTF) and Unified Theory of Acceptance and Use of Technology (UTAUT). A total of 279 licensed medical doctors in the Philippines participated in an online survey through convenience sampling. Structural equation modeling was used to analyze the relationships among constructs. Performance Expectancy and Social Influence emerged as positive significant factors of Behavioral Intention to Use. Furthermore, Task Technology Fit and Behavioral Intention to Use significantly influenced Actual Use of ChatGPT by medical doctors. The findings emphasize the importance of understanding the influencing factors in usage intention and the task-technology alignment of AI tools in driving adoption. The study provides empirical insights into exploring the potential role of ChatGPT in healthcare and discusses theoretical and practical implications.

Keywords: ChatGPT · Chatbot · Artificial Intelligence · Healthcare · Doctors

1 Introduction

The rapid advancement of technology has transformed the way we live today and continues to evolve. The development and widespread availability of Artificial Intelligence (AI) has been reported to be a transformative frontier in healthcare practice [1]. AI technology has been touted to automate and accelerate routine tasks of healthcare professionals. Moreover, AI tools and systems promise multiple applications such as the generation of patient-centric insights from large volumes of data to help improve productivity and enhance patient outcomes. These are expressed to aid healthcare workers in clinical decision support, differential diagnosis, workflow support, and medical data analysis to improve healthcare delivery [2].

E. R. Kaburuan and S. Goundar (Eds.): HIS 2025, LNCS 16392, pp. 119–131, 2026.
https://doi.org/10.1007/978-981-95-6304-3_11

Among these tools include Chatbots which are AI-powered programs that enables individuals and healthcare institutions to access information, receive support, and carry out various tasks through simple text-based conversations [3]. ChatGPT is a Generative AI chatbot that produces human-like responses to multimodal inputs. Released by OpenAI in November 2022, it has been reported to have garnered rapid and substantial growth in its user base and has been described to be the fastest uptake of users in any emerging technology [4]. The Philippines has also been featured as one of the top five users of ChatGPT with significant traffic relative to the the US which includes India, Brazil, and Indonesia offering insights to widespread interest and uptake of AI [5].

Generative AI technologies such as ChatGPT have the potential to revolutionize healthcare in developing countries such as the Philippines. However, while many studies show the promising role of AI, the usage of AI in healthcare is still in the early stage [6]. Concerns have been raised in relation to hallucinations or inaccurate information, risk of bias, privacy, ethical, and legal issues [7]. The innate resistance of the human mind to any change is thought as an evolutionary and social psychological response, therefore the concerns following the release of ChatGPT are understandable [7]. Furthermore, Healthcare is slow to adopt largely driven by user resistance by physicians to medical innovation. It has already been reported that the most important factor was physician's attitudes and perceptions toward AI, which can decide whether they would want to integrate AI in their practice or not [8].

Therefore, the aim of the study is to explore the influencing factors on medical doctors' behavioral intention to use ChatGPT. Importantly, by understanding these factors, the study aims to understand the changing demands of the healthcare sector and promote the ethical and responsible use and application of AI in healthcare.

2 Review of Related Literature

2.1 ChatGPT for Supporting Healthcare Practice

Studies have described that ChatGPT has received mixed responses expressed by arguments regarding the benefits and the risks of AI technologies [7]. The implementation of AI in clinical practice and medical research has been described as relatively restricted, but the literature remains positive that incorporating AI in various healthcare aspects can improve efficiency and accuracy. Among the benefits, ChatGPT in healthcare settings is primarily evaluated in various application-oriented scenarios such as triage, medical translation, medical research, clinical workflow, medical education, clinical consultation and multimodal applications [9].

The risks come from several limitations and ethical considerations such as information accuracy, privacy, and credibility [9, 10]. ChatGPT's lack of human connection to healthcare delivery, as well as the issue of the devaluation of human thinking are also concerns. Medico-legal accountability issues due to medical errors brought about by its use should also be considered [7]. These concerns contribute to the perception of medical doctors on the use and utility of the chatbot and AI technologies.

Related research has also suggested that there is limited quantitative evaluation data given the recency of the impact of AI in healthcare [11]. Previous studies on the acceptance of technology by healthcare professionals have mainly focused on consumer perspective and limited understanding of healthcare professionals' acceptance of innovative technology for medical use [12].

2.2 Technology Adoption Frameworks and Hypotheses Development

Various information systems theories have been used to comprehensively understand influencing factors in the individual's adoption and acceptance of technology. Studies confirm the applicability of technology acceptance models and theories on healthcare information systems adoption [13]. This supports the importance of theory-guided and user-centered design approaches to healthcare information systems. Related research in developing countries identified the use of TTF and TAM to assess ChatGPT by healthcare workers in Nigeria [26], TTF for nurses in Gaza [27], UTAUT to study healthcare workers use of e-health systems in Ethiopia [33], and the use of UTAUT for medical students in Vietnam [6].

Integrated TTF-UTAUT This research study employs an Integrated Task-Technology Fit (TTF) and Unified Theory of Use and Acceptance of Technology (UTAUT) model as illustrated in Fig. 1. UTAUT contributes an understanding of psychological and social drivers, while TTF explains the practical and technical alignment between ChatGPT as a tool and the medical practice tasks. The integrated TTF–UTAUT framework aims to form a comprehensive model that captures both why medical doctors intend to use ChatGPT and how it fits within their professional and medical workflow.

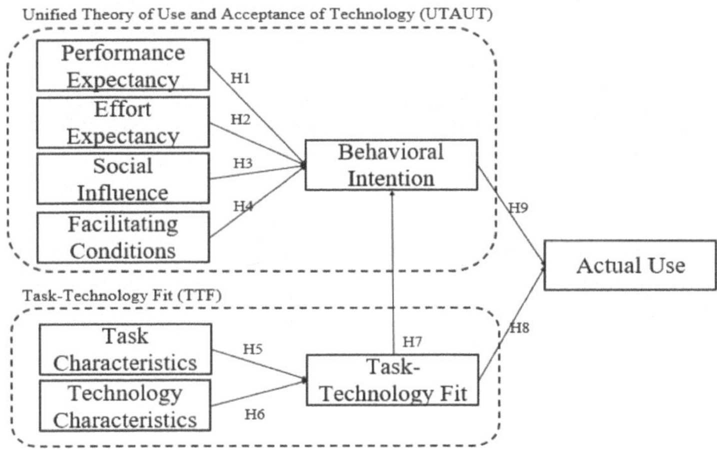

Fig. 1. Theoretical Framework using Integrated TTF-UTAUT

Unified Theory of Use and Acceptance of Technology The UTAUT is a theoretical framework developed by Venkatesh et al. (2003) that identifies four main determinants to explain how and why people adopt and use new technologies. UTAUT integrates previous technology acceptance models into one unified model [15]. Previous studies have confirmed its applicability to understand acceptance and use of AI to gain insights into what motivates early adopters and identify potential barriers [14].

Performance Expectancy (PE) refers to the degree to which an individual believes that a particular technology will help them perform their tasks more effectively or efficiently [15]. Studies on Chatbot adoption suggest that PE predicts the user acceptance and use of Chatbots. The researchers propose the hypothesis *H1*. Performance Expectancy positively influences Behavioral Intention towards ChatGPT by medical doctors.

Effort Expectancy (EE) refers to the perceived ease of using a particular technology [15]. In the case of ChatGPT, LLMs trained with a high level of effort expectancy would likely positively influence its adoption. If users perceive ChatGPT as easy to use, they are more likely to adopt and integrate it into their daily routines leading to increased usage [16]. The researchers propose the hypothesis *H2*. Effort Expectancy positively influences Behavioral Intention towards ChatGPT by medical doctors.

Social Influence (SI) refers to how an individual perceives that significant others, such as friends, family members, or colleagues, influence and believe that they should use a particular technology [15]. Positive social influence can increase the user's perception of the usefulness and ease of use of ChatGPT, reduce the perceived risks and barriers to adoption, and enhance the user's confidence in their ability to use the technology effectively [16]. The researchers propose the hypothesis *H3*. Social Influence positively influences Behavioral Intention towards ChatGPT by medical doctors.

Facilitating Conditions (FC) refers to the degree to which individuals perceive that an organizational and technical infrastructure exists to support the use of technology. It encompasses the resources, support, and technical infrastructure available to the user, such as hardware, software, technical support and training [15]. In the case of ChatGPT, if users can access the necessary facilitating conditions such as the technical resources and support, they may be more inclined to adopt ChatGPT and integrate it into their daily routines [16]. The researchers propose the hypothesis *H4*. Facilitating Conditions positively influence Behavioral Intention towards ChatGPT by medical doctors.

Behavioral intention (BI) is described as a deliberate plan to use or not to use technology in the process of performing a duty. If the adoption intention is positive, individuals shall surely use the technology and vice versa [22]. Studies have reported the effect of adoption intention on actual usage (AU) of technology. The researchers propose the hypothesis *H9*. Behavioral Intention to use ChatGPT by medical doctors has a positive effect on Actual Use.

Task-Technology Fit The TTF model is a theory that aims to explain how well a technology supports the tasks a person needs to perform. Introduced by Goodhue and Thompson (1995), it is widely used to define technology adoption and effectiveness [17]. Task-technology fit is influenced by the link between task and technology characteristics, which in turn affects user performance and the efficiency of technology in supporting healthcare tasks [18].

Task Characteristics (TAC) refer to the attributes of a task that are expected to be or can be executed using information technologies [19]. Within the context of this study, this considers the complexity and routineness of medical and clinical tasks being conducted by doctors. The researchers propose the hypothesis *H5.* Task Characteristics have a positive influence on task-technology fit of ChatGPT by medical doctors.

Technology Characteristics (TEC) refer to the aspects of technology tools that may influence technology utilization and users' perceptions [19]. Within this study, this refers to ChatGPT accuracy, responsiveness, integrability, and reliability. The researchers propose the hypothesis *H6.* Technology Characteristics have a positive influence on task-technology fit of ChatGPT by medical doctors.

Task-Technology Fit (TTF) holds that new technology is more likely to have a positive impact on individual performance and be used if the capabilities of the new technology match the tasks that the user must perform [20]. In healthcare context, the compatibility of technology with clinical activities and procedures is said to be a determining factor in the adoption of technology by healthcare users [20]. The assessment of fit among the individual, task, and technology is crucial to successful AI adoption to assess its promise of improved quality and efficiency for healthcare delivery [21]. The following two hypotheses are proposed *H7*. Task-Technology Fit has a positive effect on Behavioral Intention to use by medical doctors; and *H8*. Task-Technology Fit has a positive effect on Actual Usage of ChatGPT by medical doctors.

3 Methodology

The study used a quantitative research design. This was chosen by the researchers to be able to empirically test the influence of the independent constructs on the dependent constructs of the theoretical model using structural equation modelling (SEM).

The survey instrument was developed using measurement items for the constructs derived from questions gathered from similar studies on TTF [15, 26, 36] and UTAUT [7, 19, 35] constructs. The survey was administered online through convenience sampling. The responses were gathered through questionaries using Google Form and the links were distributed to healthcare networks and social media groups comprised by Medical Doctors in the Philippines. Participants were reminded that their responses would remain anonymous and confidential and were asked to answer a series of questions answerable by a Likert scale of 1 (Strongly Disagree) to 5 (Strongly Agree).

The population of interest was comprised of medical doctors in the Philippines. The inclusion criteria used were medical doctor (licensed physician); have used, familiar or have heard of ChatGPT; residing in the Philippines; and having a valid online account to access the survey. Exclusion criteria were medical students and allied healthcare professionals such as but not limited to nurse, pharmacist, and other healthcare workers. Participation sampling was limited to the physicians who had access and interest in completing the online survey. The data collection was conducted from February 2025 to August 2025 when GPT-4 was the large language model release by ChatGPT. The study was conducted within a limited time frame, and the findings may reflect only the sentiments during the data collection phase.

Prior complete roll-out of the survey, a pilot test was conducted with the aim of checking the internal reliability and validity within the constructs and the ease of use of the survey form. There were 58 respondents for the pilot survey. On the test of internal validity and reliability which was met with Cronbach Alpha (CA) greater than 0.7 and Average Variance Extracted (AVE) greater than 0.5. On the ease of use, the survey indicated good output with survey being easy to use and understand. This also helped the researchers for the questionnaire to have a clear, concise and neutral wording. Hence the researchers considered for rollout. Data Analysis was conducted using SmartPLS.

4 Data Analysis and Results

4.1 Participant Demographics

A total of 279 Filipino physician respondents were included in the analysis. Participants were asked about their gender, age, specialization, area of work, and region of practice.

In terms of gender, 67.38% (n = 188) are female, while 31.89% (n = 89) are male. The remaining participants (n = 2) are non-binary. This suggests majority of the respondents are female. Based on a population study of [34], the broader Philippine health profession is dominated by women and the young which may explain this sample.

In terms of age, 51.48% (n = 139) are 25 to 29 years old, 40.50% (n = 113) are 30 to 39 years old, 5.38% (n = 15) are 40 to 49 years old, and 4.30% (n = 12) are 50 years of age and above. This suggests that the sample is largely composed of early to mid-career physicians. They may reflect the representation of younger medical professionals who may be more open to technology adoption and digital innovation in healthcare.

In terms of specialization, 64.16% (n = 179) of the sample were General Practitioners while 35.84% (n = 100) have specialization working in the field of Internal Medicine (n = 22), Pediatrics (n = 15), OBGYN (n = 13), Family Medicine (n = 10), Anesthesiology (n = 7), Radiology (n = 5), Emergency Medicine (n = 5), Pathology (n = 4), Surgery (n = 4), Dermatology (n = 3), Occupational Medicine (n = 3), and Public Health (n = 2). The remaining were working in the field of Psychiatry, Cardiology, Rehabilitation, Ophthalmology, Orthopedics, ENT, and Neurology with one respondent each. Most of the respondents are GPs, showing that the sample is largely made up of frontline doctors providing primary healthcare. Specialists also contribute and add breadth allowing the study to examine ChatGPT exploration in different medical fields.

Meanwhile, for area of work 57.35% (n = 160) doctors surveyed on this study were working in private clinics or private hospitals, 23.66% (n = 66) worked for both private and public institutions, while 19.00% (n = 53) doctors worked in government or public agencies. Lastly, on the region of practice within the Philippines, the study received 50.18% (n = 140) of the doctors working in the urban National Capital Region (NCR). While the other 49.82% (n = 139) respondents are represented in the other regions. The demographic profile suggests that the study sample is composed largely by early to mid-career professionals, predominantly general practitioners likely to provide insights into how physicians drive digital adoption in healthcare in the Philippines.

4.2 Sampling Adequacy, Construct Reliability, and Validity

The Kaiser-Meyer-Olkin (KMO) factor adequacy was measured at 0.94, while the Bartlett's Test of Sphericity is p-value $< 2.2e\text{-}16$. The KMO passed the minimum value acceptable as it is > 0.6. The p value measured is also < 0.001 which means it passed the significance test. This suggests that the study has an adequate sample size and factor analysis can be done [23]. Studies for cross-sectional or descriptive studies for medical research suggests the Cochran formula [24] to calculate the sample size $n = (Z^2 * p * (1-p)) / e^2$ where Z is the Z-score at 95% confidence level and 5% margin of error, and p is the estimated proportion of 0.2 [26] to be at 246 which was met by the study.

To measure the reliability, the indicator loading was calculated as shown in Table 1. All indicator loading measures are > 0.5 which indicates that there is a good measure of latent constructs. All measured outer loading in the model are > 0.7. To measure the validity and internal consistency, Cronbach Alpha (CA) and Composite Reliability (CR) were used. All measured CA is > 0.6 suggesting acceptable internal consistency. All measured CR are > 0.7 which means adequate consistency is present. To measure the convergence among constructs, Average Variance Extracted (AVE) was also calculated. All AVE measured are > 0.5, suggesting high convergent validity [25].

Table 1. Construct Reliability and Validity Test

Construct	Item	CA	CR	AVE
Task Characteristics	TAC	0.793	0.860	0.673
Technology Characteristics	TEC	0.894	0.859	0.672
Task-Technology Fit	TTF	0.894	0.919	0.655
Performance Expectancy	PE	0.896	0.935	0.828
Effort Expectancy	EE	0.768	0.864	0.681
Social Influence	SI	0.827	0.897	0.744
Facilitating Conditions	FC	0.730	0.878	0.783
Behavioral Intention to Use	BI	0.836	0.902	0.754
Actual Use	AU	0.809	0.8897	0.725

4.3 Discriminant Validity

To check the Discriminant Validity of the model, the Heterotrait-Monotrait (HTMT) ratio score was calculated, and all measured values are < 0.90. This was further strengthened as the Fornell-Larcker criterion as shown in Table 2 which compares the square root of the AVE with the correlation of latent constructs. All measured values suggest that discriminant validity is established as the values of the main diagonal are larger than the correlation coefficient of other variables. [25].

Table 2. Fornell-Larcker Criterion

	AU	BI	EE	FC	PE	SI	TAC	TTF	TEC
AU	0.852								
BI	0.662	0.868							
EE	0.413	0.477	0.825						
FC	0.223	0.277	0.421	0.885					
PE	0.608	0.753	0.517	0.244	0.910				
SI	0.461	0.499	0.239	0.155	0.448	0.862			
TAC	0.058	0.112	0.123	0.218	0.096	0.079	0.820		
TTF	0.577	0.738	0.531	0.226	0.791	0.417	0.214	0.809	
TEC	0.465	0.566	0.522	0.321	0.544	0.376	0.122	0.583	0.820

4.4 Hypothesis Testing

Bootstrapping was conducted in SmartPLS to assess the significance of hypothesized relationships within the integrated TTF–UTAUT model are summarized in Table 3. Among the UTAUT predictors, Performance Expectancy showed the positive and significant effect on Behavioral Intention ($\beta = 0.379$, $f^2 = 0.142$, $p < 0.01$), Social Influence also was significant ($\beta = 0.172$, $f^2 = 0.067$, $p < 0.01$). In contrast, Effort Expectancy ($\beta = 0.034$, $f^2 = 0.002$, $p = 0.484$) and Facilitating Conditions ($\beta = 0.069$, $f^2 = 0.011$, $p = 0.060$) were found to be positive but not significant predictors of Behavioral Intention. On the TTF side, Technology Characteristics strongly influenced Task Technology Fit ($\beta = 0.565$, $f^2 = 0.493$, $p < 0.01$), while Task Characteristics had a positive and significant effect ($\beta = 0.145$, $f^2 = 0.033$, $p = 0.040$). Task Technology Fit significantly predicted Behavioral Intention ($\beta = 0.333$, $f^2 = 0.111$, $p < 0.01$) and had a direct effect on Actual Use ($\beta = 0.194$, $f^2 = 0.032$, $p = 0.020$). The results also indicate that Behavioral Intention significantly predicts Actual Use ($\beta = 0.519$, $f^2 = 0.225$, $p < 0.001$), confirming the role of usage intention and task-technology alignment in driving adoption behavior.

The model fit indices were within acceptable thresholds. The SRMR value (0.065) for the estimated model indicates a good model fit while the NFI (0.87) suggests acceptable fit for exploratory study [25]. The model was also found with moderate power with TTF ($R^2 = 0.361$), Intention to Use ($R^2 = 0.652$), and Actual Use ($R^2 = 0.456$).

Table 3. Hypothesis Results

Hypothesis	Path	Path Coeff	Standard Deviation	Effect Size	T-statistics	p-Value	Significance
H1	PE - > BI	0.379	0.077	0.142	4.926	0.000	Significant**
H2	EE - > BI	0.034	0.048	0.002	0.700	0.484	Not Significant

(continued)

Table 3. *(continued)*

Hypothesis	Path	Path Coeff	Standard Deviation	Effect Size	T-statistics	p-Value	Significance
H3	SI - > BI	0.172	0.046	0.067	3.769	0.000	Significant**
H4	FC - > BI	0.069	0.036	0.011	1.879	0.060	Not Significant
H5	TAC - > TTF	0.145	0.071	0.033	2.049	0.040	Significant*
H6	TEC - > TTF	0.565	0.050	0.493	11.327	0.000	Significant**
H7	TTF - > BI	0.333	0.083	0.111	4.011	0.000	Significant**
H8	TTF - > AU	0.194	0.083	0.032	2.336	0.020	Significant*
H9	BI - > AU	0.519	0.078	0.225	6.674	0.000	Significant**

Legend: * $p < 0.05$, ** $p < 0.01$

5 Discussion

5.1 Theoretical Implications

The results provide support for the relationship of task-technology fit, and most of the relationships for UTAUT extended to AI context. It also provides insights into the use of Generative AI tools specifically ChatGPT in healthcare through the perspective of Filipino physicians. The Integrated TTF-UTAUT finding suggests that even if users perceive ChatGPT as easy to use and useful (UTAUT), they are also influenced by how well the technology fits their professional context (TTF). This study suggests that ChatGPT adoption by medical doctors is not only influenced by individual usage intentions but also by their professional perception of fit of using ChatGPT with applications within their healthcare tasks, systems or processes

TTF Implications In this study, both Technology Characteristics and Task Characteristics positively and significantly influenced perceived Task-Technology Fit. This is consistent with the importance of the alignment between the task and technology features impacts the perceived fit [26]. The results are also supported by similar studies employing TTF [27, 28], highlighting the relationship of perceived fit of ChatGPT as an AI support tool to healthcare practice. Technology Characteristics was found to have a stronger effect to fit compared to the weaker effect of Task Characteristics. This may indicate that the doctor perception of ChatGPT's technological features and capabilities such as its accuracy, accessibility, speed, and responsiveness, plays a greater role in their sense of fit compared to the nature of their clinical or medical tasks. This points to opportunities for tailoring or fine-tuning ChatGPT's accuracy on medical domain increases the perception of fit and easing adoption to healthcare. Furthermore, TTF was also found to be significant predictor of intention to use and actual use with moderate explanatory power suggesting that while ChatGPT is viewed as technologically capable, the alignment to specialized clinical tasks remains limited.

UTAUT Implications In this study, the UTAUT predictors of behavioral intention were mixed in this study. Two of the UTAUT constructs, Performance Expectancy (PE) and Social Influence (SI), were found to be positive and significant while Effort Expectancy (EE) and Fa-cilitating Conditions (FC) were not significant. PE is the primary driver of adoption suggesting belief by doctors that ChatGPT can improve their work efficiency, produc-tivity, and deliver improved patient outcomes. This aligns with prior adoption re-search where performance improvements are critical in assessing the role of the digi-tal systems in e-health [30] and AI [31] and relates the perceived benefits that users expect to gain [32]. SI significantly influenced intention, indicating that endorsements from peers, colleagues, or broader professional bodies also contribute to doctor's intention to explore ChatGPT. In contrast, EE and FC were positive but not significant in this study similar to [29]. EE was not supported in this study suggesting that easiness to learn or use did not directly predict doctor's intention to use ChatGPT. Studies found that perceived risks negatively influence EE [32] highlighting ChatGPT's risks and limitations in healthcare practice. FC was also not supported suggesting that while infrastructure such as internet and devices is available, the lack of training or organizational support could still be barriers to adoption [33]. The weak relationship of EE and FC may also reflect the early to mid-career sample size with high digital literacy, implying that the perceived usefulness and social acceptance has stronger influence than perceived usability. Behavioral Intention was also found to predict Actual Use, consistent with the assumption of UTAUT. This finding suggests that once doctors form an intention to use ChatGPT, they are highly likely to translate this into actual usage [22].

5.2 Practical Implications

The findings of this study provide insights for policymakers, hospital administrators, medical associations, and academic institutions aiming to utilize ChatGPT in healthcare settings. First, the positive relationship of task and technology characteristics to fit provides support that developing ChatGPT functionalities to align with healthcare tasks can improve overall perception of fit. Second, the findings of the study emphasize the importance of highlighting the performance benefits on usage. Institutions should focus on the positive impact such as efficiency, accuracy, and integration to daily routine to lead wider adoption. Hospitals may establish standard operating protocols for the use of AI in clinical documentation and administrative support, while ensuring that all outputs remain subject to physician oversight. Policymakers can develop clear guidelines and a regulatory framework for the safe, ethical, and responsible use of generative AI such as ChatGPT in healthcare to address the risks. Third, the findings recognize that social influence contributes to positive acceptance. Medical associations and societies may play a central role in endorsing best practices of AI use. They also lead to safeguard professional standards, encouraging innovation, and ensuring safe application of AI tools in healthcare. Such measures would help foster collaboration rather than complete reliance on AI technology. Fourth, the results underscore the lack of institutional support. Investment in capacity building or training for medical professionals is recommended, ensuring that they understand both the benefits and limitations of ChatGPT.

5.3 Limitations

The study is bound by several limitations that should be acknowledged when interpreting the findings. As participation was voluntary and conducted online, the study may be subject to selection bias which could limit the generalizability of the results. As such, the findings may not fully reflect the views of all physicians and healthcare workers. The study utilized constructs derived from TTF-UTAUT framework. While the model captures key determinants of technology adoption, other relevant factors may not have been included. The study was limited to ChatGPT as one of many Generative AI tools.

6 Conclusion

The study investigated the adoption of ChatGPT by Filipino Medical doctors using the Integrated TTF-UTAUT framework. The results show that physician's intention to use ChatGPT is driven primarily and predicted by performance expectancy and social influence but did not support for the effort expectancy and facilitating conditions. The study also confirmed the Perceived Task Technology Fit on medical tasks (task characteristics) and ChatGPT as a tool to support these tasks (technology characteristics). Lastly, the perceived fit and intention to use impacts actual usage. The study provides suggestions to ease adoption in healthcare practice and promote the safe, ethical, and responsible use by understanding individual behaviors to guide healthcare institutions and policymakers on training for relevant use cases, provision of professional guidelines, and institutional endorsement while understanding the risks and limitations.

Further empirical research on the use ChatGPT and GenAI tools in healthcare is warranted, particularly studies assessing its impact on patient outcomes, clinical workflow efficiency, and medical research. The study also highlights researchers to involve locally relevant datasets to tailor and fine-tune AI models that are more attuned to respective medical contexts. Future quantitative research can consider other adoption theories and explore the current work with additional constructs or moderating factors. Future research can also employ qualitative research through the semi-structured interviews to elaborate the benefits, limitations, and barriers in local healthcare context. Future release of ChatGPT models may influence the findings suggesting longitudinal studies as technology develops to track adoption patterns over time.

References

1. Gutierrez, K.L., Viacrusis, P.M.: Bridging the Gap or Widening the Divide: A Call for Capacity-Building in Artificial Intelligence for Healthcare in the Philippines (2023)
2. Muftic, F., Kadunic, M., Musinbegovic, A., Almisreb, A.: Exploring Medical Breakthrough: A Systematic Review of ChatGPT Applications in Healthcare (2023)

3. Philippine Institute for Development Studies. Artificial Intelligence – a silver bullet to enhancing healthcare workers jobs and improving patient care in the Philippines. (2023)
4. Hu K.: ChatGPT sets record for fastest-growing user base - analyst note. Reuters (2023)
5. De Vera, B.A.: Philippines ranks 4th in global ChatGPT use – World Bank (2024)
6. Tran, A.Q., et al.: Determinants of intention to use artificial intelligence-based diagnosis support system among prospective physicians. Front. Public Health (2021)
7. Sallam, M.: ChatGPT utility in healthcare education, research, and practice: systematic review on the promising perspectives and valid concerns. Healthcare **11**, 887 (2023)
8. Petitgand, C., Motulsky, A., Denis, J.L., Régis, C.: Investigating the barriers to physician adoption of an artificial intelligence- based decision support system in emergency care: an interpretative qualitative study. Stud. Health Technol. Inform. (2020)
9. Li, J., Dada, A., Puladi, B., Kleesiek, J., Egger, J.: ChatGPT in healthcare: a taxonomy and systematic review. Comput. Meth. Prog. Biomed. (2024)
10. Kharat, A.: Artificial Intelligence and Its Role in Healthcare (2022)
11. Ali, O., Abdelbaki, W., Shrestha, A., Elbas, E., Alryalat, M., Dwivedi, Y.: A systematic literature review of artificial intelligence in the healthcare sector: benefits, challenges, methodologies, and functionalities (2023)
12. Roppelt, J.S., Kanbach, D.K., Kraus, S.: Artificial intelligence in healthcare institutions: a systematic literature review on influencing factors. Technol. Soc. **76** (2024)
13. Harst, L., Lantzsch, H., Scheibe, M.: Theories predicting end-user acceptance of telemedicine use: systematic review. J. Med. Internet Res. **21**(5), e13117 (2019)
14. Venkatesh, V.: Adoption and use of AI tools: a research agenda grounded in UTAUT. Ann. Oper. Res. **308** (2022)
15. Venkatesh, V., Morris, M., Davis G., Davis, F.: User acceptance of information technology: toward a unified view. MIS Quart. (2003)
16. Menon, D., Shilpa, K.: "Chatting with ChatGPT": analyzing the factors influencing users' intention to Use the Open AI's ChatGPT using the UTAUT model. Heliyon (2023)
17. Wang, H., Tao, D., Yu, N., Qu, X.: Understanding consumer acceptance of healthcare wearable devices: an integrated model of UTAUT and TTF (2020)
18. Spies R., Grobbelaar S., Botha A.: a scoping review of the application of the task-technology fit theory. Responsible Design, Implementation and Use of Information and Communication Technology. (2020)
19. Goodhue D.L., Thompson RL.: Task-technology fit and individual performance (1995)
20. Kang, E., Han, J.-H., Moon, S.-J.: The acceptance behavior of smart home health care services in south Korea: an integrated model of UTAUT and TTF. Int. J. Environ. Res. Public Health (2022)
21. Schnall, R., Rojas, M., Brown, W.: The Health Information Technology Usability Evaluation Model (Health-ITUEM): A theoretical framework for evaluating mobile health technology. Columbia University, New York, NY, United States (2012)
22. Slade, E.L., Dwivedi, Y.K., Piercy, N.C., Williams, M.D.: Modeling consumers' adoption intentions of remote mobile payments in the United Kingdom: extending UTAUT with innovativeness, risk, and trust. Psychol. Market. (2015)
23. Hair J.F., Black W.C., Babin B.J., Anderson R.E. Multivariate data analysis (7th ed.). Pearson Prentice Hall, Upper Saddle River, NJ (2010)
24. Charan, J., Misra, S., Kaur, R., Bhardwaj, P., Singh, K., Ambwani, S.R.: Sample size calculation in medical research: a prime. Nat. Acad. Med. Sci. (2021)
25. Hair, J.F., Risher, J.J., Sarstedt, M., Ringle, C.M.: When to use and how to report the results of PLS-SEM. Eur. Bus. Rev. **31**, 2–24 (2018)
26. Fianu, E., Amankwah - Sarfo, R., Ofori, M.: Examining the Task - Technology Fit of ChatGPT for Healthcare Services (2024)

27. Alhendawi, K.M.: Task-technology fit model: modelling and assessing the nurses' satisfaction with health information system using AI prediction models (2022)
28. Chakraborty, D., Troise, C., Bresciani, S.: Exploring consumer intentions to continue: integrating task technology fit and social technology fit in generative AI–based shopping platforms (2025)
29. Sharma, R., Khanna, T., Mehmi, S. The advancing use of fintech services among Indian adults: a study using UTAUT model. Acad. Market. Stud. J. (2023)
30. Admassu W., Gorems K.: Analyzing health service employees' intention to use e-health systems in southwest Ethiopia: using UTAUT-2 model. BMC Health Serv. Res. **24**, 1136 (2024)
31. Cornelissen L., Egher C., van Beek V., Williamson L., Hommes D.: The drivers of acceptance of artificial intelligence-powered care pathways among medical professionals: web-based survey study. JMIR (2022)
32. Dingel, J., Kleine, AK., Ceci, J., Sigl, AL., Lermer, E., Gaube, S.: Predictors of Health Care Practitioners' Intention to Use AI-Enabled Clinical Decision Support Systems: Meta-Analysis Based on the Unified Theory of Acceptance and Use of Technology (2024)
33. Prasetyo, Y.T., et al.: Determining factors affecting the acceptance of medical education eLearning platforms during the COVID-19 pandemic in the Philippines: UTAUT2 approach. Healthcare **7**, 780 (2021)
34. University of the Philippines Population Institute. Human Resource for Health in the Time of the COVID-19 Pandemic: Does the Philippines Have Enough? (2020)
35. Chen, G., Fan, J., Azam, M.: Exploring artificial intelligence (AI) chatbots adoption among research scholars using unified theory of acceptance and use of technology (2024)
36. Tao, G., Zheng, F., Li, W.: Factors affecting users' behaviour with task-oriented Chatbots: an empirical study based on the TTF and UTAUT models. (2024)

Integrating Milieu Therapy Principles into Sustainable Interior Design for Eating Disorder Rehabilitation

Annisa Zayyan Farah Yumna(✉), Andriano Simarmata, and Dini Cinda Kirana

Interior Design Department, School of Design, Bina Nusantara University, Jakarta 11480, Indonesia

zayyan.affandi@gmail.com, {andriano.simarmata, dini.kirana}@binus.ac.id

Abstract. *Eating disorders* are among the mental health conditions contributing to the highest mortality rates globally. Indonesia ranks 4th in the world in terms of the number of *eating disorde*r patients. Despite the high prevalence of *eating disorders* in Indonesia, many people still associate their causes solely with milieu and social factors. However, this assumption is incorrect, as several types of *eating disorders* have been proven to have links to the biological genes present in the human body. Individuals with eating disorders require serious and comprehensive care. The design of rehabilitation centers for eating disorder patients must be capable of responding to their cognitive conditions, including emotional states and behavioral patterns. Unfortunately, current rehabilitation facility designs often fail to fully address these individual needs. This highlights the urgency for a specific design framework that aims to produce environments that are both ideal and sustainable. Gunderson's 1978 milieu therapy principles, originally developed as behavioral treatment strategies for psychiatric wards, offer a promising foundation for addressing users' emotional and behavioral needs through healthcare instruments services. By conducting a deeper analysis of these principles and translating them into spatial elements, it is possible to formulate a design guideline that effectively responds to both the emotional and behavioral dimensions of individual users. Ultimately, this approach seeks to create a sustainable healing environment, one that not only supports therapeutic goals but also fosters long-term emotional stability and psychological recovery of the wellbeing.

Keywords: Eating disorders · mental health · highest mortality · sustainable · milieu therapy

1 Research Background

Eating disorders are a type of mental illness with a relatively high prevalence. They are characterized by abnormal eating behaviors accompanied by emotional disturbances. Individuals with eating disorders often have a problematic relationship with food and may be obsessed with body weight or physical appearance. Globally, the prevalence of

E. R. Kaburuan and S. Goundar (Eds.): HIS 2025, LNCS 16392, pp. 132–143, 2026.
https://doi.org/10.1007/978-981-95-6304-3_12

eating disorders is significant. Based on a sample of 2,980 participants, the prevalence was found to be 0.6% for anorexia nervosa, 2.8% for binge eating disorder, and 1.0% for bulimia nervosa [1]. Eating disorders are most commonly found among adolescents, who are considered a vulnerable age group. The impact of eating disorders is severe ranging from developmental delays to severe depression, which may even lead to death. One of the main triggers for eating disorders is body dissatisfaction, particularly during adolescence, a time marked by physical, cognitive, and social changes, along with strong environmental and social pressures, causing young people to become overly focused on their appearance [2].

A journal published by STIKES Kendal in 2022 based on a study conducted in Surabaya indicated a significant and positive correlation between anorexia nervosa tendencies and peer relationships. Additionally, genetic factors are known to play a role in predisposing individuals to eating disorders. While many believe mental disorders stem solely from psychological factors, eating disorders are also strongly linked to genetic and biological components. Nevertheless, it cannot be denied that sociopsychological factors such as body image perception, weight loss pressure, and fear of weight gain can trigger negative emotions that may lead to disordered eating behavior. Societal and cultural standards, especially the widespread belief that "thin is beautiful," also significantly contribute to the development of eating disorder symptoms [3].

In an interview conducted on January 19, 2024, with Dr. Rayinda Raumanen Mamahit, Sp.Kj, a psychiatrist actively practicing at three hospitals in Jakarta, she stated that most eating disorder patients are female adolescents in their teens to twenties, as well as women in their 30s. This is closely related to societal expectations placed on women at those ages. However, it is important to note that eating disorders are not exclusive to women, as cases are also found among male individuals.

To this day, eating disorders are still often underestimated by the public. Many patients only seek treatment when their symptoms have become severe. In fact, eating disorders are among the mental illnesses with the highest mortality rates, with suicide being the leading cause of death. The estimated annual mortality rate for eating disorders can reach up to 3.3 million cases. Patients with anorexia and bulimia have 2.3 and 1.4 times higher mortality risks, respectively, compared to those with other psychiatric disorders [4].

In Indonesia, treatment for eating disorder patients is typically provided by general psychiatrists, who prescribe medications alongside certain therapies. Most patients undergo outpatient treatment. However, specialized clinics for eating disorders are still very limited, and there are currently no dedicated rehabilitation center specifically designed for eating disorder recovery combined with public education facilities. In other words, treatment for eating disorders is still grouped together with other mental health issues, even though eating disorder patients require specialized treatment that differs from other mental illnesses to ensure more effective recovery.

The recovery journey for eating disorder patients is relatively long, as the illness is deeply connected to self-image and social acceptance issues that require extended and gradual healing processes. This issue has drawn the writer's interest, particularly in how treatment and recovery procedures for eating disorder patients can be integrated with the principles of milieu therapy, a therapeutic intervention focused on creating a structured environment that supports healing and personal growth.

Therefore, designing an interior rehabilitation center for eating disorder recovery based on the principles of milieu therapy can serve as a potential solution to provide healing spaces for patients in Indonesia and act as a platform to raise awareness about this serious mental health condition.

2 Literature Review

Eating disorders constitute a spectrum of psychological conditions characterized by maladaptive eating behaviors accompanied by significant emotional disturbances. These disorders pose serious risks to both physical and mental health. Although eating disorders can affect individuals across all age groups, they are most prevalent among women aged 25 to 29 years [5]. To apply the principles of milieu therapy within spatial dimensions, the author will examine and analyze the theory of milieu as proposed by Gunderson in 1978. Gunderson's model of milieu therapy consists of five key components: structure, containment, involvement, support, and validation. In the medical field, milieu therapy is recognized as a form of behavioral treatment delivered by healthcare professionals such as nurses and physicians to patients with psychiatric disorders, focusing on the creation of a therapeutic environment that supports individual healing [6, 7].

Milieu therapy can be implemented for both inpatients and outpatients. A journal published by Wiley Periodicals LLC in 2021, titled "*Effectiveness of therapeutic milieu intervention on inpatients with depressive disorder: a feasibility study from North India*", observed inpatients diagnosed with depressive disorders at the psychiatric unit of AIIMS Rishikesh, India. The study aimed to assess the effectiveness of Therapeutic Milieu Intervention (TMI) in addressing patients' low self-esteem, improving their social functioning, and reducing the level of depression [8]. This TMI program followed Gunderson's milieu therapy model (1978), which emphasizes containment, support, structure, and involvement. During the program, participants were encouraged to express their feelings and opinions within the inpatient environment. Social activities and interactions were tailored to meet the emotional and interpersonal needs of each patient. These included breathing exercises, coloring programs, and craft-making to improve self-esteem.

3 Method

This study employs a qualitative methodology to adapt and expand Gunderson's (1978) milieu therapy principles that originally developed for behavioral treatment into components with a stronger spatial dimension. The research begins by defining the five core principles of milieu therapy as outlined by Gunderson: support, involvement, validation, containment, and structure. Subsequently, an in-depth analysis of the psychological and behavioral conditions of individuals with eating disorders is conducted to identify and map their cognitive processes and emotional trajectories.

Insights derived from this user-centered analysis are then used to perform an emotional mapping, which informs the development of spatially based solutions. The findings from this analysis serve as the foundation for formulating design guidelines that integrate milieu therapy principles into the built environment. Visual elements in the built environment can serve as therapeutic intervention components within milieu therapy. These environmental interventions are expected to generate positive psychological, social, and physical responses, especially in patients with eating disorders. Also, Elements produced in the built environment can serve as therapeutic intervention components within milieu therapy. These environmental interventions are expected to generate positive psychological, social, and physical responses, especially in patients with eating disorders. Key spatial elements that can act as intervention tools include color, form, texture, spatial organization, and circulation systems. Spatial elements that can act as intervention tools include color, form, texture, spatial organization, and circulation systems.

4 Findings and Discussion

4.1 Analytical Table of Milieu Therapy Gunderson (1978) Principles into Interior Elements

This study analyzes the potential application of milieu therapy principles in the interior design of an eating disorder rehabilitation facility. The analysis begins with identifying the core aspect of the five principles, continues with a review of behavioral treatments based on milieu therapy applied in current psychiatric wards, and concludes with an analysis of their potential use in interior design (Table 1).

Based on the analysis table of the potential application of milieu therapy above (Table 1), it can be seen that the principles of milieu therapy by Gunderson (1978) have the potential to be translated into spatial elements. The next step is to analyze the behavioral patterns of the five categories of individuals with eating disorders to further assess the extent to which the application of milieu therapy principles can address the challenges they face.

Table 1. Analysis of the application of milieu therapy in the interior space.

Gunderson 1978 "Milieu Therapy"					
	Support	Containment	Involvement	Structure	Validation
Key Aspects	Support, Provision, Guidance [6]	Safety, limitation, management, and safeguarding [6]	Engagement, interaction, stimulation, and compromise[6]	Structured, organized, connected[6]	Individual rights. Personal boundaries and honor[6]
Behavioral treatment aspects	Providing support through supporting subjects such as healthcare professionals and family members, as well as fulfilling the patients' needs in accordance with agreed-upon terms. [9]	Establishing "house rules" that must be followed by patients, implementing curfews, designated mealtimes, and rest periods, as well as conducting regular monitoring by staff to observe the patients' condition[10]	Providing activities that enhance patients' practical and social skills, while also offering opportunities for them to make their own decisions [8]	Creating a structured and consistent activity schedule for patients to follow [8]	Affirming the individuality of each patient by providing them with a comfortable space and clear personal boundaries [8]
Potential form of spatial application	Color, shape and circulation	Safety aspect, Space, material, shape and color	Spatial Programming, Shape and material	Layout, Circulation	Spatial Programming, Shape, Color

4.2 Psychological Condition Analysis of Individuals with Eating Disorders

The author attempts to gather data through several interviews with an psychiatrist based in Jakarta and patients with eating disorders, as well as through research by comparing various documented journals concerning the psychological and physiological conditions of individuals with eating disorders.

In this study, five categories of eating disorders are included as key aspects of the research. These categories are formally recognized and identified in the DSM-5, namely Anorexia Nervosa, Bulimia Nervosa, Binge Eating Disorder, Avoidant/Restrictive Food Intake Disorder (ARFID), and Pica.

Table of psychological condition analysis of individuals with eating disorders

	Social Condition	Psychological Condition	Physical Condition	Emotional Response	Spatial Response	Milieu Principle Applied
Anorexia Nervosa	Avoidant, Difficulty socializing - vulnerable to bullying, family or partner conflict, lack of support, social environmental pressure, inherent socio-cultural constructs, lack of knowledge.	Excessive anxiety, depression, self-hate, low self-esteem, burdened, ashamed, suicidal, overwhelmed, feeling worthless, compensatory behavior, social problems.	Weak, helpless, underweight, gastrointestinal disorders, organ system failure, malnutrition and up to certain level risk of death.	Provide, comfort, soothing.	Color ; blueish & green color[12]	Support
				Safe environment.	Shape : rounded & minimize ligature[13], high Visibility [10].	Containment, support.
				Accsessible, Familiar.	Spatial programming : typical layout, repetitive [14]	Structure, support.
				Relaxing ambience.	Spatial Programming; Special chamber to regulating their emotions[10].	Support
				Stimulate appetite.	Color: color with red spectrum.	Support
				Evoking individual to create connection.	Materiality	Envolvement
Bulimia Nervosa	Avoidant, interpersonal disorders, - Feelings of low self-esteem, mood disorders, prone to depression, social and cultural pressures, self-destructive behavior, experiences of violence such as (victims of sexual violence)	Excessive anxiety, depression, self-hate, self-sabotage, feelings of worthlessness, emotional overwhelm, suicidal, interpersonal problems,	Gastrointestinal disorders, tooth enamel damage, jaw swelling, chemical imbalances in the body, nutritional deficiencies. Weakness.	Provide, comfort, soothing.	Color ; Blueish & green color[12]	Support
				Safe environment.	Shape: Rounded and Minimize ligature[13]. High Visibility [10]	Containment, Support
				Accsessible, Familiar.	Material : High Visibility Material [10] Spatial Programming: Typical Layout [14]	Containment, structure
				Engaging activity.	Color ; Bright Color[12] Light : Natural Light [15]	Support
				High Visibility.	Material : High Visibility material[10]	Containment
				color interventions that support the digestive system by activating the parasympathetic nervous system and helps with nausea.	Color : Red Spectrum and yellow spectrum[16]	Support
Binge Eating Disorder	Avoidant-prone to bullying, family conflict, stress and depression. Interpersonal relationships.	Excessive anxiety, low self-esteem, emotional overwhelm, self-hate. Lazy to move, unproductive.	Obesity, risk of type 2 diabetes, risk of organ failure, risk of death.	Provide, comfort, soothing.	Color ; Blueish & green color[12].	Support
				Relaxing ambience.	Spatial programming : special chamber to regulating their emotion[10].	Support

(*continued*)

(continued)

				Evoking individual to create connection.	Materiality	Envolvement
				Facilitating user's ability to regulate their emotion that led to positive impact.	Yellowish accent to stimulates positive emotion[12]	Support
				Establishing a spatial atmosphere aimed at appetite control.	Soft lighting , diffused. [15]	Support
PICA	Avoidant, Difficulty socializing- emotional triggers, relationships with family and partners.	Anxiety, embarrassment, stress.- interpersonal problems, emotional triggers.	Chemical imbalance in the body, malnutrition, weakness.	Provide, comfort, soothing.	Color ; Blueish & green color[12].	Support
				Evoking individual to create connection.	Materiality	Envolvement
				High Visibility	Material : High Visibility material[10]	Containment
				Accessible	Spatial programming : Typical layout, repetitive[14].	Structure,support.
ARFID	Isolating oneself, difficulty socializing,	Stress, anxiety, low self-esteem, ashamed of yourself.	Malnutrition, weakness, chemical imbalance in the body.	Enhances accessibility	Accessible, High visibility, minimized spatial ligature [10].	Containment, Support.
				Relaxing ambience.	Spatial programming : special chamber to regulating their emotion[10].	Support
				Evoking individual to create connection	Materiality	Envolvement
				Relaxing ambience.	Spatial programming : special chamber to regulating their emotion[10].	Support

From the table above (Table 2), the results highlight the potential of milieu therapy applications with interior design elements.

5 Prospect of Sustainability Within Its Design

The spatial principles of milieu therapy strongly support the creation of a sustainable healing environment. Most spatial analysis results indicate an ecosystem that benefits both healthcare efficiency and patient psychological and behavioral well-being. Sustainability is further reinforced through renewable material use, layouts that optimize natural ventilation to reduce cooling needs, and flexible programming adaptable over time.

6 Design Implementation

The milieu therapy design approach aims to create an ideal healing environment that fosters psychological well-being while maintaining a sustainable relationship between users and their surrounding environment. In this context, the design implementation and spatial responses are carefully adjusted based on specific therapeutic criteria, particularly in layout organization and color selection. For instance, the dining area in the rehabilitation facility (as shown in Fig. 1) demonstrates how spatial arrangement and color palette can support both comfort and behavioral recovery within a sustainable therapeutic setting.

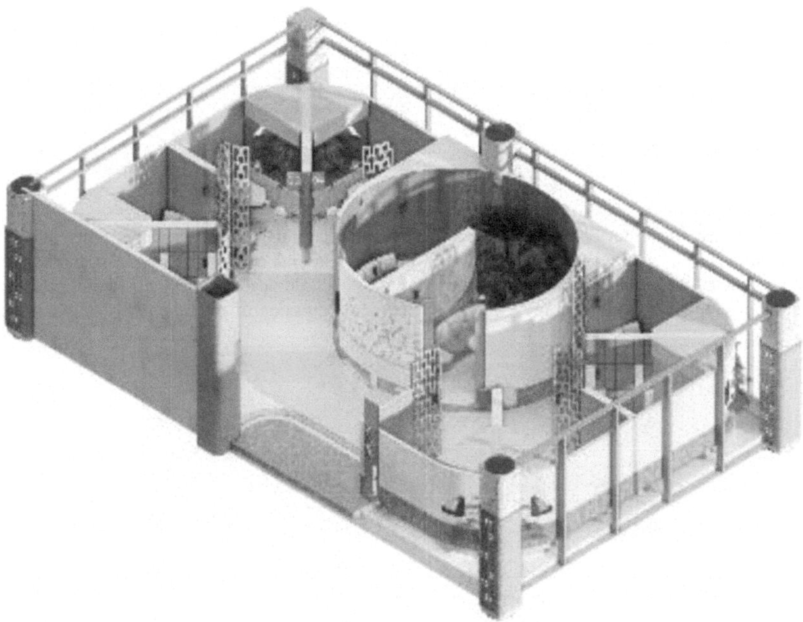

Fig. 1. Milieu Therapy Design Implementation Into Dining Area

The dining area in the rehabilitation facility features eating pods for patients who feel distressed or uncomfortable eating in groups. Reflecting the principle of *validation*, the pods accommodate individual emotional needs by offering a comfortable, private dining experience. Arranged to face one another, they balance privacy with subtle social connection, while surrounding greenery enhances calm and tranquility.

The dining area uses diffused lighting to create bright, even illumination that fosters comfort and reassurance, reflecting the *support* principle. Green acoustic panels reduce noise, while semi-transparent pod walls provide privacy without compromising safety, embodying containment. Varied materials around the pods encourage sensory engagement, supporting *involvement*. A calming palette of greens and blues is balanced with subtle yellow and red accents to boost confidence, productivity, and appetite while maintaining harmony. The modular and familiar layout promotes order, predictability, and

Table of rendered visual of milieu therapy principles application on the interior design of eating disorder rehabilitation based on previous analysis.

Interior Element Implemented	Description
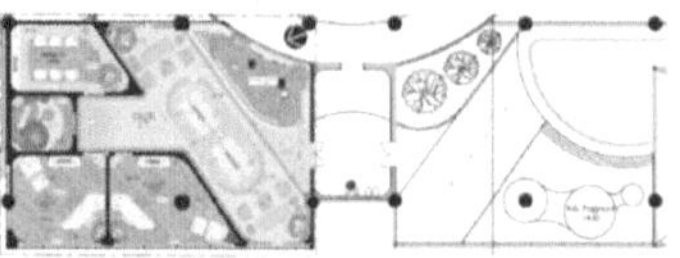	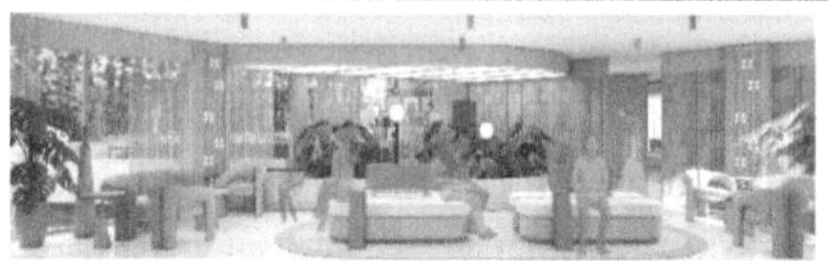
Different room with typical layout and design (structure)	Rooms with standardized layouts and typical design configurations particularly in areas such as individual counseling rooms can help reduce feelings of uncertainty and excessive anxiety commonly experienced by individuals with eating disorders. In addition, the use of consistent spatial design enhances the efficiency and effectiveness of healthcare professionals in carrying out their duties.
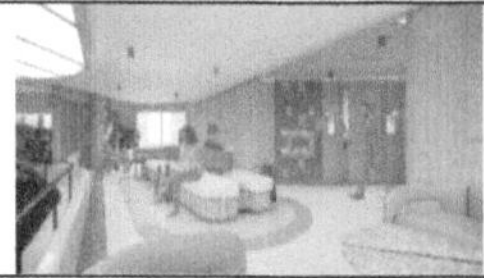	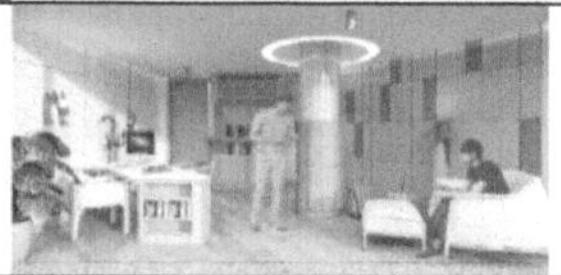
The strategic use of dominant colors and specific materials for targeted certain positive emotion impact within the user reflects the principle of support in milieu therapy	The use of dominant green and blue tones in clinic waiting areas and counseling rooms is intended to provide psychological support by offering a calming effect an expression of the *Support* principle within milieu therapy.
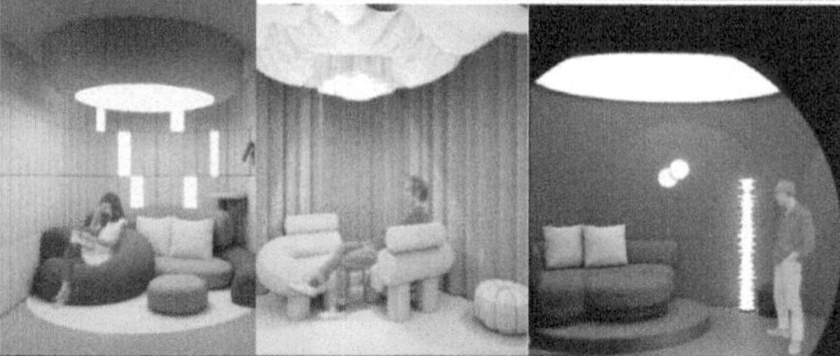	
The use of high-visibility materials serves specific purposes, particularly in supporting the principles of *Containment* and *Support*.	The provision of dedicated spaces designed to help individuals independently regulate their emotions and reduce feelings of fear or anxiety is a crucial aspect of therapeutic environments. These rooms can be intentionally designed with rounded and organic forms, minimizing sharp corners. These spaces should foster a sense of emotional acknowledgment while encouraging gentle engagement with the environment. Soft, diffused lighting and warm color temperatures can contribute to a soothing atmosphere, helping users feel seen, supported, and empowered to participate in their healing process.to evoke a sense of safety and nurture. The use of specific materials with tactile textures encourages users to engage in tactile interaction with the space, promoting grounding and sensory comfort. Additionally, diffused lighting can create a warm, homelike atmosphere that contributes to a sense of safety and helps alleviate stress experienced by users.

(*continued*)

(*continued*)

<table>
<tr><td colspan="2">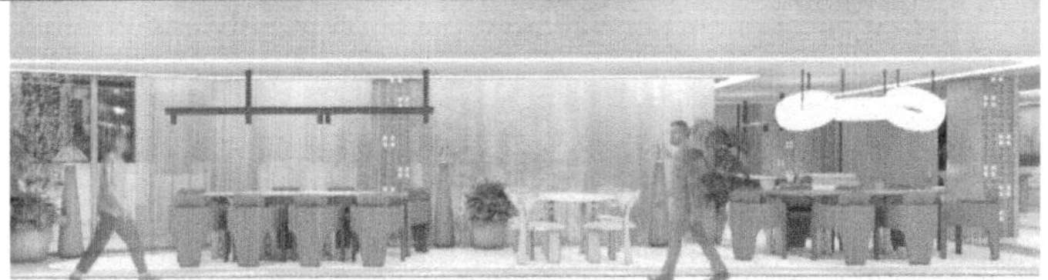</td></tr>
<tr><td>The use of specific color accents is intended to create a positive psychological impact, reflecting the Support principle.</td><td>The dining area serves as a central meeting point for patients in an eating disorder rehabilitation facility, and as such, it can be a particularly sensitive and complex space to design. The use of bold accent colors within the red spectrum (such as red-orange) can help stimulate appetite in individuals. However, to balance the psychological intensity of these strong colors, carefully considered spatial forms such as rounded corners and organic shapes in decorative elements should be introduced to create a softer and more emotionally supportive atmosphere. In addition, the integration of varied textures can encourage sensory engagement and stimulate interpersonal interaction among patients during mealtime, further supporting emotional and social recovery goals.</td></tr>
<tr><td colspan="2">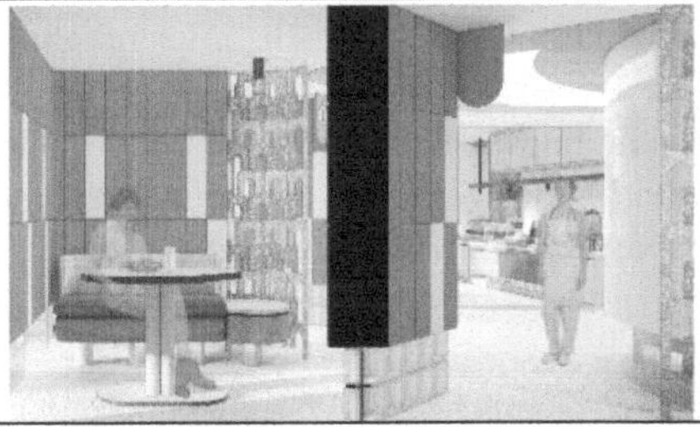</td></tr>
<tr><td>The provision of a dedicated area for patients experiencing moments of emotional distress reflects the principle of Validation, by acknowledging and responding to their behavioral and emotional states. These spaces are designed to offer comfort and psychological support during vulnerable periods. At the same time, the application of carefully selected materials ensures not only the safety and well-being of the individual but also supports the operational effectiveness of healthcare professionals. This aligns with the principle of Containment, which emphasizes structured safety and functional oversight within therapeutic environments.</td><td>A dedicated space in the form of semi-enclosed individual dining pods can provide support for individuals who may be experiencing emotional difficulty during mealtimes. To ensure comfort, the layout is designed so that pods face one another, encouraging a sense of presence and connection, while still allowing for personal space and ease of access.
The lower portion of each pod is constructed using transparent materials to uphold individual safety without compromising the patient's right to privacy. This design approach balances therapeutic oversight with emotional sensitivity, offering a more humane and responsive dining environment for those in recovery.</td></tr>
</table>

psychological stability, aligning with the *structure* principle. Table 3 below presents several implementations derived from the author's analysis of the application of Gunderson's 1978 milieu therapy principles.

The application of milieu therapy in design is carried out holistically through components such as color, material, texture and ambience, creating spaces that support patient healing and healthcare component service both psychologically and practically.

7 Conclusion

Eating disorders, as one of the most prevalent mental health conditions, require substantive and effective interventions to reduce their increasing incidence. The creation of a healing environment that is responsive to the psychological, physical, and social conditions of patients is expected to significantly enhance the recovery process.

The implementation of milieu therapy principles within the interior design of healthcare facilities is both feasible and impactful. Gunderson's five core principles of milieu therapy (1978) support, validation, involvement, containment, and structure are capable of addressing users behavioral and emotional needs. These principles can be spatially interpreted to influence nearly all interior design elements, including color, lighting, form, texture, circulation, materials, and space programming. When these spatial applications are integrated with the behavioral implementation of milieu therapy by healthcare professionals, they have the potential to optimize the healing process for individuals with eating disorders.

Furthermore, the spatial application of Gunderson's milieu principles holds broader potential and can be extended beyond eating disorder rehabilitation centers to other healthcare contexts. However, further research and in-depth studies are necessary to strengthen and validate the findings collected thus far. Such continued investigation will ensure that the implementation of milieu therapy principles in design practice is both evidence-based and capable of delivering meaningful benefits within the healthcare sector.

Authorship Statement. Annisa Zayyan Farah Yumna (Interior Design, BINUS University, Bandung Campus) served as the student member and corresponding author, responsible for conceptualization, data curation, drafting the manuscript, prototyping, and creating de-sign illustrations. Andriano Simarmata, S.Ds., M.Ds. (Lecturer, Interior De-sign, BINUS Bandung) acted as the research leader, guiding the methodology, supervising students, methodology development, and reviewing and editing the manuscript. Dini Cinda Kirana S.Ds., M.Ds. (Lecturer, Interior Design, BINUS Bandung) contributed to data curation, and refinement of the literature review. All authors actively discussed, provided critical feedback, and approved the final manuscript

Data Availability. This research used qualitative methods by combining literature review and observation with design-based approaches to study visual impairment experi-ences. The datasets generated are qualitative in nature and contain sensitive information from participants. Therefore, the data is not publicly available due to privacy and ethical considerations. However, anonymized excerpts may be made available from the corresponding author upon reasonable request.

References

1. Hudson, J.I., Hiripi, E., Pope, H.G., Kessler, R.C.: The prevalence and correlates of eating disorders in the national comorbidity survey replication. Biol. Psychiatry, **61**(3), 348–358 (2007)
2. Permanasari, K., Arbi, D.K.A.: Pengaruh ketidakpuasan tubuh terhadap kecenderungan gangguan makan pada remaja. Buletin Riset Psikologi dan Kesehatan Mental (BRPKM), **2**(1), 776–788 (2022)
3. Mardiah, K., Nurmala, I.: Hubungan antara Teman Sebaya dan Kecederungan Anoreksia Nervosa pada Remaja Surabaya. PSKM. **12**(4), 979–988 (2022). https://journal2.stikeskendal.ac.id/index.php/PSKM/article/view/228. Accessed 30 June 2025
4. van Hoeken, D., Hoek, H.W.: Review of the burden of eating disorders: mortality, disability, costs, quality of life, and family burden. Curr. Opin. Psychiatry **33**(6), 521–527 (2020). https://www.ncbi.nlm.nih.gov/pmc/articles/PMC7575017/
5. Santomauro, D.F., Melen, S., Mitchison, D., Vos, T., Whiteford, H., Ferrari, A.J.: The hidden burden of eating disorders: an extension of estimates from the Global Burden of Disease Study 2019. Lancet Psychiatry **8**(4) (2021)
6. Abroms, G.M.: Defining milieu therapy. Arch. Gen. Psychiatry. **21**(5), 553–560 (1969). https://jamanetwork.com/journals/jamapsychiatry/article-abstract/490104
7. Gunderson, J.G.: Defining the therapeutic processes in psychiatric milieus. Psychiatry **41**(4), 327–335 (1978)
8. Chellappan, X.B., Rentala, S., Das, A.: Effectiveness of therapeutic milieu intervention on inpatients with depressive disorder: a feasibility study from North India. Perspect. Psychiatric Care. **57**(4) (2021)
9. Oeye, C., Bjelland, A.K., Skorpen, A., Anderssen, N.: User participation when using milieu therapy in a psychiatric hospital in Norway: a mission impossible? Nurs. Inq. **16**(4), 287–296 (2009)
10. Curtis, S., et al.: Compassionate containment? Balancing technical safety and therapy in the design of psychiatric wards. Soc. Sci. Med. **97**, 201–209 (2013)
11. Rodríguez-Labajos, L., Kinloch, J., Grant, S., O'Brien, G.: The role of the built environment as a therapeutic intervention in mental health facilities: a systematic literature review. HERD: Health Environ. Res. Des. J. **17**(2) (2024)
12. Jannesari, A., Darvish, B., Saghafi, M.R.: To evaluate the effectiveness of the therapeutic effect of color and health centers. **36**(3) (2015)
13. Kakkar, G.: Architectural psychology: the impact of architecture in human psyche. Int. J. Hous. Hum. Settl. Plann. **8**(1) (2022)
14. Sari, A.O.B., Jabi, W.: Architectural spatial layout design for hospitals: a review. J. Build. Eng. **97**, 110835–5 (2024). https://www.sciencedirect.com/science/article/pii/S2352710224024033?via%3Dihub
15. Mathiasen, N., Øien, T.B., Volf, C.: Empathic lighting design for healthcare environments. In: IOP Conference Series Earth and Environmental Science vol. 1320(1), pp. 012031–1 (2024)
16. Healing Hues: Color Your Life With Chromotherapy | beem® Light Sauna [Internet]. beem® Light Sauna (2023). https://beemlightsauna.com/healing-hues-chromotherapy/. Accessed 30 June 2025

Simultaneous Anonymization of Electronic Health Records: A Multi-Privacy-Model Optimization Approach

Mingshan You[1], Yong-Feng Ge[1(✉)], Jiao Yin[1], Kate Wang[2], and Hua Wang[1]

[1] Institute for Sustainable Industries and Liveable Cities, Victoria University, Melbourne, VIC 3011, Australia
mingshan.you@live.vu.edu.au, {yongfeng.ge,jiao.yin,hua.wang}@vu.edu.au
[2] School of Health and Biomedical Sciences, RMIT University, Melbourne, VIC 3064, Australia
kate.wang@rmit.edu.au

Abstract. Releasing electronic health records (EHRs) typically requires trialing multiple, complementary privacy models—k-anonymity, l-diversity, and t-closeness—before publication, with model and parameter choices selected to fit the release context by balancing each model's privacy protection level against task-specific data utility. However, most methods optimize these models in isolation, limiting effectiveness and efficiency. We formalize their joint execution as multi-task optimization (MTO) over a shared anonymization plan spanning per-attribute generalization and record suppression. Further, we present multi – task anonymization by differential evolution (MTADE), a differential evolution (DE) framework that coevolves three privacy model related populations with distributed evaluation and an elite-migration/weak-replacement knowledge transfer policy, enabling cross-task reuse while curbing negative transfer. Across 16 healthcare datasets and six DE backbones, MTADE attains higher utility under equal privacy thresholds and converges faster than per-model single-task optimizers, yielding robust anonymization plans. This formulation and algorithm provide a principled route to simultaneously satisfying k-anonymity, l-diversity, and t-closeness for EHR release within a unified optimization pipeline, avoiding fragmented per-model tuning.

Keywords: Multi-task optimization · Knowledge transfer · Privacy preserving data publication · Data anonymization

1 Introduction

Timely access to high – quality electronic health records (EHRs) enables clinical decision support, population health surveillance, and AI model development. However, sharing EHRs introduces re-identification risks via quasi-identifier (QI)

E. R. Kaburuan and S. Goundar (Eds.): HIS 2025, LNCS 16392, pp. 144–155, 2026.
https://doi.org/10.1007/978-981-95-6304-3_13

linkage and attribute disclosure, and must comply with regulatory expectations (e.g., GDPR, HIPAA) [19,23]. Technical mitigations span access control [24,29], vulnerability management [25,26], secure computation [4,17], differential privacy (DP), and schema-preserving data anonymization [6,8,20]. Anonymization remains widely used because it preserves table structure, is auditable, and integrates with existing analytics pipelines [1,5,6,11].

In practice, data publishers routinely trial multiple, complementary privacy models—k-anonymity, l-diversity, and t-closeness—before release [14,15,21]. Practitioners then choose the model(s) and parameter settings to fit the release context, balancing each model's privacy protection level against task-specific data utility—for example, stricter t for public releases, moderate l for cross-institutional collaboration, or higher k for internal testing. Tuning generalization and suppression to meet these guarantees while maximizing utility is combinatorial and typically handled model-by-model, which forgoes opportunities for coordinated search.

Most prior methods optimize a single privacy model in isolation [9,10,12, 27,28] or use a hierarchical (bi-level) scheme in which a greedy outer loop for k-anonymization invokes inner-loop optimization l-diversity and t-closeness [16]. To our knowledge, no method jointly optimizes k-anonymity, l-diversity and t-closeness as parallel tasks over a shared anonymization decision space. However, tasks explore the same space and tend to concentrate near overlapping high-utility regions, suggesting benefits from principled cross-task reuse.

We formalize simultaneous satisfaction of $k/l/t$ as a multi-task optimization (MTO) problem over the shared plan $\theta = (g, z)$ (generalization levels and record suppression). We propose multi – task anonymization by differential evolution (MTADE), a differential evolution (DE) framework that co-evolves three task populations with distributed evaluation and an elite-migration/weak-replacement knowledge transfer policy to enable reuse while curbing negative transfer. MTADE is utility-agnostic; in experiments we instantiate transparency degree (TD) [5]. Across 16 healthcare datasets and six DE backbones, MTADE attains higher utility under equal privacy thresholds and faster convergence than per-model single-task optimizers.

Contributions.

1. **Formulation.** We formalize the joint execution of k-anonymity, l-diversity, and t-closeness as a MTO problem over a shared anonymization search space with task-specific objectives and constraints; to our knowledge, this setting has not been explicitly defined.
2. **Algorithm.** We introduce MTADE, a multi-task anonymization DE framework with distributed evaluation and an elite-migration/weak-replacement knowledge-transfer mechanism that enables effective cross-task reuse while mitigating negative transfer.
3. **Evaluation.** Empirical evidence on 16 healthcare datasets and six DE backbones showing higher utility at equal privacy and faster convergence than per-model single-task optimizers.

2 Problem Formulation

We formalize anonymization as choosing an anonymization plan that preserves data utility while satisfying one or more privacy models.

Data Model. Let $T = \{r_i\}_{i=1}^n$ be a table with QIs $X_1, \ldots, X_m$ and a sensitive attribute S. Each record is $r_i = (x_{i,1}, \ldots, x_{i,m}, s_i)$ with $x_{i,j} \in \mathrm{Dom}(X_j)$ and $s_i \in \mathrm{Dom}(S)$.

Operations: Generalization and Suppression. For each QI X_j, let $\mathcal{G}_j$ be a rooted taxonomy tree whose leaves are raw values and internal nodes are generalized values [13]. We denote by $\mathrm{Nodes}(\mathcal{G}_j)$ the set of all taxonomy nodes and define a per-attribute generalization mapping

$$g_j : \mathrm{Dom}(X_j) \to \mathrm{Nodes}(\mathcal{G}_j), \qquad x \mapsto v_{g_j}(x),$$

which maps a leaf value to one of its ancestors $v_{g_j}(x)$. Write $|v|$ for the number of leaf descendants of a node $v \in \mathcal{G}_j$ (coarser nodes have larger $|v|$). Let $g = (g_1, \ldots, g_m)$ collect all generalizations. Record-level suppression is $z = (z_1, \ldots, z_n) \in \{0,1\}^n$ with $z_i = 0$ removing r_i. The decision variables are $\theta = (g, z)$, and the released dataset is

$$T'(\theta) = \left\{ r_i' = (v_{g_1}(x_{i,1}), \ldots, v_{g_m}(x_{i,m}), s_i) \ : \ z_i = 1 \right\}. \tag{1}$$

Equivalence Classes and Distributions. Records in $T'(\theta)$ that share the same generalized QI vector form an equivalence class; let $\mathcal{E}(T')$ be the set of all classes and $E \in \mathcal{E}(T')$ a class with size $|E|$. The empirical sensitive-value distribution in E is

$$P_E(s) = \frac{1}{|E|} \sum_{r' \in E} \mathbf{1}\{s_{r'} = s\}, \quad s \in \mathrm{Dom}(S),$$

where $\mathbf{1}\{\cdot\}$ is the indicator. The overall distribution on $T'(\theta)$ is $P_{T'}$.

Utility (Transparency Degree). We measure retained information via TD [5]:

$$\mathrm{TD}\big(T'(\theta)\big) = \sum_{r' \in T'(\theta)} \sum_{j=1}^{m} \frac{1}{|v_{g_j}(x_{r',j})|}. \tag{2}$$

Smaller taxonomy cells (finer generalization) contribute more to TD.

Privacy Constraints. All constraints are expressed over $\mathcal{E}(T')$, class sizes $|E|$, and distributions P_E and $P_{T'}$.

k-anonymity. Every class must contain at least k records [21]:

$$\forall E \in \mathcal{E}\big(T'(\theta)\big) : \quad |E| \geq k. \tag{3}$$

l-diversity. Each class must exhibit sufficient sensitive-value diversity [15]. Let $\mathcal{D}(\cdot)$ be a diversity functional on distributions over $\mathrm{Dom}(S)$:

$$\forall E \in \mathcal{E}(T'(\theta)) : \quad \mathcal{D}(P_E) \geq l. \tag{4}$$

t-closeness. Each class's sensitive-value distribution must be close to the global distribution [14]. Fix a statistical distance $D(\cdot, \cdot)$ on probability distributions:

$$\forall E \in \mathcal{E}(T'(\theta)) : \quad D(P_E, P_{T'(\theta)}) \leq t. \tag{5}$$

Three Related Optimization Subtasks. This shared-space formulation is illustrated in Fig. 1. Each privacy model induces a task that optimizes the same decision variables $\theta = (g, z)$ for TD subject to task-specific feasibility:

$$\textbf{Task } (\mathsf{K}) \max_{\theta} \ \mathrm{TD}(T'(\theta)) \qquad \text{s.t. (3)} \tag{6}$$

$$\textbf{Task } (\mathsf{L}) \max_{\theta} \ \mathrm{TD}(T'(\theta)) \qquad \text{s.t. (4)} \tag{7}$$

$$\textbf{Task } (\mathsf{T}) \max_{\theta} \ \mathrm{TD}(T'(\theta)) \qquad \text{s.t. (5)} \tag{8}$$

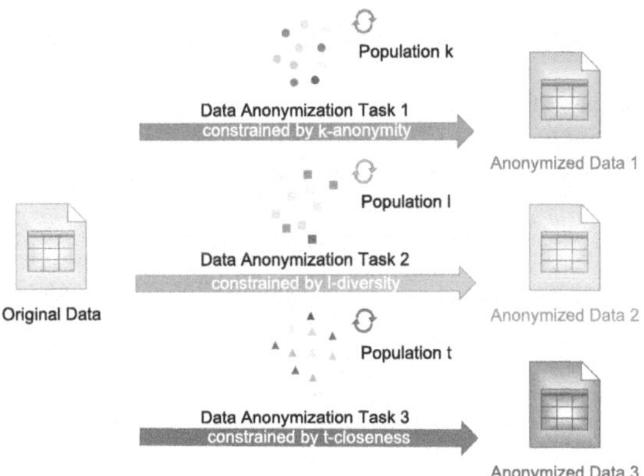

Fig. 1. Shared-space formulation: the anonymization plan $\theta = (g, z)$ is evaluated against the three task-specific feasibility sets (k-anonymity, l-diversity, t-closeness) while maximizing the same utility TD.

3 Methodology

This section presents MTADE for the multi-task instance in Sect. 2. We retain notation: a candidate plan $\theta = (g, z) \in \Theta$, tasks $\tau \in \{\mathsf{K}, \mathsf{L}, \mathsf{T}\}$, and utility $f_\tau(\theta) = \mathrm{TD}(T'(\theta))$. We also use a task-specific feasibility predicate $\mathrm{Feas}_\tau(\theta) \in \{0, 1\}$ indicating whether the constraints of (3) – (5) hold for task τ.

3.1 Overview and Algorithm

Tasks (K), (L), (T) share the decision variables and utility (2) but differ in feasibility; high-TD candidates from one task often lie near feasible regions of others, so controlled transfer can accelerate search while curbing negative transfer [3, 22]. MTADE maintains one DE population per task, $P_\tau^{(t)} = \{\theta_{\tau,i}^{(t)}\}_{i=1}^N \subseteq \Theta$, evolved in parallel. Every κ generations, tasks exchange elites via weak replacement (Sect. 3.3; cadence in (11)).

Algorithm 1. MTADE (condensed): Multi-Task Anonymization by DE with Elite-Migration / Weak-Replacement

Require: T, taxonomies $\{\mathcal{G}_j\}_{j=1}^m$, privacy params (k, l, t), pop. size N, generations $T_{\max}$, fixed DE params (F_τ, C_τ), migration interval κ.
Ensure: Best feasible plans $\theta_{\mathsf{K}}^\star, \theta_{\mathsf{L}}^\star, \theta_{\mathsf{T}}^\star$.

Init (parallel over $\tau \in \{\mathsf{K}, \mathsf{L}, \mathsf{T}\}$): sample $P_\tau^{(0)} \subseteq \Theta$, project Π_Θ, evaluate $\mathrm{Feas}_\tau(\cdot)$ and masked utility $\tilde{f}_\tau(\cdot)$ per (9).
for $t \leftarrow 0$ **to** $T_{\max} - 1$ **do**
  DE (for each τ and $i \in \{1, \ldots, N\}$; all in parallel):
  Mutation. Pick a mutation strategy;
  cross. $\hat{\theta} \leftarrow \mathrm{BinomialCrossover}(\theta_{\tau,i}^{(t)}, \tilde{\theta}; C_\tau)$; project $\hat{\theta} \leftarrow \Pi_\Theta(\hat{\theta})$.
  Eval. Compute $\mathrm{Feas}_\tau(\hat{\theta})$ and $\tilde{f}_\tau(\hat{\theta})$ (Eq. (9)).
  Select. $\theta_{\tau,i}^{(t+1)} \leftarrow \mathrm{SELECT}_\tau(\theta_{\tau,i}^{(t)}, \hat{\theta})$ using the three-case rule in §3.2 with mono_τ (Eq. (10)).
  if $(t+1) \bmod \kappa = 0$ **then** ▷ Migration cadence per (11)
    Elite-migration/weak-replacement:
    (i) For each τ, define elite $e_\tau^{(t+1)}$ under the same order as selection (feasible $\Rightarrow$ highest $\tilde{f}_\tau$; else $\Rightarrow$ highest mono_τ).
    (ii) For each ordered pair (τ, τ'), $\tau \neq \tau'$, evaluate $e_\tau^{(t+1)}$ under task τ' and weakly replace the M worst individuals in $P_{\tau'}^{(t+1)}$ ranked by the same order (we use $M{=}2$).
  end if
end for
Return $\theta_\tau^\star$ as the best *feasible* plan in $P_\tau^{(T_{\max})}$ by $\tilde{f}_\tau$.

3.2 Representation, Objective, and Feasibility

Encoding and projection. For QI X_j with taxonomy depth L_j, encode generalization by $h_j \in \{0, \ldots, L_j\}$ (0=leaf/raw, L_j=root); let $h = (h_1, \ldots, h_m)$. Suppression is $z \in \{0,1\}^n$. A search point is $\theta = (h, z)$; a fixed decoder maps h to g used in (1). Projection Π_Θ rounds h_j to $[0, L_j]$ and clips z_i to $\{0, 1\}$.

Utility and Masked Utility. For task τ, $f_\tau(\theta) = \mathrm{TD}\big(T'(\theta)\big)$ and $\mathrm{Feas}_\tau(\theta) \in \{0, 1\}$. For selection we use the masked utility

$$\tilde{f}_\tau(\theta) = \begin{cases} \mathrm{TD}\big(T'(\theta)\big), & \mathrm{Feas}_\tau(\theta) = 1, \\ 0, & \mathrm{Feas}_\tau(\theta) = 0, \end{cases} \tag{9}$$

i.e., utilities of infeasible candidates are treated as zero.

Selection with Feasibility and Task-Specific Monotone Scores. Let $\mathcal{E}(T'(\theta))$ be the set of equivalence classes induced by plan θ. Define per-task privacy scores that align with the constraints:

$$\begin{aligned} k_{\min}(\theta) &:= \min_{E\in\mathcal{E}(T'(\theta))} |E|, \\ l_{\min}(\theta) &:= \min_{E\in\mathcal{E}(T'(\theta))} \mathcal{D}(P_E), \\ t_{\max}(\theta) &:= \max_{E\in\mathcal{E}(T'(\theta))} D\big(P_E, P_{T'(\theta)}\big). \end{aligned}$$

Define the infeasible-regime task-aligned *monotone score* (higher is better).

$$\text{mono}_\tau(\theta) = \begin{cases} k_{\min}(\theta), & \tau = \mathsf{K}\ (k\text{-anonymity}), \\ l_{\min}(\theta), & \tau = \mathsf{L}\ (l\text{-diversity}), \\ -t_{\max}(\theta), & \tau = \mathsf{T}\ (t\text{-closeness}). \end{cases} \tag{10}$$

Given an incumbent θ and a trial $\hat{\theta}$ for task τ, selection follows the three-case rule (ties keep the incumbent):

$$\theta^{\text{next}} = \begin{cases} \arg\max\limits_{\xi\in\{\theta,\hat{\theta}\}} \text{mono}_\tau(\xi), & \text{if } \text{Feas}_\tau(\theta) = \text{Feas}_\tau(\hat{\theta}) = 0, \\ \arg\max\limits_{\xi\in\{\theta,\hat{\theta}\}} \text{Feas}_\tau(\xi), & \text{if } \text{Feas}_\tau(\theta) \neq \text{Feas}_\tau(\hat{\theta}), \\ \arg\max\limits_{\xi\in\{\theta,\hat{\theta}\}} \tilde{f}_\tau(\xi), & \text{if } \text{Feas}_\tau(\theta) = \text{Feas}_\tau(\hat{\theta}) = 1, \end{cases}$$

where the masked utility $\tilde{f}_\tau$ credits utility only when feasible (Eq. (9)).

3.3 Evolutionary Update and Knowledge Transfer

Within-Task DE. Each task uses `DE` with fixed (F_τ, C_τ) [18]. Mutation, crossover, projection, and selection operate in the encoded space; decoding to g occurs only for evaluating feasibility and f_τ (or $\tilde{f}_\tau$).

Elite-Migration/Weak-Replacement. Every κ generations, each task exports its elite $e_\tau^{(t)}$. Migrants are evaluated under the receiver's constraints and weakly replace the receiver's worst M individuals under that order, bounding negative transfer while preserving diversity [2,7] (Fig. 2).

3.4 Execution, Cadence, Termination

Parallel Evaluation. Computing $T'(\theta)$, forming equivalence classes, and evaluating feasibility and f_τ factorize over individuals and tasks (parallel map; synchronize at generation and migration barriers).

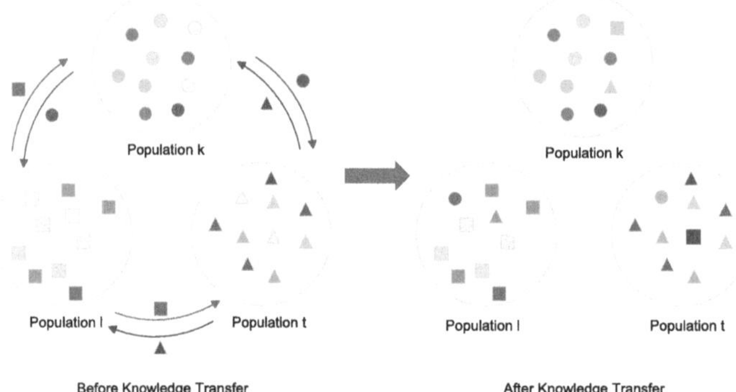

Fig. 2. Knowledge transfer schematic. At a migration generation, each task exports its elite $e_{\mathcal{T}}^{(t)}$ to the other tasks. Migrants are evaluated under the receiver's constraints and ranked consistently with selection: feasible candidates by masked utility (9), otherwise by the monotone score (10). They weakly replace the receiver's worst M individuals under the same order (we use M=2).

Migration Cadence. We set the exchange interval to a fraction of the per-task evaluation budget:

$$\kappa = \left\lfloor \alpha_{\text{mig}} \cdot \frac{\text{NFE}_{\max}}{|\mathcal{T}|\, N} \right\rfloor = \left\lfloor \alpha_{\text{mig}} \cdot \frac{\text{NFE}_{\max}}{3N} \right\rfloor, \tag{11}$$

with $\alpha_{\text{mig}} \in (0, 1]$ the migration fraction, N population per task, $|\mathcal{T}| = 3$, and $\text{NFE}_{\max} = 3nm$ for n records, m quasi-identifiers.

Termination. After $T_{\max}$ generations, return $\theta_{\mathcal{T}}^{\star}$ as the best *feasible* plan in $P_{\mathcal{T}}^{(T_{\max})}$ by $\tilde{f}_{\mathcal{T}}$; if no feasible candidate exists, report that no solution satisfies (k, l, t) under the given budget.

4 Experiment Evaluation

We evaluate MTADE on 16 healthcare test cases derived from the SPARCS 2015 de-identified inpatient dataset.[1]

4.1 Experimental Setup

Datasets. Following [28], we construct 16 cases across four themes by varying QIs, retained attributes, and record counts (n_R). To save space while preserving detail, Table 1 lists tuples *(nQI, attributes,*n_R) per scenario.

[1] https://health.data.ny.gov/Health/Hospital-Inpatient-Discharges-SPARCS-De-Identified/82xm-y6g8.

Table 1. Test cases by scenario; each tuple is *(nQI, attributes, n_R)*.

Emergency	D_1 (6,6,706); D_2 (6,6,1396); D_3 (10,8,695); D_4 (10,8,1394)
Mental Health	D_5 (6,6,699); D_6 (6,6,1359); D_7 (10,8,676); D_8 (10,8,1409)
HIV	D_9 (5,5,727); D_{10} (5,5,1066); D_{11} (9,7,698); D_{12} (9,7,993)
Respiratory	D_{13} (6,6,683); D_{14} (6,6,1431); D_{15} (10,8,687); D_{16} (10,8,1440)

Baselines. Six DE variants with different mutation strategies run without transfer: **DE/best/1**, **DE/best/2**, **DE/current-to-best/1**, **DE/rand/1**, **DE/rand/2**, **DE/current-to-rand/1**. For each backbone, we compare "kernel only" vs. "kernel + MTADE" to isolate the effect of cross-task transfer.

Settings. Unless noted: population N=30, crossover C_r=0.3, mutation scale F=1.6; fixed privacy thresholds (k=4, $l=\max\{2, \lfloor 0.5|\text{supp}(P_T)|\rfloor\}$, t=0.3) with $D(P,Q) = \|P - Q\|_2$; evaluation budget per run $\text{NFE}_{\max} = 3nm$ (with n records and m quasi-identifiers); migration fraction α_{mig}=0.05 and migration interval $\kappa = \lfloor \alpha_{\text{mig}} \cdot \frac{\text{NFE}_{\max}}{3N} \rfloor$; weak-replacement size M=2; identical random

Table 2. Comprehensive data utility across all cases for DE/best/1, DE/best/2, and DE/current-to-best/1. Baseline (kernel-only) vs. MTADE (kernel + transfer). †: Mann – Whitney U p<0.05 (Holm-corrected).

Case	DE/best/1			DE/best/2			DE/curr-to-best/1		
	Baseline	MTADE	Δ (%)	Baseline	MTADE	Δ (%)	Baseline	**MTADE**	Δ (%)
D_1	1366.97	**1670.44**†	22.2%	1150.30	**1351.07**†	17.5%	957.48	**1105.13**†	15.4%
D_2	3348.03	**3547.51**†	6.0%	2868.06	**3089.82**†	7.7%	2210.20	**2515.48**†	13.8%
D_3	1162.06	**1869.54**†	60.9%	989.09	**1471.59**†	48.8%	680.77	**1136.76**†	67.0%
D_4	2505.81	**3864.47**†	54.2%	2431.12	**3369.38**†	38.6%	1849.45	**2673.11**†	44.5%
D_5	1518.74	**1784.84**†	17.5%	1234.12	**1410.97**†	14.3%	986.07	**1143.17**†	15.9%
D_6	3069.14	**3152.01**†	2.7%	2564.80	**2711.24**†	5.7%	2031.62	**2239.31**†	10.2%
D_7	1225.66	**1818.62**†	48.4%	997.10	**1487.06**†	49.1%	753.50	**1161.86**†	54.2%
D_8	2736.56	**4021.67**†	47.0%	2581.96	**3481.93**†	34.9%	1943.56	**2777.69**†	42.9%
D_9	1691.67	**1756.55**†	3.8%	1372.15	**1454.08**†	6.0%	1130.95	**1268.49**†	12.2%
D_{10}	2631.75	**2691.36**†	2.3%	2081.56	**2119.11**†	1.8%	1671.07	**1908.43**†	14.2%
D_{11}	1648.54	**2166.54**†	31.4%	1310.34	**1637.01**†	24.9%	1036.44	**1378.96**†	33.0%
D_{12}	2376.92	**2821.91**†	18.7%	1993.29	**2246.51**†	12.7%	1525.11	**1933.69**†	26.8%
D_{13}	1122.10	**1387.66**†	23.7%	971.14	**1106.30**†	13.9%	753.66	**920.62**†	22.2%
D_{14}	3110.82	**3211.92**†	3.2%	2577.04	**2764.93**†	7.3%	1964.43	**2225.06**†	13.3%
D_{15}	1133.72	**1693.75**†	49.4%	901.11	**1321.49**†	46.7%	668.76	**1082.38**†	61.8%
D_{16}	2514.22	**3686.97**†	46.6%	2250.73	**3166.59**†	40.7%	1645.10	**2520.68**†	53.2%

seeds across competing methods for variance reduction. The global evaluation counter (NFE) includes initialization, trial evaluations, and migrant evaluations.

Protocol and Statistics. For each case/method we run 25 trials and report means (where space permits). Significance is assessed with a two-sided *Mann – Whitney U* (Wilcoxon rank-sum) test at $\alpha = 0.05$ with Holm correction; markers in result tables indicate cases where MTADE outperforms its paired backbone under this test.

4.2 Results

Utility Under Equal Privacy. Tables 2 and 3 report comprehensive utility (mean TD across the three privacy tasks) per case and backbone, contrasting baseline vs. MTADE and the relative gain Δ (%). Across all 16 cases, MTADE improves comprehensive utility on average by 27.4% (DE/best/1), 23.2% (DE/best/2), 31.3%(DE/current-to-best/1), 23.8% (DE/rand/1), 23.6% (DE/rand/2), and 27.2% (DE/current-to-rand/1), with the largest gains in higher-dimensional nQI settings.

Table 3. Comprehensive data utility across all cases for DE/rand/1, DE/rand/2, and DE/current-to-rand/1. Notation as in Table 2.

Case	DE/rand/1			DE/rand/2			DE/curr-to-rand/1		
	Baseline	MTADE	Δ (%)	Baseline	MTADE	Δ (%)	Baseline	MTADE	Δ (%)
D_1	1105.27	**1270.24**†	14.9%	1077.95	**1238.14**†	14.9%	728.39	**842.61**†	15.7%
D_2	2523.77	**2733.24**†	8.3%	2427.34	**2573.80**†	6.0%	1658.78	**1795.89**†	8.3%
D_3	893.24	**1362.45**†	52.5%	841.22	**1300.18**†	54.6%	534.92	**838.33**†	56.7%
D_4	2148.66	**2982.68**†	38.8%	1920.46	**2747.57**†	43.1%	1191.75	**1803.95**†	51.4%
D_5	1173.66	**1325.53**†	12.9%	1130.85	**1278.19**†	13.0%	759.94	**852.33**†	12.2%
D_6	2270.48	**2449.02**†	7.9%	2166.60	**2298.68**†	6.1%	1575.10	**1667.40**†	5.9%
D_7	936.32	**1382.44**†	47.6%	869.02	**1302.18**†	49.8%	564.94	**870.43**†	54.1%
D_8	2247.57	**3100.38**†	37.9%	2170.87	**2885.25**†	32.9%	1395.84	**1967.71**†	41.0%
D_9	1264.77	**1364.56**†	7.9%	1241.82	**1329.72**†	7.1%	897.48	**997.60**†	11.2%
D_{10}	1891.28	**1960.16**†	3.6%	1847.51	**1906.75**†	3.2%	1307.10	**1405.62**†	7.5%
D_{11}	1255.54	**1515.27**†	20.7%	1198.13	**1456.62**†	21.6%	802.36	**1021.07**†	27.3%
D_{12}	1787.02	**2054.31**†	15.0%	1734.36	**1957.43**†	12.9%	1209.29	**1403.24**†	16.0%
D_{13}	901.36	**1055.38**†	17.1%	848.58	**998.55**†	17.7%	583.37	**711.22**†	21.9%
D_{14}	2264.89	**2401.61**†	6.0%	2167.19	**2268.25**†	4.7%	1495.90	**1582.94**†	5.8%
D_{15}	851.17	**1271.83**†	49.4%	783.82	**1188.74**†	51.7%	501.24	**802.36**†	60.1%
D_{16}	2025.71	**2853.70**†	40.9%	1888.81	**2603.13**†	37.8%	1267.63	**1772.16**†	39.8%

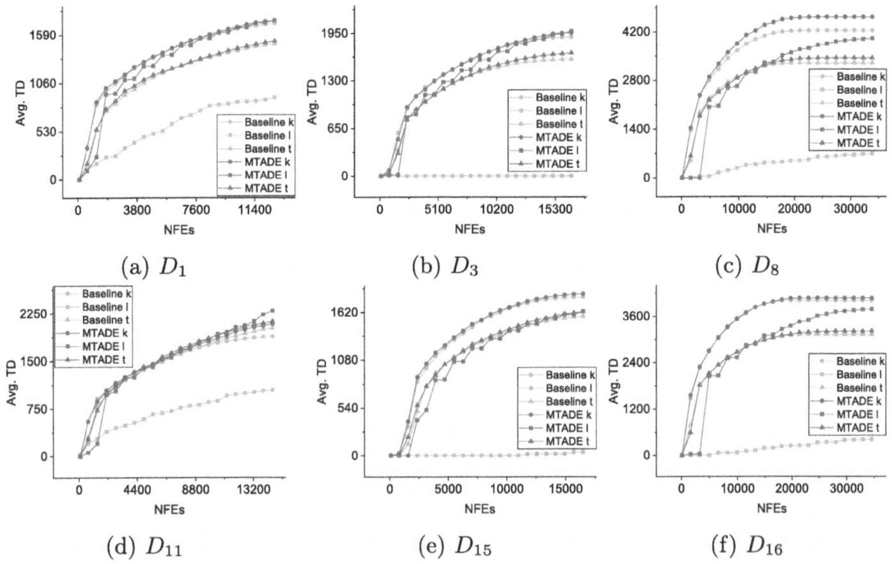

Fig. 3. Convergence under three privacy models across six representative cases. Each subpanel shows Avg. TD (y-axis) against NFEs (x-axis). Legends denote Baseline-k, l, t and MTADE-k, l, t for the three tasks.

Convergence. Figure 3 reports convergence in terms of average TD (Avg. TD) versus number of evaluations (NFEs) for six representative cases D_1, D_3, D_8, D_{11}, D_{15} and D_{16}. For each privacy model we plot both the kernel-only baseline and its MTADE variant. Curves show the mean over 25 independent runs. Across all panels, MTADE reaches feasibility earlier and continues to improve TD more rapidly. The advantage of MTADE is particularly evident in l-diversity.

4.3 Efficiency and Scalability

We compare wall-clock runtimes for single-task kernels executed serially across tasks vs. MTADE's parallel coevolution. Speedup (WS $= T_{\text{serial}}/T_{\text{parallel}}$) ranges from **1.18×** (D_9) to **3.68×** (D_{14}) and is $\geq 2\times$ **in 10/16 cases**. Full per-case WS values are preserved concisely in Table 4.

Table 4. Per-case speedup WS $= T_{\text{serial}}/T_{\text{parallel}}$ (higher is better). Compact layout retains all values.

D_1	1.37	D_2	1.40	D_3	1.30	D_4	2.33	D_5	2.18	D_6	2.47	D_7	2.20	D_8	1.89
D_9	1.18	D_{10}	1.54	D_{11}	2.20	D_{12}	2.31	D_{13}	2.21	D_{14}	3.68	D_{15}	3.17	D_{16}	2.57

5 Conclusion

We presented MTADE, a multi-task DE framework that optimizes k-anonymity, l-diversity, and t-closeness over a shared anonymization space. Each task evolves its own population while periodically exchanging elites via a weak-replacement policy, enabling cross-task reuse without eroding task-specific adaptation. Across 16 SPARCS-derived cases and six DE backbones, MTADE yielded higher utility under equal privacy than kernel-only baselines, with average gains between 23% and 31% and maxima up to 66.98%. Convergence curves show earlier feasibility and faster utility growth. In addition, parallel coevolution reduced end-to-end runtime with speedups up to 3.68×.

References

1. Alkhathami, M., Ge, Y.F., Wang, H.: A variation-based genetic algorithm for privacy-preserving data publishing. In: 2024 11th International Conference on Machine Intelligence Theory and Applications (MiTA), pp. 1–8. IEEE (2024)
2. Araujo, J.N.R., Batista, L.S.: A diversity-driven migration strategy for distributed evolutionary algorithms. Swarm Evol. Comput. **82**, 101361 (2023). https://doi.org/10.1016/j.swevo.2023.101361
3. Bali, K.K., Ong, Y.S., Gupta, A., Tan, P.S.: Multifactorial evolutionary algorithm with online transfer parameter estimation: Mfea-ii. IEEE Trans. Evol. Comput. **24**(1), 69–83 (2020). https://doi.org/10.1109/TEVC.2019.2906927
4. Chen, G., Tong, M., Yin, J., Wang, M., Cao, J., Wang, H.: Securegraphfl: A privacy-preserving and attack-resilient federated learning framework for traffic prediction. IEEE Internet Things J. (2025)
5. Fung, B.C.M., Wang, K., Chen, R., Yu, P.S.: Privacy-preserving data publishing: A survey of recent developments. ACM Comput. Surv. **42**(4) (2010). https://doi.org/10.1145/1749603.1749605
6. Garfinkel, S.L.: De-identifying government data sets and documents. Technical Report, NIST Special Publication 800-188 (2016). https://csrc.nist.gov/pubs/sp/800/188/final
7. Ge, Y.F., Bertino, E., Wang, H., Cao, J., Zhang, Y.: Distributed cooperative coevolution of data publishing privacy and transparency. ACM Trans. Knowl. Discov. Data **18**(1), 1–23 (2023)
8. Ge, Y.F., Wang, H., Bertino, E., Cao, J., Zhang, Y.: Multiobjective privacy-preserving task assignment in spatial crowdsourcing. IEEE Trans. Cybern. (2025)
9. Ge, Y.F., Wang, H., Cao, J., Zhang, Y.: An information-driven genetic algorithm for privacy-preserving data publishing. In: International Conference on Web Information Systems Engineering, pp. 340–354. Springer (2022)
10. Ge, Y.F., Wang, H., Cao, J., Zhang, Y., Jiang, X.: Privacy-preserving data publishing: an information-driven distributed genetic algorithm. World Wide Web **27**(1), 1 (2024)
11. Ge, Y.F., Wang, H., Cao, J., Zhang, Y., Kambourakis, G.: Federated genetic algorithm: Two-layer privacy-preserving trajectory data publishing. In: Proceedings of the Genetic and Evolutionary Computation Conference, pp. 749–758 (2024)
12. Kohlmayer, F., Prasser, F., Eckert, C., Kemper, A., Kuhn, K.A.: Flash: efficient, stable and optimal k-anonymity. In: 2012 International Conference on Privacy, Security, Risk and Trust and 2012 International Conferenece on Social Computing, pp. 708–717. IEEE (2012)

13. LeFevre, K., DeWitt, D.J., Ramakrishnan, R.: Incognito: Efficient full-domain k-anonymity. In: Proceedings of the 2005 ACM SIGMOD International Conference on Management of data, pp. 49–60 (2005). https://doi.org/10.1145/1066157.1066164
14. Li, N., Li, T., Venkatasubramanian, S.: t-closeness: Privacy beyond k-anonymity and ℓ-diversity. In: Proc. IEEE ICDE, pp. 106–115 (2007). https://www.cs.purdue.edu/homes/ninghui/papers/t_closeness_icde07.pdf
15. Machanavajjhala, A., Kifer, D., Gehrke, J., Venkitasubramaniam, M.: ℓ-diversity: Privacy beyond k-anonymity. ACM Trans. Knowl. Discovery Data **1**(1) (2007)
16. Mauger, C., Mahec, G.L., Dequen, G.: Multi-criteria optimization using l-diversity and t-closeness for k-anonymization. In: International Workshop on Data Privacy Management, pp. 73–88. Springer (2020)
17. Ning, D., Ge, Y.F., Wang, H., Zhou, C.: Cadif-osn: Detecting cloned accounts with missing profile attributes on online social networks. In: Proceedings of the 33rd ACM International Conference on Information and Knowledge Management, pp. 1795–1803 (2024)
18. Price, K.V., Storn, R.M., Lampinen, J.A.: Differential Evolution: A Practical Approach to Global Optimization. Natural Computing Series, Springer, Berlin, Heidelberg (2005). https://doi.org/10.1007/3-540-31306-0
19. Regulation, P.: General data protection regulation. Intouch **25**, 1–5 (2018)
20. Rieke, N., Hancox, J., Li, W., et al.: The future of digital health with federated learning. NPJ Digital Med. **3**(119) (2020). https://www.nature.com/articles/s41746-020-00323-1.pdf
21. Sweeney, L.: k-anonymity: A model for protecting privacy. Internat. J. Uncertain. Fuzziness Knowledge-Based Systems **10**(5), 557–570 (2002). https://doi.org/10.1142/S0218488502001648
22. Tan, Z., Luo, L., Zhong, J.: Knowledge transfer in evolutionary multi-task optimization: A survey. Appl. Soft Comput. **138**, 110182 (2023). https://doi.org/10.1016/j.asoc.2023.110182
23. U.S. Department of Health and Human Services: Guidance regarding methods for de-identification of PHI under HIPAA (2012). https://www.hhs.gov/hipaa/for-professionals/special-topics/de-identification/index.html
24. Yin, J., Chen, G., Hong, W., Cao, J., Wang, H., Miao, Y.: A heterogeneous graph-based semi-supervised learning framework for access control decision-making. World Wide Web **27**(4), 35 (2024)
25. Yin, J., Chen, G., Hong, W., Wang, H., Cao, J., Miao, Y.: Empowering vulnerability prioritization: A heterogeneous graph-driven framework for exploitability prediction. In: International Conference on Web Information Systems Engineering, pp. 289–299. Springer (2023)
26. Yin, J., Hong, W., Wang, H., Cao, J., Miao, Y., Zhang, Y.: A compact vulnerability knowledge graph for risk assessment. ACM Trans. Knowl. Discov. Data **18**(8), 1–17 (2024)
27. You, M., Ge, Y.F., Wang, K., Wang, H., Cao, J., Kambourakis, G.: Tlef: Two-layer evolutionary framework for t-closeness anonymization. In: Zhang, F., Wang, H., Barhamgi, M., Chen, L., Zhou, R. (eds.) Web Information Systems Engineering - WISE 2023, pp. 235–244. Springer Nature Singapore, Singapore (2023)
28. You, M., Ge, Y.F., Wang, K., Wang, H., Cao, J., Kambourakis, G.: Hierarchical adaptive evolution framework for privacy-preserving data publishing. World Wide Web **27**(4), 49 (2024)
29. You, M., Yin, J., Wang, H., Cao, J., Miao, Y.: A minority class boosted framework for adaptive access control decision-making. In: International Conference on Web Information Systems Engineering, pp. 143–157. Springer (2021)

Blockchain-Based Telemedicine in Cross-Border Medical Tourism Post-Treatment Care

Angelina Marlina Fatmawati(✉) and Pan Lindawaty Suherman Sewu(✉)

Universitas Kristen Maranatha, Bandung, Indonesia
angelina.mf@maranatha.edu, lindawaty.ss@law.maranatha.edu

Abstract. The rapid expansion of medical tourism has been accompanied by an increasing reliance on telemedicine for pre-operative consultations and post-treatment follow-up care across jurisdictions. While this integration presents promising continuity of care and improvement in patient convenience, it also exposes significant legal gaps in legal liability, regulatory compliance, and data governance. This paper examines the intersection of medical tourism and telemedicine, emphasizing how the absence of harmonized legal frameworks between host and home countries creates challenges for both healthcare providers and patients. Utilizing a normative juridical method combined with a comprehensive legal analysis of prominent medical tourism destinations, the study extracts insights from a thorough literature review to analyse regulatory frameworks in key medical tourism hubs and patient-exporting countries, aiming to identify areas of misalignment and legal ambiguity. It advocates for the establishment of international legal instruments and bilateral agreements that delineate provider responsibilities, ensure informed consent, and protect patient rights in transnational care arrangements. By proposing a model for cross-border legal alignment in telemedicine-based follow-up care, this paper aims to ensure legal certainty, safeguard patient welfare, and create a safer, more coherent system for global healthcare delivery in the era of digital medicine.

Keywords: Medical Tourism · Telemedicine · Blockchain · Post-Treatment Care · Cross-Border

1 Introduction

In each passing year, people are increasingly interested in overseas medical and healthcare services, longing for better medical care options. The phenomenon of patients travelling across national borders to seek healthcare services is commonly referred to as medical tourism [1]. The growth of medical tourism popularity depends on various factors, such as the availability of better paramedical staff and healthcare practitioners abroad, the unavailability of certain treatments or procedures, and the need for better facilities. The effectiveness of the leading healthcare systems in specific countries influences patients' decisions when considering cross-border medical procedures [2].

The convenience of medical tourism presents a significant challenge, particularly when patients require post-treatment care from local medical services. It is important to

E. R. Kaburuan and S. Goundar (Eds.): HIS 2025, LNCS 16392, pp. 156–166, 2026.
https://doi.org/10.1007/978-981-95-6304-3_14

note that not all medical procedures are concluded with a single treatment [3]. Some cases require additional follow-up care to ensure optimal outcomes, such as those involving chronic diseases or complicated surgeries, which necessitate ongoing care, monitoring, and potential adjustments by local medical professionals upon return [4]. In such cases, healthcare providers may encounter difficulties in obtaining the necessary medical records due to varying regulations across different jurisdictions [5]. This issue can hinder the delivery of appropriate follow-up care and may impact patient outcomes, including the potential for misdiagnosis, which could result in the delivery of inadequate care [6].

The absence of universally standardized post-operative care protocols also presents a significant gap in the medical tourism realm, which leads local healthcare providers to become reluctant to assume responsibility for managing complications arising from medical procedures performed abroad [7]. Communication and delivery of medical records obtained abroad to the local healthcare facilities system are still poorly coordinated. Additionally, differences in medical practice standards and the management of medical records across various countries can pose challenges towards the respective providers when encountering unfamiliar protocols and procedures.

The advancement of telemedicine now has the potential to address issues related to communication and the delivery of medical records that arise during medical tourism. This technology may facilitate the transfer of information required for follow-up care in local healthcare facilities, thereby improving the overall patient experience and continuity of care [8].

This paper aims to elucidate the significance of remote consultations and telemedicine services in promoting cost-effectiveness, enhancing accessibility, and ensuring continuity of follow-up care for medical tourism patients. It particularly focuses on the collaboration between healthcare providers in the destination country and the home country regarding the management and transfer of medical records. Literature research will contribute to the discussion on the effective management of electronically obtaining medical records for patients involved in medical tourism. Further emphasize the importance of ensuring privacy and secure access to this information by utilizing a blockchain-based telemedicine platform. Moreover, a comprehensive analysis of the potential benefits and obstacles associated with implementing blockchain technology as a transformative force in the medical tourism sector will be presented.

2 Literature Review

While considerable research has been conducted on blockchain-based smart contracts for electronic medical record management, extensive studies on the specific application of telemedicine for medical tourism follow-up remain limitedly unexplored. This section will further emphasize potential utilization of blockchain-based smart contracts in a telemedicine platform, particularly highlighting the management of authorized access to Electronic Health Records (EHRs) for medical tourism follow-ups across borders. This approach will further delve into leveraging potential security issues that may arise, as well as ensuring seamless collaboration among healthcare providers across jurisdictions.

2.1 Continuum of Post-Treatment Care in Medical Tourism Landscapes

Medical tourism, in general, can be defined as patients travelling beyond their home country's borders to seek healthcare services [9]. Consequently, a significant concern associated with cross-border medical procedures lies in ensuring the continuity of post-treatment care. Depending on the clinical case, medical treatment typically involves several stages and might require repeated interventions [10]. For instance, Vequist, in his research, argues that in the context of medical tourism, the absence of a continuum of care may raise additional ethical issues for providers and increase the risk of complications for patients [7]. The complexities of communication between international providers and domestic healthcare systems are insufficiently addressed, leading to delays in identifying post-treatment complications and, in some cases, inappropriate treatment decisions [11].

2.2 Electronic Health Records in Post-Treatment Care

The adoption of Electronic Health Records (EHRs) has been widely implemented among hospitals, resulting in a more effective healthcare management ecosystem [12]. EHRs can be defined as an inter-organizational system that serves as a comprehensive digital repository for patient information. EHRs typically comprise a clinical data repository to ensure that healthcare providers make well-informed decisions, supporting clinical decision support, controlled medical vocabulary, order entry, pharmacy management, and clinical documentation applications. This system enables the secure maintenance and sharing of health data, ensuring it is accessible to numerous authorized users, such as healthcare providers and specialists [13]. By facilitating the flow of information across different organizations, EHRs can also enhance collaboration among healthcare teams in providing patient care while safeguarding confidential information related to patients' medical histories [14]. However, due to the sensitive and confidential nature of data contained in EHRs, such systems become susceptible to threats related to security, privacy, and malicious sharing.

2.3 Blockchain-Based Smart Contracts in the Health Sector

The vulnerability of EHR systems poses significant risks to data integrity, confidentiality, and reliability. To address the respective concerns, blockchain technologies have been increasingly recognized as viable solutions to enhance the security, traceability, and resilience of EHR systems. Additionally, a blockchain-based system enables patients to enhance control over their medical records while maintaining the accuracy and accessibility of the respective data [15].

Blockchain is a technology that stores data through the utilization of decentralized nodes, with each node holding linked blocks that record valid transactions [16]. Each of the chains in a blockchain-based technology features integrated hash chains with a consensus mechanism to establish a reliable and verifiable understanding of the data recorded on each chain [17]. Its transparency, decentralization, and verifiability make it a promising tool for managing electronic health records (EHRs) in medical organizations, enabling data sharing while maintaining integrity [18]. These characteristics of blockchain technology are compelling infrastructure for managing the access control of medical records using a decentralized ledger that tracks and verifies access information [19]. Despite the promising potential of blockchain-based technology for electronic medical records, its widespread adoption in EHR systems remains underexplored due to significant challenges in the general standardization of medical record formats, interoperability, and authorization [20].

Further advancement of blockchain technology is the creation of smart contracts, aiming for the automated execution of the pre-consented conditions [21]. The application of smart contracts is indeed essential, particularly when autonomous operations, such as clinical data sharing, are involved [22]. In this regard, smart contracts serve as the key to defining digital access and rights to the medical data demanded [23].

3 Discussion

Healthcare institutions can systematically manage patients' treatment information, including medical records, accident history, physiological profiles, diagnoses, disease history, and prior health screenings to support more accurate clinical decision-making and enhance the overall quality of care accordingly. By leveraging an integrated system that provides access to important medical information, providers are better equipped to identify and anticipate complications, as well as tailor appropriate and adequate interventions to individual patient needs. As the complexity of electronic medical data systems continues to grow, the development of a secure, interoperable, and ethically governed infrastructure is essential, particularly for the medical tourism industry.

3.1 Current Challenges on the Regulatory Frameworks on EHRs Access and Interoperability

Interoperability Data Control and Privacy Concerns

While the integration of blockchain into the EHR system presents promising opportunities, numerous studies have identified major challenges related to interoperability, privacy, and authorization [24]. A critical policy priority lies in addressing interoperability due to the lack of harmonized data management practices and standardised protocols for medical records, which hinder the exchange of health information [25]. The interoperability of medical records is predominantly circulated and restricted to the originating system; for instance, hospital-issued medical records are generally accessible within the hospital's internal system [23]. This makes cross-institutional exchange of medical data severely challenging due to diverse procedures and governance regulations, computational algorithmic complexity, and prohibitive data-sharing agreements [26]. Moreover, the absence of universally accepted standards of data exchange continues to hinder secure and effective interoperability as well [27].

In many developing countries, the accessibility of EHRs remains a challenge due to the lack of coordinated care systems and a shortage of adequately trained healthcare professionals in utilizing such systems [27]. In Indonesia, the efforts toward regulatory harmonization of EHRs are still hindered by significant challenges, such as inadequate compatibility between the issuing systems, insufficient infrastructure, particularly in remote areas, and the absence of applicable laws governing data accessibility [28].

In other regions, efforts to promote cross-border integration and enhanced accessibility of EHRs are beginning to be strived for. A notable example is the European Union (EU), which has initiated various frameworks aimed at the digital transformation of healthcare systems to elevate cross-border interoperability and access to EHRs [29]. The EU Digital Decade report particularly emphasises challenges concerning cross-institutional data access and interoperability of EHRs. It highlighted the restrictive barriers that impede access to and data sharing between EHRs of private-run healthcare services and public healthcare authorities [30].

Furthermore, the protection of medical digital records is governed by the General Data Protection Regulation (GDPR) [31]. The regulation particularly denoted the importance of transparent data processing, ensuring lawful practices, and maintaining the confidentiality of patients' EHRs in order to protect against unauthorised access, loss, alteration, or damage of sensitive data [32]. Furthermore, GDPR specifically emphasize the essentiality of the patient's informed consent and agreement between healthcare providers and the respective patient for the use of the medical data records [33].

Blockchain-based EHRs indeed offer significant potential for improving healthcare, yet their adoption is impeded by interoperability gaps and regulatory complexities, particularly hindering cross-institutional data access and data privacy protection.

Telemedicine Role in Cross-Border Medical Tourism.

Telemedicine in medical tourism can play two important roles: connecting patients with the appropriate specialist to discuss their problem prior to travelling abroad and providing postoperative home monitoring after the medical trip [34]. Despite their role in shaping patients' decision-making, numerous medical tourism websites present an imbalanced narrative, highlighting advantages while offering minimal to no information on potential risks associated with certain medical procedures. Furthermore, critical details such as surgical risks, postoperative treatments, and legal protections are frequently absent from these platforms [35].

This lack of transparency not only hinders patients from adequate informed consent but also raises potential complications for patients' transition care upon returning home. Inadequate information and documentation will also significantly hinder the ability of domestic healthcare providers to deliver appropriate post-treatment care. Comprehensive medical records will be essential, especially when the patient returns to their country of residence and requires postoperative treatment in local healthcare facilities. In this regard, telemedicine platforms serve a pivotal role in enabling the secure, timely, and accessible exchange of on-demand, authoritative medical records between international and local healthcare providers, thereby delivering appropriate post-treatment care [36].

The pertinent patient information will be further organized within Electronic Health Records (EHRs). This will include comprehensive details related to the medical history, diagnoses, imaging results (including CT scans and X-rays), laboratory reports, and records of treatments administered [37]. However, access to patients' EHR data is usually limited due to the lack of interoperability among various medical organizations, particularly across different jurisdictions [38]. Privacy and security concerns remain significant challenges in enhancing accessibility for the exchange of EHR among multiple authorized healthcare providers [39]. Inherently, this also influences the improvement of the telemedicine role in medical tourism.

In that regard, a blockchain-based smart contract operating system is proposed for the telemedicine platform as a solution to ensure the accountability of all authorized stakeholders involved in providing post-treatment care in medical tourism.

3.2 Blockchain-Based Smart Contracts Utilization in Telemedicine for Medical Tourism Platform

The decentralized architecture of blockchain technology, characterized by its resistance to unauthorized modification, provides a potential framework for secure data exchange among authoritative stakeholders, enabling enhanced collaborative clinical decision-making in both telemedicine and precision medicine [40]. Initially, a blockchain-based smart contract was designed as an encoded agreement between parties with an automated execution system [41]. This architecture is operationalized through a private blockchain framework, which is defined by limited participation and restricted authority management of data access [42].

Within this framework, the smart contract functions as a programmable contract that manages access rights to the beneficiary's medical data, enabling real-time management and control over data sharing [43]. With a nature-permissioned blockchain-based function, the authorization of access to the network will be restricted to individuals or organizations involved in the contract [44]. To establish patient identity, we will leverage critical personal information, including social security numbers, birthdates, names, and zip codes. This data will undergo comprehensive encryption and be integrated into the blockchain algorithm to ensure security and privacy [45]. Consequently, only consortium members are enabled to perform validation, review, and grant access to the preselected blockchain-based network.

The decentralisation of blockchain technology further enhances stakeholders' accessibility to the EHR ledger. Simultaneously, the immutable nature of the blockchain ledger ensures data integrity by making it nearly impossible to alter medical records without the unanimous authorisation of all stakeholders. The censorship-resistant attribute allows all related parties to access all timestamped records while maintaining anonymity through a generated address [43].

EHR management and interoperability for clinical data sharing could be achieved by applying smart contracts on the Ethereum blockchain, which is referred to as Fast Health Interoperability Records and Blockchain (FHIRChain) [46]. The chain will respectively secure access to the database while facilitating retrieval of the requested data. This framework will ensure seamless interactions among stakeholders for medical data, while maintaining robust security and privacy measures in compliance with healthcare standards [46].

In the notion of telemedicine frameworks tailored to support the continuum of care for medical tourism, telemedicine services are designed to ensure remote monitoring capabilities and enhance data interoperability required by home healthcare services, particularly in the delivery of post-treatment care [47]. For example, in Dubai Healthcare City (DHCC), a pioneer in telehealth regulation, there is significant empowerment in integrating blockchain-based telemedicine. This system enables physicians and medical experts to compile comprehensive patient histories that combine data from various treatment stages and laboratory results, irrespective of the locations of the patient and healthcare provider [47].

The initiatives integrating telemedicine with blockchain-based smart contracts are promising, particularly in ensuring the continuity of post-treatment care for medical tourism patients.

3.3 Patient-Driven Interoperability with Blockchain-Based Smart Contracts Architecture for EHRs in Medical Tourism Telemedicine

Although there is no specific international regulatory framework for electronic medical data, the World Health Organisation has previously issued a medical records manual for developing countries. This guidance highlights that the integration and management of EHRs must ensure an accurate, timely, and accessible record, particularly to facilitate the easy exchange of data between healthcare professionals, thereby leveraging continuity of care [48].

Furthermore, the integration and interoperability of medical data shall be in compliance with the World Medical Association (WMA) Declaration on Ethical Considerations Regarding Health Databases and Biobanks, specifically related to the storage and use of data and biological material. It is regulated that collection and utilisation must be supported by informed consent from the respective individuals, ensuring privacy and confidentiality in accordance with the Declaration of Helsinkiv[49].

In healthcare frameworks, obtaining patient consent is crucial for ensuring that individuals are adequately informed and give their informed consent to the proposed treatments, procedures, or participation in clinical trials. With the application of smart contracts, the registration of all entities and stakeholders involved in the post-treatment medical tourism chain, along with their respective medical data and records, will be verified.

The integration of telemedicine with blockchain-based data interchange can be implemented by developing a smart contract that includes access conditions unanimously agreed upon by all stakeholders involved [47]. In this regard, significant parties include the patient, the doctor at the medical tourism destination, the doctor overseeing the patient's post-treatment care in the patient's local healthcare services, the pharmacy involved in medication prescription, and, alternatively, the medical insurance provider.

Interoperability and access to the data exchange could be integrated by utilizing blockchain's public-key infrastructure (PKI). The utilization of PKI involves the management of cryptographic key pairs that are securely held by significant individuals or entities related to the network, which is particularly verified through a digital certificate [50]. This mechanism provides a decentralised identification method, where an individual's public key serves as a unique identifier that links a particular patient's records across various healthcare institutions, eliminating the need for third-party certifying authorities [51]. Consent for interoperability and access to EHRs will be integrated through blockchain-based smart contracts that serve as an informed consent agreement of all respective stakeholders.

The telemedicine interfacing portal can be leveraged through application or web-based configurations during the implementation of FHIRChain. This setup facilitates seamless integration and interoperability in healthcare data exchange. Therefore, while blockchain-enabled PKI and smart contract agreements offer a promising pathway toward secure and decentralized patient identification that may enhance interoperability across healthcare systems, their practical adoption remains contingent upon addressing critical challenges, including scalability constraints, governance complexities, and alignment with diverse regulatory frameworks.

4 Conclusion

This study highlights the critical need for a cohesive legal and regulatory framework to govern blockchain-based telemedicine in cross-border medical tourism landscapes, particularly concerning post-treatment care. While blockchain and smart contracts offer promising opportunities for secure data governance with transparent provider-patient arrangements, they are inherently constrained by inadequate regulations due to varying standards of liability and an inconsistent approach to data protection. Although existing legal frameworks, such as GDPR, HIPAA, and WMA guidelines, offer a perspective of guidance, their comprehensive applicability across jurisdictions remains limited. To ensure patient safety, legal certainty, and ethical compliance, an international binding standard is indispensable, particularly in the notion of cross-border landscapes involving patients' electronic health records. Ultimately, to create a seamless, integrated and patient-centred global digital healthcare ecosystem, it is crucial to address and bridge the existing regulatory gaps.

References

1. Labonte R., et al.: Government roles in regulating medical tourism: evidence from guatemala. Inter. J. Equity in Health **17**, 150, 1–10 (2018) https://doi.org/10.1186/s12939-018-0866-1
2. Lianto, M., Suprapto, W., Mel, M.: The analysis factor of medical tourism in Singapore. In: SHS Web of Conference, pp. 1–9 (2020) https://doi.org/10.1051/shsconf/20207601028
3. Helble, M.: The Movement of Patients Across Borders: Challenges and Opportunities for Public Health. Bulletin of the World Health Organization. 89:1 https://link.gale.com/apps/doc/A252190655/HRCA?u=txshracd2623&sid=HRCA&xid=4680131b. In: David, G., Vequist, IV.: The Continuum of Care in Cross-Border Health Travel: Implications for Medical Tourism Standards. Journal of Healthcare Management Standards (2021). https://doi.org/10.4018/JHMS.2021010101
4. Nadella, N, et al.: Medical tourism: patients without borders. Global J. Med. Students (2024). https://doi.org/10.25259/GJMS_3_2024
5. Cynthia, A.N.: Ethical Dilemmas in International Medical Health Tourism: A Critical Commentary. SSM – Health Systems 5 (2025). https://doi.org/10.1016/j.ssmhs.2025.100111
6. Davison, et.al.: The Price of Medical Tourism: The Legal Implications of Surgery Abroad. Plastic and Reconstructive Surgery. 142:4 (2018) https://doi.org/10.1097/PRS.0000000000004816. In Cynthia, AN.: Ethical Dilemmas in International Medical Health Tourism: A Critical Commentary. SSM – Health Systems 5 (2025). https://doi.org/10.1016/j.ssmhs.2025.100111
7. David, G., Vequist, I.V.: The continuum of care in cross-border health travel: implications for medical tourism standards. J. Healthcare Manag. Standards. (2021). https://doi.org/10.4018/JHMS.2021010101

8. Garshnek, V., Hassell, L.H.: Rethinking telemedicine evaluation for a new technological Era. Int. J. Healthc. Technol. Manag. **2**, 271–280 (2000). https://doi.org/10.1504/IJHTM.2000.001073
9. Crist M., Appiah, G., Leidel, L., Stoney, R.: Medical Tourism CDC Yellow Book 2024 (2023). https://wwwnc.cdc.gov/travel/yellowbook/2024/health-care-abroad/medical-tourism. (Accessed 5 August 2025)
10. Helble, M.: The Movement of Patients Across Borders: Challenges and Opportunities for Public Health. Bulletin of the World Health Organization. 89(1) https://link.gale.com/apps/doc/A252190655/HRCA?u=txshracd2623&sid=HRCA&xid=4680131b. In: David, G., Vequist IV.: The Continuum of Care in Cross-Border Health Travel: Implications for Medical Tourism Standards. Journal of Healthcare Management Standards (2021). https://doi.org/10.4018/JHMS.2021010101
11. Cynthia, A.N.: Ethical dilemmas in international medical tourism: a critical commentary. SSM Health Syst. **5** (2025). https://doi.org/10.1016/j.ssmhs.2025.100111
12. Miller-Jacobs, H., Smelcer, J.: Usability of blockchain medical record system: an application in its infancy with a crying need. In: Smith, M.J., Salvendy, G. (eds.) Human Interface and the Management of Information. Interacting in Information Environments. Human Interface 2007. LNCS, vol. 4558. Springer, Heidelberg (2007). https://doi.org/10.1007/978-3-540-73354-6_83
13. Anshari, M.: Redefining Electronic Health Records (EHR) and Electronic Medical Records (EMR) to promote patient empowerment. IJID Inter. J. Inform. Develo. **8**(1), 35–39 (2019) https://doi.org/10.14421/ijid.2019.08106
14. Shahnaz, A., Qamar, U., Khalid, A.: Using blockchain for electronic health records. IEEE Access **7**, 147782–147795 (2019)
15. Shahnaz, U., Qamar, A., Khalid, A.: Using blockchain for electronic health records. IEEE Access **7**, 147782–147795 (2019). https://doi.org/10.1109/ACCESS.2019.2946373
16. Tawfik, A.M., Al-Ahwal, A., Eldien, A.S.T. et. al.: Blockchain-based access control and privacy preservation in healthcare: a comprehensive survey. Cluster Comput. **28**(529) (2025) https://doi.org/10.1007/s10586-025-05308-x
17. Griggs, K.N., Ossipova, O., Kohlios, C.P., Baccarini, A.N., Howson, E.A., Hayajneh, T.: Healthcare blockchain system using smart contracts for secure automated remote patient monitoring. J. Med. Syst. **42**(7), 1–7 (2018)
18. Ettaloui, N., Arezki, S., Gadi, T.: Blockchain-based electronic health record: systematic literature review. Hum. Behav. Emerging Technol.. (2024). https://doi.org/10.1155/hbe2/4734288
19. Niesya, N., Sayeed, M.S.: Adoption of blockchain technology in healthcare supply chain management: a review. HighTech Innovation J. **5**(4), 1154–1169 (2024) https://doi.org/10.28991/HIJ-2024-05-04-019
20. Ettaloui, N., Arezki, S., Gadi, T.: An overview of blockchain-based electronic health records and compliance with GDPR and HIPAA. Data Metadata **2**(166) (2023) https://doi.org/10.56294/dm2023166
21. Hawashin, D., Salah, K., Jayaraman, R., Yaqoob, I., Musamih, A.: A blockchain-based solution for mitigating overproduction and underconsumption of medical supplies. IEEE Access **10**, 71669–71682 (2022). https://doi.org/10.1109/ACCESS.2022.3188778
22. Kamel Boulos, M.N., Wilson, J.T., Clauson, K.A.: Geospatial blockchain: promises, challenges, and scenarios in health and healthcare. Inter. J. Health Geograp. 5,17(1), 25 (2018). https://doi.org/10.1186/s12942-018-0144-x
23. Gordon, W.J., Catalini, C.: Blockchain technology for healthcare: facilitating the transition to patient-driven interoperability. Comput. Struct. Biotechnol. J. **16**, 224–230 (2018). https://doi.org/10.1016/j.csbj.2018.06.003

24. Mayer, A.H., da Costa, C.A., da Rosa Righi, R .: Electronic health records in a blockchain: a systematic review. Health Inform. J. **26**(2), 1273–1288 (2019) https://doi.org/10.1177/1460458219866350
25. Ekblaw, A., Azaria. A., Halamka, J.D., Lippman, A.: A case study for blockchain in healthcare: "medrec" prototype for electronic health records and medical research data. In: Proceedings IEEE Open Big Data Conference, vol. 13(13) (2016)
26. Downing, N.L., Adler-Milstein, J., Palma, J.P., Lane, S., Eisenberg, M., Sharp, C., et.al.: Health information exchange policies of 11 diverse health systems and the associated impact on volume of exchange. J. Am. Med. Inform. Associat. **24**, 113–122 (2017). https://doi.org/10.1093/jamia/ocw063
27. Omotosho, A., Ayegba, P.: Current state of ICT in healthcare delivery in developing countries. Inter. J. Online Eng. (iJOE). **15**(8), 91–107 (2019). https://doi.org/10.3991/ijoe.v15i08.10294
28. Simandjuntak, M.E.: Implementation of E-medical record regulation: issues and challenges in Indonesia. In: E-Proceedings of the 3rd Health Law International Online Seminar 2022, "Digital Healthcare Transformation: Electronic Medical Record and Personal Data Protection (2022). https://repository.unika.ac.id/36051/7/Paper%20-%20Implementation%20of%20E-Medical%20Record%20Regulation_%20Issues%20and%20Challenges%20in%20Indonesia.pdf
29. European Court of Auditors. Special Report on Digitalisation of Healthcare: EU Support for Member States Effective Overall, but Difficulties in Using EU Funds (2024). https://www.eca.europa.eu/ECAPublications/SR-2024-25/SR-2024-25_EN.pdf
30. European Commission. Directorate-General for Communications Networks, Content and Technology, empirica Gesellschaft für Kommunikations- und Technologieforschung mbH, PredictBy, Deimel, L., Hentges, M. et al.: Digital Decade e-Health Indicators Development – Annexes, Publications Office of the European Union (2023). https://data.europa.eu/doi/ https://doi.org/10.2759/931828
31. Regulation (EU) 2016/679 of the European Parliament and of the Council of 27 April 2016 on the protection of natural persons with regard to the processing of personal data and on the free movement of such data and repealing Directive 95/ 46/EC (General Data Protection Regulation). in: O.J.E. U., ed., 2016, L119:111–188
32. Solvang, O.S., Cassidy, S., Granja, C., Solvoll, T.: Healthcare professionals' cross-organisational access to electronic health records: a scoping review. Int. J. Med. Inform. **193**, 105688 (2025). https://doi.org/10.1016/j.ijmedinf.2024.105688
33. Regulation (EU) 2016/679 of the European Parliament and of the Council of 27 April 2016 on the protection of natural persons with regard to the processing of personal data and on the free movement of such data and repealing Directive 95/ 46/EC (General Data Protection Regulation). in: O.J.E. U., ed., L119: 111–188 (2016)
34. Brebner, J., Brebner, E., Ruddick-Bracken, H., Wootton, R.: The development of a pilot telemedicine network in scotland: lessons learned. J. Telemed. Telecare **7**, 83–84 (2001). https://doi.org/10.1258/1357633011937254
35. Lee, H., Kevin, B., Wright, O'Connor, M., Wombacher, K.: Health Communication. Framing Medical Tourism: An Analysis of Persuasive Appeals, Risks and Benefits, and New Media Features of Medical Tourism Broker Websites, Health Communication (2013) https://doi.org/10.1080/10410236.2013.794412
36. Gu, D., Humbatova, G., Xie, Y., Yang, X., Zolotarev, O., Zhang, G.: Different roles of telehealth and telemedicine on medical tourism: an empirical study from Azerbaijan. Healthcare J. **9**(1073) (2021). https://doi.org/10.3390/healthcare9081073
37. Mayer, A.H., Andre´da Costa, C., da Rosa Righi, R.: Electronic health records in a blockchain: a systematic review. Health Inform. J. **26**(2), 1273–1288 (2020). https://doi.org/10.1177/1460458219866350

38. Zhang, R., Xue, R., Liu, L.: Security and privacy for healthcare blockchains. IEEE Trans. Serv. Comput. (2021). https://doi.org/10.1109/TSC.2021.3085913
39. Badve, O., Gupta, B.B., Gupta, S.: Reviewing the security features in contemporary security policies and models for multiple platforms. In: Handbook of Research on Modern Cryptographic Solutions for Computer and Cyber Security, pp. 479–504 (2016). https://doi.org/10.4018/978-1-5225-0105-3.ch020
40. Cheng EC., Le, Y., Zhou, J., et. al.: Healthcare services across China — on implementing an extensible universally unique patient identifier system. Inter. J. Healthcare Manag. **11**(3), 210–216. (2018). https://doi.org/10.1080/20479700.2017.1398388
41. Tresnawati, Fatmawati, A.F.: Blockchain-based smart contract: advancing digital consumer protection and preventing private international law e-commerce cases. Yustisia Law J. **10**(3), (2021). https://doi.org/10.20961/yustisia.v10i3.54891
42. Ichikawa, D., Kashiyama, M., Ueno, T.: Tamper-resistant mobile health using blockchain technology. J. Med. Internet Res. mHealth Uhealth. **5**(7), E111 (2017). https://doi.org/10.2196/mhealth.7938
43. Fekih, R.B., Lahami, M.: Application of blockchain technology in healthcare: a comprehensive study. In: Jmaiel, M., Mokhtari, M., Abdulrazak, B., Aloulou, H., Kallel, S. (eds.) The Impact of Digital Technologies on Public Health in Developed and Developing Countries. ICOST 2020, LNCS, vol. 12157. Springer, Cham (2020). https://doi.org/10.1007/978-3-030-51517-1_23
44. Ettaloui. N., Arezki, S., Gadi, T.: An overview of blockchain-based electronic health records and compliance with GDPR and HIPAA. Data Metadata **2**(166) (2023). https://doi.org/10.56294/dm2023166
45. Dubovitskaya, A., Xu, Z., Ryu, S., Schumacher M., Wang, F.: Secure and Trustable Electronic Medical Records Sharing using Blockchain. arXiv preprint arXiv:1709.06528, (2017)
46. Zhang, P., White, J., Schmidt, D.C., Lenz, G., Rosenbloom, S.T.: FHIRChain: applying blockchain to securely and scalably share clinical data. Comput. Structural Biotechnol. J. **16**, 267–278, (2018). In: Fekih, RB., Lahami, M.: Application of Blockchain Technology in Healthcare: A Comprehensive Study. (2020). In: Jmaiel, M., Mokhtari, M., Abdulrazak, B., Aloulou, H., Kallel, S. (eds.) The Impact of Digital Technologies on Public Health in Developed and Developing Countries. ICOST 2020, LNCS, vol. 12157. Springer, Cham (2020). https://doi.org/10.1007/978-3-030-51517-1_23
47. Abugabah, A., Nizamuddin, N., Alzubi, AA.: Decentralized telemedicine framework for smart healthcare ecosystem. IEEE Access. **8** (2020) https://doi.org/10.1109/ACCESS.2020.3021823
48. World Health Organization.: Medical Records Manual: A Guide for Developing Countries. WHO Library Cataloguing in Publication Data (2006). https://iris.who.int/handle/10665/208125
49. World Medical Association. Handbook of WMA Policies (2025). https://www.wma.net/wp-content/uploads/2025/05/HB-E-Version-2025.pdf
50. Mjeat, SN., Yousif, M., Bader, S., Mohammed, O., Saeed, AH.: A public key infrastructure based on blockchain for IoT-based healthcare systems. J. Cybersec. Inform. Manag. **15**(1), 233–243 (2025). https://doi.org/10.54216/JCIM.150118
51. Tahir, N.U.A., Rashid, U., Hadi, H.S., et.al.: Blockchain-based healthcare records management framework: enhancing security, privacy, and interoperability. Technol. **12**(9) (2024). https://doi.org/10.3390/technologies12090168

Design and Implementation of an Intelligent Medical Record Review Assistant Based on Large Language Models

Xuguang Zhu, Siyan Wu, Pengtao Li, Chunxiao Xing, and Yong Zhang(✉)

Tsinghua University, Beijing 100084, China
zhangyong05@tsinghua.edu

Abstract. Traditional manual review methods are plagued by issues such as being time-consuming, labor-intensive, and prone to inconsistent standards. To overcome these limitations, an intelligent medical record review assistant was developed in conjunction with the cardiac surgery department of a tertiary Grade A hospital, leveraging the advanced text comprehension and reasoning of large language models (LLMs). This assistant, built on the Dify platform, employs the divide-and-conquer strategy that structures the review into a three-stage visual workflow: text structuring, multi-dimensional parallel analysis, and results aggregation. During the parallel analysis stage, prompt engineering techniques, including Expert Mimicry and Chain-of-Thought, direct multiple LLM nodes to independently assess records across four key dimensions: medical terminology, content completeness, diagnostic rationale, and the appropriateness of the treatment plan. Experimental results demonstrate that LLMs outperform both traditional machine learning and deep learning methods in medical record reviewing, and that the divide-and-conquer strategy yields better outcomes than using a single LLM.

Keywords: Large Language Model · Medical Record Review · Prompt Engineering · Divide-and-Conquer

1 Introduction

Medical records serve as critical documentation of patient conditions, diagnostic processes, and treatment plans, playing a central role in modern healthcare systems. High-quality medical documentation supports accurate clinical decision-making and directly influences hospitals' ability to enhance patient safety, improve quality management, and comply with healthcare reimbursement policies. Medical record review, by systematically examining the standardization, accuracy, and completeness of medical record content, plays an irreplaceable role in safeguarding patient safety and enhancing the quality of healthcare services.

Currently, medical record review is primarily conducted manually. This approach is not only time- and labor-intensive but is also susceptible to subjective interpretation, which may lead to oversights and inconsistencies. With the continuous growth of medical

E. R. Kaburuan and S. Goundar (Eds.): HIS 2025, LNCS 16392, pp. 167–178, 2026.
https://doi.org/10.1007/978-981-95-6304-3_15

data, manual review has become increasingly inadequate, creating an urgent need for intelligent solutions for automated medical record reviewing.

In recent years, generative artificial intelligence technologies, particularly large language models (LLMs), have achieved breakthrough progress [1]. Equipped with advanced natural language understanding, logical reasoning, and text generation capabilities, LLMs have demonstrated significant potential in numerous medical applications—including medical text analysis, diagnostic assistance, and information extraction—offering new opportunities for developing intelligent medical record review systems. In this context, prompt engineering serves as one of the key technologies for interacting with LLMs.

Using the example of an cardiac surgery outpatient medical record review system, this paper explores the design and implementation of an LLM-based reviewing system employing prompt engineering. The aim is to improve the efficiency and accuracy of medical record reviews, thereby strengthening healthcare safety and service quality.

2 Related Work

The following section will review related work from two perspectives: the applications of LLMs in medical field, and prompt engineering as a key technical approach for leveraging LLMs.

2.1 Applications of LLMs in the Medical Field

LLMs have advanced rapidly in recent years, demonstrating powerful language processing capabilities across various healthcare-related tasks such as medical text comprehension, question answering, summarization, and information extraction [2–7]. For instance, Sonoda et al. reported that the Claude 3 Opus model performed exceptionally well in the "Diagnosis Please" case-based diagnostic task [2]. Research by Akyon et al. confirmed that models like GPT-4 and Claude exhibit strong performance in understanding medical literature [3]. In a study evaluating both general-purpose and medically specialized LLMs, Ntinopoulos et al. found that these models excel at entity extraction and classification within electronic health records (EHR) [4]. The DeepSeek model series has also shown considerable potential in medical applications. In practical settings, these models have been successfully deployed for various EHR-related functions—such as predicting prescription medications, identifying drug interactions, and generating patient education materials with high readability—offering efficient intelligent solutions for resource-constrained healthcare environments [5]. These advancements provide a solid technical foundation for developing intelligent and automated medical record review tools.

Although LLMs demonstrate strong performance in medical tasks, their complex development processes, high deployment barriers, and limited user-friendliness for medical professionals pose challenges to widespread adoption. Furthermore, ensuring data privacy in clinical settings remains a critical concern [8], often motivating the adoption of local deployment strategies. To facilitate practical implementation, foundational platforms for LLM applications can be employed to achieve faster development and more flexible deployment.

Dify is an open-source platform for developing LLM applications that integrates concepts of Backend as a Service (BaaS) and LLM Operations (LLMOps). Recognized for its engineering capabilities and support for private deployment, it is gaining increasing attention in data-sensitive industries such as healthcare. Within specific nodes of the Dify workflow, developers are required to apply prompt engineering techniques to optimize input instructions and fully leverage the model's potential.

2.2 Prompt Engineering

Prompt engineering is one of the key techniques in the practical application of LLMs. Its core idea is to use carefully designed prompts to guide the model toward generating outputs that better align with expectations without modifying the model's core parameters [9]. With the advancement of AI, prompt engineering has become essential for enhancing a model's adaptability across various scenarios, mitigating model bias and hallucinations, and promoting the expansion of automated applications [10].

In the medical field, prompt engineering is increasingly integrated throughout the clinical process. It plays a significant role in multiple healthcare scenarios—improving doctor-patient communication, streamlining clinical documentation and administrative tasks, supporting medical education and training, and facilitating personalized medicine and shared decision-making—thereby creating new opportunities for the healthcare industry [11]. In clinical text processing, Hu et al. developed a prompt framework consisting of four components—annotation guidelines, error analysis instructions, and few-shot examples—for clinical named entity recognition. Using this framework, they evaluated the zero-shot and few-shot performance of GPT-3.5 and GPT-4 on clinical text entity recognition tasks. The results showed that GPT-4's performance under the relaxed-match criteria was close to that of the fine-tuned BioClinicalBERT model, offering an efficient solution for accurate clinical information extraction [12]. To address challenges in diagnostic reasoning, the Clinical Chain-of-Thought (Clinical CoT) framework encourages the model to integrate multimodal data and generate diagnostic reasoning pathways. These reasoning capabilities are then transferred to smaller models via knowledge distillation, improving diagnostic accuracy and interpretability, and demonstrating strong potential in few-shot scenarios [13]. For multi-round diagnostic consultation, the Diagnostic-Reasoning Chain-of-Thought (DR-CoT) prompt template guides InstructGPT to progressively narrow down differential diagnoses by explicitly structuring a differential diagnosis list, simulating clinicians' diagnostic reasoning process. This approach has been shown to significantly enhance diagnostic accuracy in few-shot settings [14].

However, prompt engineering still faces several challenges in practical use. On one hand, prompt design is highly sensitive to wording and structure, where minor changes can lead to significant variations in model output [15]. On the other hand, prompts often lack transferability and are difficult to reuse across different tasks or models [16]. Furthermore, with the growing complexity of reasoning and multi-step tasks, prompt engineering must also address new issues such as context length limitations and control of reasoning pathways. Therefore, systematically exploring effective prompt techniques remains an essential path toward improving the efficiency of model capability utilization.

3 System Architecture

The following sections elaborate on the design of the reviewing assistant from three perspectives: basic approach, architectural framework, and workflow design.

3.1 General Approach

Medical record review that relies solely on the direct output of an LLM may suffer from breaks in logical reasoning or the omission of critical details, making it difficult to ensure comprehensiveness and depth. To address this limitation, the Divide-and-Conquer (DaC) strategy from multiple-prompt techniques shows promising potential.

The core idea of DaC is to break down a large or complex task into smaller, more manageable, and often independent subtasks. The LLM is guided to process each subtask individually, after which the results are integrated to form a final output. This approach is particularly suitable for processing long texts, multi-fact verification, or tasks involving repetitive operations. By decomposing the problem, the DaC strategy significantly reduces the model's cognitive load, allowing it to focus more effectively on local information within each subtask. This helps mitigate issues such as information omission, factual confusion, or error propagation caused by excessively long contexts. Research by Zhang et al. [17] provides solid theoretical and empirical support for the effectiveness of the DaC prompting strategy. They emphasize that DaC offers theoretical advantages and substantially improves model performance in scenarios involving numerous parallel subtasks and potentially deceptive content.

Within individual nodes, several single-prompt techniques are integrated to stabilize outputs and enhance professionalism:

1. Expert Mimicry: In medical research and practice, this technique is applied in scenarios such as medical question answering. By simulating the reasoning logic and professional judgment processes of medical experts, the model leverages expert knowledge and clinical experience to generate medically accurate and trustworthy responses [18].
2. Chain-of-Thought (CoT): This approach guides the model to first articulate a detailed, step-by-step reasoning process before presenting the final conclusion. As noted by Wei et al. [19], this technique decomposes complex problems into smaller, more manageable logical units, helping the model construct a coherent reasoning chain. For instance, when solving multi-step math word problems, the model can—under guided prompting—parse the problem conditions, establish relationships among variables, compute intermediate results, and ultimately derive the correct answer. Experiments in the medical domain have also confirmed that CoT enhances model accuracy in handling complex clinical questions [18].
3. Zero-Shot Learning: This allows the LLM to perform new tasks without task-specific fine-tuning or examples. Its main advantages are simplicity and efficiency; by eliminating the need for example construction, it reduces token usage, making it especially suitable for applications with input length constraints.
4. Structured Output Guidance: This method uses explicit instructions to compel the model to organize its output in specific machine-readable formats (e.g., JSON).

This approach not only facilitates subsequent programmatic processing and data integration but also supports systematic evaluation and analysis of model outputs.

3.2 Architectural Framework

As shown in Fig. 1, the system is structured into four hierarchical layers, from top to bottom: the Application Layer, the Service Layer, the Model Layer, and the Infrastructure Layer.

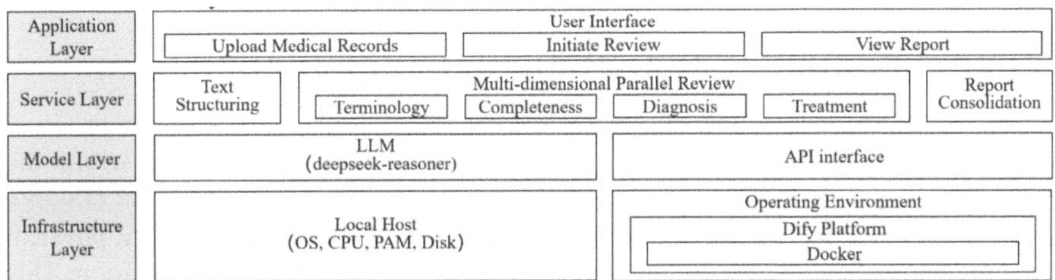

Fig. 1. Medical Record Reviewing System Architecture Diagram

The application layer provides users with an intuitive and streamlined interface that supports three core functions: medical record upload, review initiation, and report viewing. At the service layer, the central function involves orchestrating and managing the entire reviewing process using the visual workflow platform provided by Dify. The model layer serves as the intelligent core of the system, supplying the essential cognitive and reasoning capabilities required by the service layer. The system employs deepseek-reasoner as its primary inference engine. The infrastructure layer delivers the underlying hardware and environmental support necessary for stable system operation. Deployed on local servers with containerized management via Docker, the system achieves enhanced reliability and maintainability.

3.3 Workflow Design

Guided by a DaC approach, the process of developing the medical record reviewing assistant using Dify workflows is illustrated in Fig. 2. The overall design follows a "structuralization – parallel review – aggregation" pattern, which consists of three core stages. The first stage involves structuralizing the medical text, where unstructured raw medical records are parsed into a standardized data format including key fields such as chief complaint, present illness, and diagnosis. This initial data preparation step echoes the principles of the data enhancement framework by Sheng et al. [20], and provides a consistent and processable input for subsequent parallel operations. The second stage conducts multi-dimensional parallel reviewing, inspired by multi-agent collaboration. Four parallel "expert agent" LLM nodes simultaneously review the record from the following perspectives: medical terminology, content completeness, diagnostic rationality, and treatment plan rationality. The third stage aggregates the review results and generates a report. Findings from each parallel node are merged and processed through a final summarization node to produce a logically organized, human-readable comprehensive review report, thereby completing the entire process.

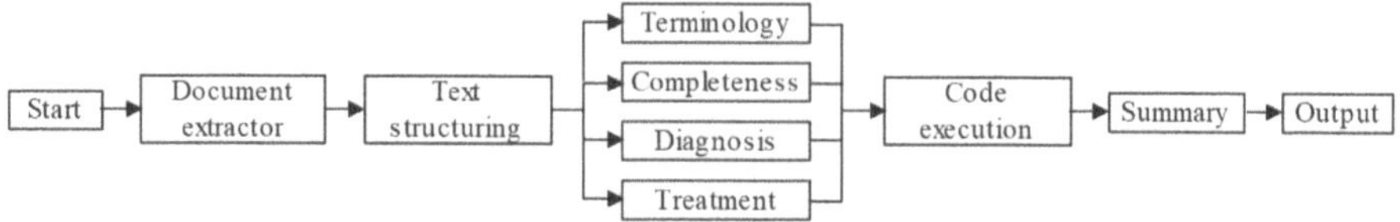

Fig. 2. Intelligent Medical Record Reviewing Assistant Workflow Orchestration

1. Start Node: Receives the raw outpatient medical record text input by the user.
2. Text Structuralization Node: This node serves as the preprocessing step within the assistant. It parses free-text medical records into a structured data format (JSON), extracting key fields including chief complaint, present illness, past history, physical examination, diagnosis, treatment plan, and other relevant clinical information. This step supplies standardized and easily processable input for subsequent parallel review.
3. Parallel Review: The structured medical record is simultaneously distributed to four specialized review agents, each conducting an independent assessment from a different dimension:
   (1) Medical Terminology Review Node: Focuses on identifying typos, non-standard medical terms, or abbreviations.
   (2) Content Completeness Review Node: Checks for missing key items (e.g., allergy history, chief complaint, diagnosis) based on predefined required fields and guidelines.
   (3) Diagnostic Rationality Review Node: Evaluates whether the diagnosis is consistent with the patient's chief complaint, present illness, and physical signs, and identifies any logical contradictions.
   (4) Treatment Plan Rationality Review Node: Reviews prescribed medications for compatibility with the diagnosis, checks for drug interactions or inappropriate dosages, and concurrently assesses the rationality of non-pharmacological treatments.
4. Code Execution Node: performs a preliminary merge of the review results (in JSON) from the four parallel agents into a unified data structure.
5. Summarization Node: Receives the merged preliminary results, interprets, organizes, and polishes the information to generate a coherent, uniformly formatted, and highly readable comprehensive review report.
6. Result Output Node: Delivers the final review report.

4 System Implementation and Experimental Validation

The system was designed in response to practical requirements from a tertiary Grade A hospital. With annual outpatient visits and hospital discharges ranking among the highest nationwide, the hospital generates a massive volume of medical documents and patient records daily. This leads to a substantial burden in medical record review. Consequently, the development of an intelligent tool capable of automated and efficient medical record reviewing is of significant practical value for enhancing the hospital's medical quality management and reducing the workload of healthcare professionals.

4.1 System Implementation

Testing Environment

The target production environment for the system is a private on-premises server equipped with dual Intel Xeon 4314 processors and high-performance graphics cards. For the purpose of this study, testing was conducted on a device with a 13th Gen Intel® Core™ i7-13700H processor and 32 GB of RAM. Dify version 4.2.6 was deployed locally, and the DeepSeek-R1–0528 model was used to build and execute the medical record reviewing workflow.

System Functional Testing

To evaluate the functionality of the intelligent medical record reviewing assistant, de-identified medical record samples were used for testing. The samples were divided into two categories: positive samples with no critical issues, and negative samples containing known serious errors.

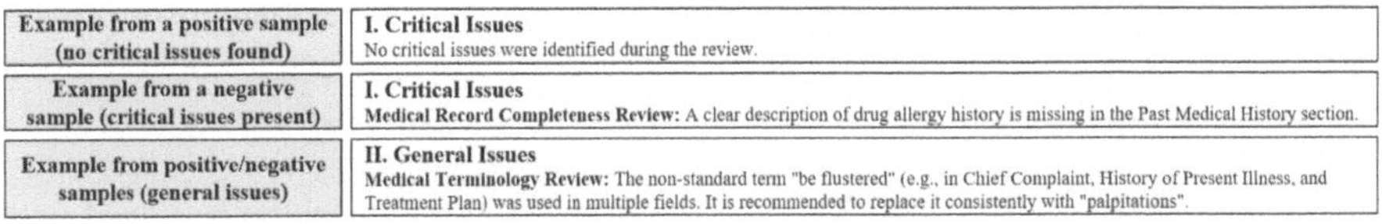

Example from a positive sample (no critical issues found)	**I. Critical Issues** No critical issues were identified during the review.
Example from a negative sample (critical issues present)	**I. Critical Issues** **Medical Record Completeness Review:** A clear description of drug allergy history is missing in the Past Medical History section.
Example from positive/negative samples (general issues)	**II. General Issues** **Medical Terminology Review:** The non-standard term "be flustered" (e.g., in Chief Complaint, History of Present Illness, and Treatment Plan) was used in multiple fields. It is recommended to replace it consistently with "palpitations".

Fig. 3. Test Result Example

The test results clearly demonstrate the system's effectiveness: For positive samples, the system confirmed the absence of serious issues while providing only minor optimization suggestions. For negative samples, the system accurately identified and listed critical errors requiring correction, with findings largely consistent with predefined errors. It also highlighted additional advisory notes. These outcomes fully affirm the assistant's practical capability to help correct medical errors and enhance healthcare safety. A sample test result is shown in Fig. 3.

4.2 Experiments

To further evaluate the performance advantages of the system in the domain of medical record reviewing, two comparative experiments were designed and conducted.

Experiment 1

Objective. To verify whether LLMs outperform traditional machine learning and deep learning models in medical text comprehension.

Data Source. A total of 100 medical question-answering instances in cardiac surgery were randomly selected from the CCKS 2019 Chinese Electronic Medical Record dataset [21]. Using these as reference, five different LLMs (Kimi, Doubao, ChatGLM, ChatGPT, Gemini) were employed to generate 10 sets of texts with correct diagnoses and 10 sets with incorrect diagnoses each. This process resulted in a final dataset containing 100 instances of "patient information + diagnosis + correctness label".

Experimental Design

This experiment focused on a key step in medical record reviewing—diagnostic rationality verification. The binary classification task of determining whether a diagnosis is clinically logical was addressed. The models compared included two machine learning models (logistic regression, LR; multinomial Naive Bayes, MNB), two deep learning models (TextCNN and Chinese-BERT-wwm), and the DeepSeek LLM.

For both machine learning and deep learning approaches, the dataset was partitioned into training and test sets in an 8:2 ratio. In the traditional machine learning setup, textual data was segmented using the jieba tokenizer and represented with TF-IDF features. Hyperparameter tuning was performed via five-fold cross-validation, with the macro-average F1-score set as the optimization objective. In the deep learning experiments, input texts were uniformly truncated or padded to a length of 512 tokens. All models used cross-entropy loss and the Adam optimizer with a batch size of 8. The TextCNN model was trained for 5 epochs with a learning rate of 1e-3, while the BERT-based model was trained for 10 epochs with a learning rate of 2e-5.

For the DeepSeek model, a concise classification prompt was utilized. The prompt instructed the model to adopt the persona of a chief cardiac surgeon and to evaluate the logical consistency between the patient's information and the given diagnosis, providing a binary "correct/incorrect" judgment. It processed all 100 samples, and relevant evaluation metrics were calculated.

Experimental Environment

The experiments were conducted on a cloud-based virtual machine equipped with an Intel(R) Xeon(R) 2.00 GHz CPU, along with an NVIDIA Tesla T4 GPU (16 GB VRAM, Driver Version 550.54.15, CUDA 12.4). The operating environment was a Linux container with Python 3.12.11, and the deep learning framework used was PyTorch 2.8.0 + cu126.

For the LLM experiment segment, a device with a 13th Gen Intel® Core™ i7-13700H processor and 32 GB RAM was used. Inference was performed via the official web interface of DeepSeek. All input prompts were constructed using a unified template and applied with consistent interaction methods.

Results. The experimental outcomes were analyzed based on four metrics: accuracy, precision, recall, and F1-score. The results are summarized in Table 1.

The results indicate that the DeepSeek significantly outperforms traditional machine learning and deep learning models in medical text analysis, confirming the strong advantage of LLMs for this task.

Experiment 2

Objective. To verify whether an LLM workflow employing a DaC strategy outperforms a single LLM in medical record reviewing.

Data Source. A total of 100 medical question-answering instances in cardiac surgery were randomly selected from the CCKS 2019 Chinese Electronic Medical Record dataset [21]. Using these as reference, five different LLMs (Kimi, Doubao, ChatGLM, ChatGPT, Gemini) were used to generate 10 standard medical records and 10 records containing

Table 1. Performance Comparison of Diagnostic Text Classification Models

	Accuracy	Precision	Recall	F1-score
LR	0.8000	0.8125	0.8000	0.7980
MNB	0.7500	0.7747	0.7500	0.7742
TextCNN	0.7000	0.8120	0.7000	0.6700
Chinese-BERT-wwm	0.7500	0.7530	0.7500	0.7490
DeepSeek	0.9300	0.9778	0.8800	0.9263

issues related to medical terminology, content completeness, diagnostic rationality, and treatment plan rationality. After manual verification, a final set of 100 instances of "patient information + diagnosis + correctness label" was obtained, comprising 50 problematic records and 50 standard records. The problematic records contained a total of 101 critical errors.

Experimental Design

Using the Dify platform, two medical record reviewing workflows were constructed: one implemented the proposed DaC strategy, distributing the reviewing task across multiple independent LLM nodes; the other was designed as a single-LLM workflow, where one node performed all four aspects of reviewing (medical terminology, content completeness, diagnostic rationality, and treatment rationality). The core prompt frameworks for the two workflows are illustrated in Fig. 4. Both workflows processed the same medical record dataset and were evaluated based on three aspects: problem detection accuracy, error localization accuracy, and explanation reasonableness. Problem detection accuracy was measured per medical record, assessing whether the system correctly identified the presence of issues. The latter two aspects were evaluated per error instance through manual scoring (1 point for correct identification/localization), normalized to a maximum score of 100.

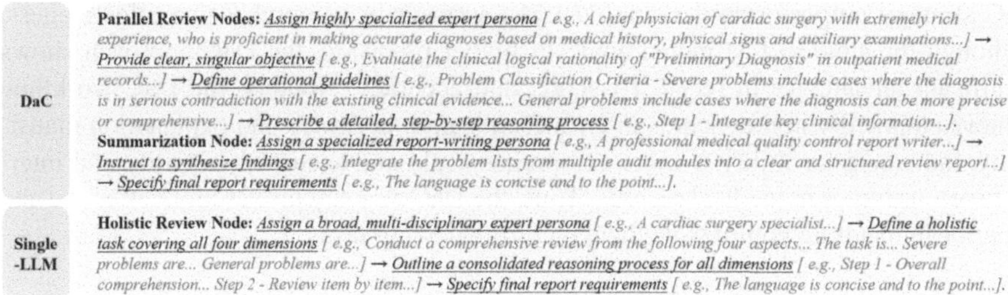

Fig. 4. Prompt Frameworks for the Two Workflows

Experimental Environment

The experiment was conducted on a device with a 13th Gen Intel® Core™ i7-13700H processor and 32 GB RAM. Dify 4.2.6 was deployed locally, and the DeepSeek-R1–0528 model was used to implement and test the medical record reviewing workflow.

Results

The performance comparison of the two workflows in terms of problem detection accuracy is shown in Table 2.

Table 2. Comparison of Problem Detection Accuracy

	Accuracy	Precision	Recall	F1-score
Single-LLM	0.8600	1.0000	0.7200	0.8372
DaC	0.9000	0.8846	0.9200	0.9020

The results for error localization accuracy and explanation reasonableness are presented in Table 3.

Table 3. Scores for Error Localization Accuracy and Explanation Reasonableness

	Localization Accuracy	Explanation Reasonableness
Single-LLM	82.18	76.24
DaC	89.11	86.63

* All metrics are on a scale with a total possible score of 100.

Furthermore, the DaC medical record reviewing workflow generally identifies a larger number of errors compared to the single-LLM workflow. It often detects subtle issues beyond predefined errors and provides more reasonable explanations. In contrast, the single-LLM workflow tends to output fewer errors and generate shorter review results, making it more prone to underreporting and insufficient explanations.

Overall, the experimental results demonstrate that the workflow employing the DaC strategy outperforms the single-LLM approach in comprehensive effectiveness. Although the single-LLM model achieves higher precision, the DaC approach shows significant advantages in recall, F1-score, and accuracy. Notably, the DaC workflow achieves markedly higher scores in error localization accuracy and explanation plausibility, indicating its ability to more comprehensively and accurately identify and interpret various issues in medical records. Thus, the DaC strategy proves more effective and superior in handling complex medical record reviewing tasks.

5 Conclusion

This paper elaborates on the design and implementation of an intelligent medical record reviewing assistant based on LLMs. Developed on the Dify platform, the system adopts a DaC strategy to construct an automated workflow consisting of "structuralization – parallel review – aggregation". By decomposing the complex task of medical record review into four independent reviewing dimensions—medical terminology, content completeness, diagnostic rationality, and treatment plan rationality—and leveraging prompt engineering techniques such as Expert Mimicry and Chain-of-Thought, the system achieves precise and in-depth analysis across each dimension, and demonstrates superior overall performance compared to single-LLM and traditional methods.

Despite these results, we acknowledge several limitations. Primarily, the scale of our experiments was constrained by limited computational resources, which restricted the throughput of our validation. Additionally, the inherent risk of LLM 'hallucinations' persists, and biases present in the model's training data may propagate into the review process, potentially affecting the objectivity and fairness of the assessment. In future work, we plan to acquire a large-scale dataset, comprising thousands of anonymized, real-world medical records from diverse clinical scenarios, to conduct more comprehensive validation. Furthermore, we aim to extend the application of this assistant to other medical departments. This will allow us to rigorously evaluate its cross-domain generalizability and robustness, paving the way for wider clinical adoption.

References

1. Liu, Y., Jin, C, Yang, S, et al.: The journey of language models in understanding natural language. Web Information Systems and Applications. In: WISA (2024)
2. Sonoda, Y., Kurokawa, R., Nakamura, Y., et al.: Diagnostic performances of GPT-4o, Claude 3 Opus, and Gemini 1.5 Pro in "Diagnosis Please" cases. Jpn. J. Radiol. **42**, 1231–1235 (2024)
3. Akyon, S.H., Akyon, F.C., Camyar, A.S., et al.: Evaluating the capabilities of generative AI tools in understanding medical papers: qualitative study. JMIR Med. Inform. **12**, e59258 (2024)
4. Ntinopoulos, V., Rodriguez Cetina Biefer, H., Tudorache, I., et al.: Large language models for data extraction from unstructured and semi-structured electronic health records: a multiple model performance evaluation. BMJ Health Care Inform. **32**(1), e101139 (2025)
5. Deng, Z., Ma, W., Han, Q.L., et al.: Exploring DeepSeek: a survey on advances, applications, challenges and future directions. IEEE/CAA J Autom Sinica **12**(5), 872–893 (2025)
6. Shool, S., Adimi, S., Saboori Amleshi, R., et al.: A systematic review of large language model (LLM) evaluations in clinical medicine. BMC Med. Inform. Decis. Mak. **25**, 117 (2025)
7. Li, Y.L., Wu, P.C., Zheng, A.Z., et al.: UniMRE: a unified framework for zero-shot medical relation extraction with large language models. Health Inf Sci Syst **13**, 43 (2025)
8. Zhao, L.T., Xie, H.R., Zhong, L., et al.: Explainable federated learning scheme for secure healthcare data sharing. Health Inf Sci Syst **12**, 49 (2024)
9. Huang, J., Lin, F., Yang, J., et al.: Prompt engineering for large generative AI models: methods, status, and prospects. Journal of Intelligent Science and Technology **6**(2), 115–133 (2024). [in Chinese]
10. S N, B P, P R, et al.: A comprehensive study on prompt engineering. Inter. J. Adv. Res. Sci. Commun. Technol., 420–425 (2025)
11. Patil, R., Heston, T.F., Bhuse, V.: Prompt engineering in healthcare. Electronics **13**(15), 2961 (2024)
12. Hu, Y., Chen, Q., Du, J., et al.: Improving large language models for clinical named entity recognition via prompt engineering. J. Am. Med. Inform. Assoc. **31**(9), 1812–1820 (2024)
13. Kwon, T., Ong, K.T., Kang, D., et al.: Large language models are clinical reasoners: reasoning-aware diagnosis framework with prompt-generated rationales. In: Proceedings of the AAAI Conference on Artificial Intelligence, vol. 38(16), pp. 18417–18425 (2024)

14. Wu, C.K., Chen, W.L., Chen, H.H.: Large language models perform diagnostic reasoning[J/OL]. (2023). arXiv:2307.08922
15. Sahoo, P., Singh, A.K., Saha, S., et al.: A systematic survey of prompt engineering in large language models: techniques and applications[J/OL]. arXiv preprint arXiv:2402.07927, (2024)
16. Liu, P., Yuan, W., Fu, J., et al.: Pre-train, prompt, and predict: a systematic survey of prompting methods in natural language processing. ACM Comput. Surv. **55**(9), 195 (2023)
17. Zhang, Y., Du, L., Cao, D., et al.: An examination on the effectiveness of divide-and-conquer prompting in large language models[J/OL] (2024). arXiv:2402.05359
18. Naderi, N., Atf, Z., Lewis, P., et al.: Evaluating Prompt Engineering Techniques for Accuracy and Confidence Elicitation in Medical LLMs[J/OL] (2025). https://doi.org/10.48550/arXiv.2506.00072
19. Wei, J., Wang, X., Schuurmans, D., et al.: Chain-of-thought prompting elicits reasoning in large language models. Adv. Neural Inform. Process. Syst. **35**, 24824–24837 (2022)
20. Sheng, M., Wang, S.L., Zhang, Y., et al.: A multi-source heterogeneous medical data enhancement framework based on lakehouse. Health Inf Sci Syst **12**, 37 (2024)
21. CCKS 2019. CCKS 2019 Evaluation Task: Chinese Electronic Medical Records [EB/OL] (2019). https://github.com/Toyhom/Chinese-medical-dialogue-data

Federated Deep Learning Framework for EEG Classification in BCI Applications

Taslima Khanam[1(✉)], Siuly Siuly[1], Kate Wang[2], Frank Whittaker[3], and Hua Wang[1]

[1] Institute for Sustainable Industries and Liveable Cities, Victoria University, Melbourne, Australia
taslima.khanam@live.vu.edu.au
[2] RMIT University, Melbourne, Australia
[3] Nexus Research Institute Pty Ltd, Melbourne, Australia

Abstract. Electroencephalography (EEG)-based Brain – Computer Interface (BCI) systems enable direct communication between the brain and external devices, facilitating neurorehabilitation. Motor imagery (MI) classification and event-related potential (ERP) detection are two critical paradigms for developing efficient EEG-based BCIs. While deep learning enhances decoding accuracy, centralized training poses significant risks to user privacy, data ownership, and regulatory compliance. Especially the following three challenges remain unsolved in the existing research work: (1) lack of mechanisms for privacy-preserving feature extraction, (2) poor handling of inter-subject heterogeneity, and (3) minimal evaluation of privacy risks alongside model performance. To address these challenges, we propose FedDeepAutoCloAk a novel Federated learning framework that integrates local Deep Autoencoder-based unsupervised feature extraction and KMeans Cluster Optimization with Adaptive Knowledge for improving MI and ERP classification while minimizing information loss and strengthening privacy protection for stroke patient data. In this framework raw EEG data stay local, with cluster centroids homomorphically encrypted before secure server-side aggregation, ensuring confidentiality. The framework was evaluated on two post-stroke publicly available EEG datasets, achieved better classification performance using three deep learning models. This work provides a scalable, secure, and personalized solution for decentralized EEG-based BCIs, advancing both technical robustness and ethical integrity in neurotechnology.

Keywords: Brain – Computer Interface · electroencephalography · motor imagery · event-related potential

1 Introduction

Brain – Computer Interface (BCI) systems enable direct communication between the human brain and external devices, bypassing traditional neuromuscular path-

E. R. Kaburuan and S. Goundar (Eds.): HIS 2025, LNCS 16392, pp. 179–190, 2026.
https://doi.org/10.1007/978-981-95-6304-3_16

ways [16,20,22]. These systems have proven especially valuable in neurorehabilitation, assistive technologies, and human-computer interaction [21].Among signal acquisition methods, electroencephalography (EEG)-based BCIs are prominent due to their non-invasiveness, affordability, portability, and high temporal resolution [7,9]. EEG captures brain activity through surface electrodes and supports real-time applications like motor imagery (MI), event-related potential (ERP) detection, cognitive workload monitoring, and emotion detection [8,10–12]. In MI-based BCIs, users control devices by imagining movements such as moving their left hand or foot. This allows them to operate prosthetics, control robots, or support motor rehabilitation after a stroke [26]. Conversely, ERP-based BCIs exploit time-locked neural responses to external stimuli, such as visual or auditory events, which are crucial for paradigms like the P300 speller and decision-making tasks [1]. While MI and ERP paradigms target different aspects of brain function, combining them enhances the flexibility and efficiency of BCI systems. However, decoding MI signals remains difficult due to EEG's low signal-to-noise ratio, high dimensionality, and inter/intra-subject variability [2]. Effective MI classification thus requires sophisticated models that capture both spatial and temporal features [25]. Recent advances in deep learning, particularly convolutional neural networks (CNNs), have led to significant improvements in EEG signal decoding. Architectures like EEGNet, DeepConvNet, and ShallowNet outperform traditional methods by learning task-relevant features directly from raw EEG [4,13].

Despite these advances, most EEG-based MI and ERP classification frameworks rely on centralized training, where raw EEG data are aggregated on a single server. This approach raises serious privacy, security and data ownership concerns, as EEG signals contain highly sensitive neurological information and can expose personal cognitive states. Storing EEG data centrally increases the risk of data breaches and may violate data protection regulations such as General Data Protection Regulation (GDPR) [11,19]. Therefore, there is a growing demand to develop machine learning approaches that protect user privacy while ensuring high classification performance in MI classification and ERP detection [5]. Federated Learning (FL) addresses this by training models locally and sharing only model updates, preserving data privacy. FL has shown success in various healthcare applications [14]. However, it remains underexplored in EEG-based BCIs, particularly with deep, unsupervised models. Existing FL-EEG studies often use shallow architectures or handcrafted features, assume homogeneous clients, and fail to balance privacy, personalization, and performance trade-offs [6,24]. In clinical datasets such as post-stroke MI and ERP EEG recordings, subject heterogeneity, varying recording conditions, and high sensitivity to data sharing make these challenges even more significant [15]. Especially, the following three challenges remain unsolved in the existing research work: (1) lack of mechanisms for privacy-preserving feature extraction, (2) poor handling of inter-subject heterogeneity, and (3) minimal evaluation of privacy risks alongside model performance.

Motivated by current limitations, we propose FedDeepAutoCloAk, a novel

Federated learning framework that integrates local Deep Autoencoder (Deep-Auto) -based unsupervised feature extraction and KMeans Cluster Optimization (Clo) with Adaptive Knowledge (Ak) protection framework for improving MI and ERP classification while minimizing information loss and strengthening privacy preservation for stroke patient data. This architecture integrates deep autoencoder-based unsupervised feature extraction, KMeans clustering for personalization, and homomorphic encryption for secure aggregation. We chose this framework because its architectural advantage lies in combining federated deep autoencoders with cluster-based personalization and privacy-preserving mechanisms.

Unlike traditional FL frameworks, FedDeepAutoCloAk learns discriminative latent representations locally, adapts to client heterogeneity using clustering, and ensures end-to-end security through homomorphic encryption (HE) of model updates and cluster centroids. In this framework, raw EEG data remain local and cluster centroids are encrypted using the Cheon – Kim – Kim – Song (CKKS) based HE scheme prior to secure aggregation on the server [3]. The framework is evaluated on two Publicly available EEG based BCI datasets: the CBCIC-Stroke MI dataset and the GIB-UVA ERP-BCI dataset, using three deep learning classifiers ShallowNet, EEGNet, and DeepConvNet. This scalable approach advances decentralized privacy-aware EEG classification in neurorehabilitation and BCI research. The major contributions of this work are as follow:

- Developing a novel FedDeepAutoCloAk federated learning framework that integrates deep autoencoder-based unsupervised feature extraction with HE to ensure privacy-preserving EEG analysis.
- Incorporating KMeans-based cluster-aware personalization to address inter-subject heterogeneity and enhance model adaptability for both MI and ERP classification tasks.
- Benchmarking of three popular deep classifiers on two publicly available post-stroke MI and ERP based EEG datasets, demonstrating significant improvements in classification performance and privacy protection.

The remainder of this paper is organized as follows: Sect. 2 presents the proposed methodology in detail. Section 3 discusses the evaluation results, and Sect. 4 compares our method with a centralized baseline technique. Section 5 concludes with future directions.

2 Methodology

This study introduces FedDeepAutoCloAk, a federated deep learning framework designed for the classification of MI and ERP based EEG signals collected from stroke patients. In the proposed FedDeepAutoCloAk framework, model training occurs in a federated learning environment where raw EEG data remain securely

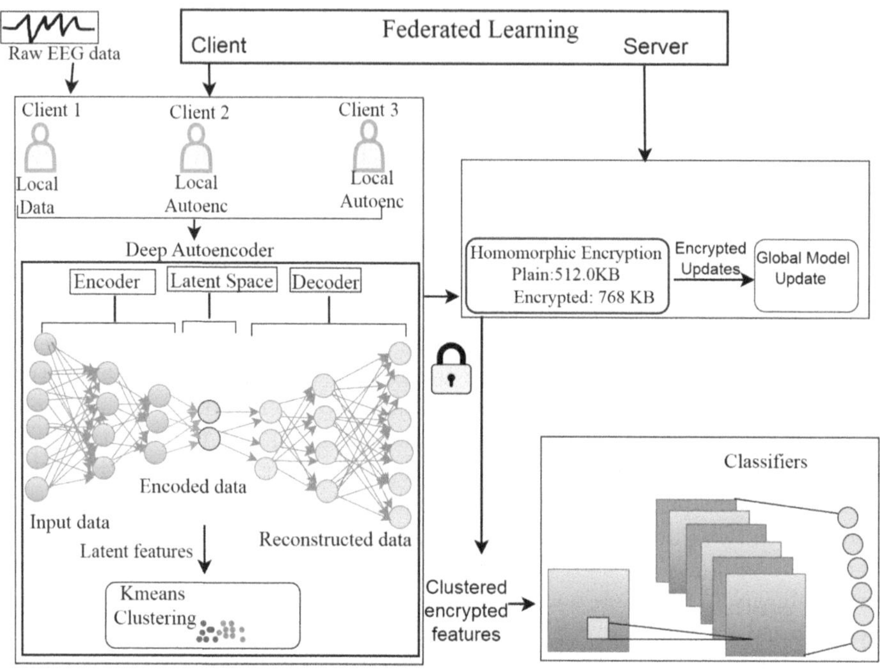

Fig. 1. An overview of the proposed method. The process begins with local EEG data on each client device, where raw trials are standardized using Z-score normalization. Features are then extracted using a deep autoencoder and grouped via K-means clustering to enhance task-specific representation. After clustering, model updates are secured using homomorphic encryption before being transmitted to the central server. The server performs federated averaging to aggregate encrypted updates and build a global model. Finally, the aggregated model is used for EEG classification with three deep learning models.

on the client devices, ensuring privacy preservation. After feature extraction using the deep autoencoder and task-specific clustering via K-means, each client trains a local model using its clustered EEG representations. Before transmitting model updates, the gradients are encrypted using HE to prevent potential data leakage. These encrypted updates are then transmitted to the central server, where federated averaging (FedAvg) is performed to aggregate client-side models into a single global model without accessing any individual-level raw data. Once the global model is updated, it is redistributed back to each client, where the model is fine-tuned using the client's local clustered features. This iterative process continues until convergence. Classification of EEG signals is then performed using three deep learning models. Figure 1 shows the architectural overview of the proposed framework. The developed framework integrates four key components, which are given below along with datasets:

2.1 Datasets

This study utilizes two publicly available post-stroke EEG-based BCI datasets: GIB-UVA ERP-BCI Stroke Dataset (D1): This data set includes P300-based ERP recordings of 73 participants: 42 healthy controls and 31 individuals diagnosed with amyotrophic lateral sclerosis (ALS) or other severe motor disabilities [17]. EEG was recorded using 16 active electrodes placed according to the 10 – 20 system at a 256 Hz sampling rate. Stimuli were presented using a 6×6 visual speller matrix, where target and non-target flashes elicited ERP responses, particularly the P300 component. Data are organized into session files containing preprocessed epochs labeled as target (class 1) or non-target (class 0).
CBCIC Stroke Dataset (D2): This dataset contains EEG recordings from 10 hemiparetic stroke patients without prior BCI experience [27]. EEG was recorded using 12 electrodes at a 512 Hz sampling rate. Each subject performed 120 motor imagery trials, where they imagined moving either the left or right hand. Of these, 80 trials were used for training and 40 trials for evaluation. The recorded channels included F3, FC3, C3, CP3, P3, FCz, CPz, F4, FC4, C4, CP4, and P4. Each trial contained 4096 samples (8 s × 512 Hz).

2.2 Data Preprocessing

For dataset D1 has a shape of (701615, 128, 8), for 73 subjects indicating that there are 701,615 ERP samples, each consisting of 128 time steps recorded from 8 EEG channels. The labels have a shape of (701615,), meaning each ERP sample corresponds to a binary classification label (target or non-target). For a single subject, the dataset D2 has a shape of (40, 12, 4096), where: total number of trials = 40, number of EEG channels recorded per trial = 12, and number of time samples per channel =4096 in each trial, with sampling rate at 512 Hz. When EEG data from 10 subjects are combined for model training, the total dataset consists of 400 trials with a final combined shape of (400, 12, 4096) and a label vector of (400,). For both datasets raw EEG trials were standardized per channel using Z-score normalization, ensuring zero mean and unit variance. These features are fed into the feature extraction stage.

2.3 Federated Deep Autoencoder-Based Feature Extraction

After data preprocessing, the next stage is feature extraction. Feature extraction was conducted through a federated deep autoencoder (FedAutoencode). The t-sne visualization of the extracted features for both datasets is shown in Fig. 2. The steps are as follows:

- Local Training: EEG data was distributed among simulated clients. For the CBCIC dataset and the GIB-UVA dataset, each subject corresponded to a client. Each client trains a deep autoencoder locally to extract low-dimensional latent features from raw EEG signals. This process ensures that

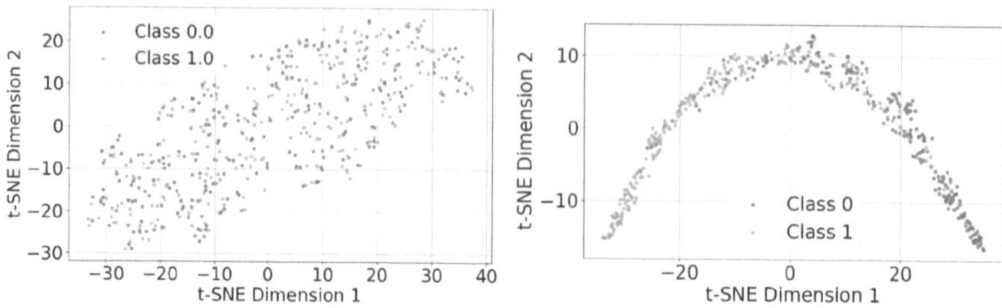

Fig. 2. t-SNE visualization of FedDeepAutoCloAk, for datasets a) D1 (left) and b) D2 (right).

raw EEG data never leave the client device.

- Share of secure models: After learning local features, only the parameters of the autoencoder model are encrypted and transmitted to the central server.
- Global Aggregation: A secure global model was computed using FedAvg, integrating all client-side updates without exposing raw EEG signals.

2.4 Cluster-Based Feature Aggregation

After feature extraction, the framework applies KMeans clustering to improve personalization and reduce inter-subject variability. KMeans clustering was applied locally in each client to group trials into clusters of similar neurophysiological patterns. The EEG embeddings of each subject were first projected into a lower-dimensional feature space, where clustering was performed to identify meaningful structures in the data. The optimal number of clusters (k) was chosen to match the number of MI or ERP task classes (e.g., k = 2 or 3 depending on the dataset), ensuring both interpretability and task-relevance. To secure cluster-level information, all KMeans centroids were encrypted using the CKKS based HE scheme implemented via TenSEAL.

2.5 Privacy-Preserving Secure Aggregation

The CKKS-based HE implemented via TenSEAL was applied after feature extraction and clustering but before sending updates to the server. This protects against privacy threats such as gradient inversion and membership inference. Despite encryption overhead, model sizes remained computationally feasible (e.g., D1: 1.03 to 1.55 MB and D2: 49.8 to 74.8MB).

2.6 Federated Model Training and Classification

After secure aggregation, encrypted updates are then transmitted to the central server, where FedAvg is used to aggregate client-side models into a single global model without accessing individual-level raw data. Once the global model is updated, it is redistributed back to each client for local fine-tuning and classification. This iterative process continues until convergence. The classification of EEG signals is then performed using three popular deep learning architectures: ShallowNet (lightweight and fast), EEGNet (moderate depth and generalization), and DeepConvNet (deeper with stronger representational power) [13, 18]. We compared FedDeepAutoCloAk with a centralized baseline using 5-fold cross-validation and ten iterations with 50 epochs [23]. Performance metrics included accuracy, standard deviation, information loss, and convergence curve [7]. Hyper-parameters were empirically tuned per data set, with learning rates of 1e-3 and early stopping to prevent overfitting.

3 Results

This study proposes a FedDeepAutoCloAk-based network model for classifying post-stroke MI and ERP based EEG signals. Research focuses on improving classification accuracy while minimizing information loss and strengthening privacy preservation of stroke patient data. To achieve this, the framework first applied FL and then CKKS of HE to encrypt both model updates and cluster centroids before transmission to the server, enabling secure aggregation without exposing sensitive data or intermediate representations. Within this encrypted federated environment, three deep learning classifiers are trained on clustered features to improve MI and ERP classification performance.

Table 1 presents the overall classification accuracy and standard deviation of three deep learning models under the proposed framework and a traditional cen-

Table 1. Overall accuracy (%) and standard deviation (Std.) of three deep learning models under the proposed FedDeepAutoCloAk and centralized frameworks across two EEG datasets.

Dataset	Framework	Model	Accuracy (%)	Std.
D1	FedDeepAutoCloAk	ShallowNet	83.40	1.13
		EEGNet	83.17	1.07
		DeepConvNet	81.87	0.90
	Centralized	ShallowNet	82.90	0.03
		EEGNet	82.00	0.02
		DeepConvNet	82.80	0.01
D2	FedDeepAutoCloAk	ShallowNet	63.18	8.53
		EEGNet	60.79	6.63
		DeepConvNet	61.78	8.28
	Centralized	ShallowNet	63.00	2.57
		EEGNet	51.50	4.83
		DeepConvNet	61.50	6.19

tralized framework in two EEG datasets, D1 (ERP dataset) and D2 (MI dataset). For data set D1, the FedDeepAutoCloAk + ShallowNet model achieved the highest accuracy of 83.40% (± 1.13), outperforming EEGNet (83.17% ± 1.07) and DeepConvNet (81.87% ± 0.90) within the same framework. This represents an improvement of 0.23% over EEGNet and 1.53% over DeepConvNet. Compared to the centralized configuration, where ShallowNet reached 82.90% (± 0.03), FedDeepAutoCloAk achieved a modest 0.5% increase in mean accuracy, confirming that privacy preservation did not compromise performance. For data set D2, FedDeepAutoCloAk + ShallowNet again performed the best among the federated models, reaching 63.18% (± 8.53), slightly higher than EEGNet (60.79% ± 6.63) and DeepConvNet (61.78% ± 8.28), an improvement of 2.39% and 1.40%, respectively. Although the gain over the centralized ShallowNet (63.00% ± 2.57) was only 0.18%, this configuration demonstrated strong generalization with higher variability due to client diversity. In general, FedDeepAutoCloAk + ShallowNet consistently outperformed the other classifiers in both datasets, showing that the proposed federated framework improves accuracy while maintaining privacy in decentralized EEG learning.

Table 2 presents the classification performance and information loss of the proposed FedDeepAutoCloAk framework in three deep learning models of ShallowNet, EEGNet and DeepConvNet over the first ten training iterations for both datasets. Across ten iterations, FedDeepAutoCloAk + ShallowNet consistently achieved the highest and most stable performance on both datasets. For D1, ShallowNet reached an accuracy of 83.40% ± 0.03, surpassing EEGNet (83.17% ± 0.03) by 0.23% and DeepConvNet (81.87% ± 0.03) by 1.53%, while maintaining the same low information loss (IL = 0.16). For D2, ShallowNet reached the highest accuracy of 64.24% ± 6.37, outperforming EEGNet (61.15% ± 9.04) by 3.09% and DeepConvNet (61.12% ± 10.36) by 3.12%, with the lowest IL (0.35). These results demonstrate that ShallowNet provides the best balance between accuracy, stability, and privacy preservation within the FedDeepAutoCloAk framework, outperforming the other models across both datasets.

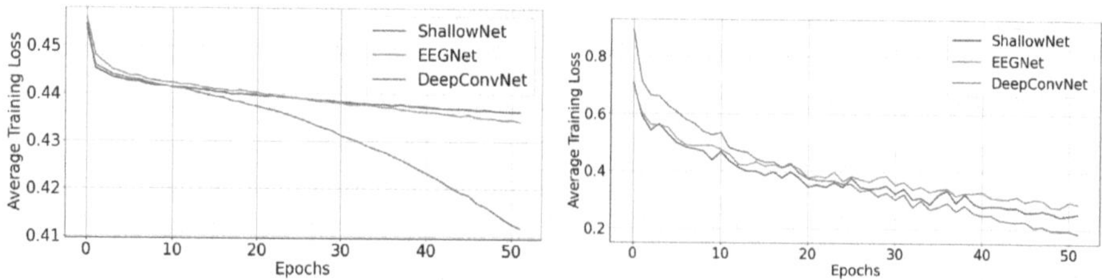

Fig. 3. Convergence graph of three classifiers based on training loss over 50 epochs for (a) Dataset D1 (left) and (b) Dataset D2 (right).

Figure 3 illustrates the average training loss curves for three deep learning models ShallowNet, EEGNet, and DeepConvNet under the FedDeepAutoCloAk

Table 2. Performance comparison (Accuracy ± Std.)of FedDeepAutoCloAk framework using ShallowNet, EEGNet, and DeepConvNet classifiers across 10 iterations (It) for datasets D1 and D2, along with information loss (IL).

It	Dataset	ShallowNet			EEGNet			DeepConvNet		
		Acc. (%)	± Std.	IL	Acc. (%)	± Std.	IL	Acc. (%)	± Std.	IL
1	D1	83.37	0.03	0.16	83.08	0.03	0.16	81.38	0.03	0.16
	D2	58.03	9.50	0.41	55.98	9.96	0.44	47.72	11.00	0.52
2	D1	83.37	0.03	0.16	83.11	0.03	0.16	81.38	0.03	0.16
	D2	58.90	6.79	0.41	55.41	6.92	0.44	47.07	8.60	0.52
3	D1	83.38	0.03	0.16	83.38	0.03	0.16	83.38	0.03	0.16
	D2	58.14	6.17	0.41	55.63	7.09	0.44	52.25	10.72	0.47
4	D1	83.37	0.03	0.16	83.05	0.03	0.16	81.38	0.03	0.16
	D2	58.85	7.60	0.41	58.82	9.13	0.41	57.41	8.12	0.42
5	D1	83.37	0.03	0.16	83.00	0.03	0.16	81.38	0.03	0.16
	D2	59.24	7.52	0.40	60.46	8.79	0.39	55.75	9.26	0.44
6	D1	83.38	0.03	0.16	83.09	0.03	0.16	81.38	0.03	0.16
	D2	57.97	6.28	0.42	59.14	9.96	0.40	54.74	9.17	0.45
7	D1	83.37	0.03	0.16	83.16	0.03	0.16	81.38	0.03	0.16
	D2	57.17	5.91	0.42	56.10	5.50	0.43	57.46	9.78	0.42
8	D1	83.37	0.03	0.16	83.03	0.03	0.16	81.38	0.03	0.16
	D2	60.89	6.75	0.39	58.95	7.13	0.41	58.87	9.70	0.41
9	D1	83.36	0.03	0.16	83.08	0.03	0.16	81.38	0.03	0.16
	D2	61.02	5.09	0.38	62.23	10.00	0.37	59.68	9.57	0.40
10	D1	83.40	0.03	0.16	83.17	0.03	0.16	81.87	0.03	0.16
	D2	64.24	6.37	0.35	61.15	9.04	0.38	61.12	10.36	0.38

framework over 50 training epochs, comparing data set D1 (ERP based EEG, left) and data set D2 (MI based EEG, right). In the convergence analysis, DeepConvNet showed the fastest convergence and the lowest training loss on D1 (ERP dataset), while ShallowNet achieved superior performance on D2 (MI dataset) with smoother and more stable loss reduction. EEGNet demonstrated balanced but comparatively moderate performance in both datasets.

4 Discussion

This study introduces FedDeepAutoCloAk, a new privacy-preserving federated learning framework that integrates deep autoencoder-based unsupervised feature extraction, KMeans cluster optimization, and adaptive knowledge protection for robust EEG classification. Compared to conventional centralized training, FedDeepAutoCloAk maintained or improved classification accuracy, particularly when paired with ShallowNet. ShallowNet consistently achieved the highest accuracy, 83.40% for D1 and 60.79% for D2, while preserving low variability and minimizing information loss. Although DeepConvNet demonstrated strong ERP decoding capabilities and EEGNet showed stable generalization, none matched the robustness of ShallowNet. The use of KMeans clustering helped mitigate inter-subject variability, and CKKS-based homomorphic encryption ensured that model updates remained secure during aggregation. Furthermore, convergence analysis confirmed that ShallowNet is a stable learning dynamics, with smoother and faster loss reduction across datasets. Collectively, these findings indicate that FedDeepAutoCloAk-ShallowNet is a scalable and secure solution for collaborative EEG research in clinical neurorehabilitation. To our knowledge, no existing study has reported comparable performance in the two post-stroke EEG datasets: D1 (ERP-based EEG) and D2 (MI-based EEG), while preserving privacy, limiting direct comparisons with state-of-the-art methods.

5 Conclusion

This study introduced FedDeepAutoCloAk, a novel privacy-preserving federated learning framework for EEG-based BCI applications. By integrating deep autoencoder-based feature extraction, KMeans-driven representation optimization, and homomorphic encryption, the framework enables secure and collaborative model training without sharing raw EEG data. Experimental results in two benchmark datasets demonstrate that FedDeepAutoCloAk combined with ShallowNet consistently achieves the highest accuracy and stability compared to EEGNet and DeepConvNet, while maintaining minimal information loss. This finding demonstrates the potential of FedDeepAutoCloAk to enable secure, scalable, and efficient EEG classification without compromising data privacy, providing significant advances for clinical and real-time BCI applications. Future work will explore extending the framework to cross-dataset generalization, multimodal EEG fusion, and adaptive privacy mechanisms to further enhance performance in real-world BCI applications.

References

1. Ahmed, S.F.B., et al.: Recent trends in eeg-based p300, neuromarketing, and e-sports brain-computer interface applications. Adv. Electr. Anal. Methods, 1st Edition, 282 (2024)
2. Alvi, A.M., Siuly, S., Wang, H.: Neurological abnormality detection from electroencephalography data: a review. Artif. Intell. Rev. **55**(3), 2275–2312 (2022)
3. Cha, D., Sung, M., Park, Y.R., et al.: Implementing vertical federated learning using autoencoders: practical application, generalizability, and utility study. JMIR Med. Inform. **9**(6), e26598 (2021)
4. Dharia, S.Y.: Advancing EEG-Based Emotion Recognition: Multimodal Techniques, Channel Optimization, and Insights into Subjective Emotion Perception. Ph.D. thesis, University of Winnipeg (2024)
5. Jahan, S., Ge, Y.F., Wang, H., Kabir, E.: Adaptive-parameter memetic algorithm for privacy-preserving trajectory data publishing: A multi-objective optimization approach: S. jahan et al. Computing **107**(7), 151 (2025)

6. Kairouz, P., McMahan, H.B., Avent, B., Bellet, A., Bennis, M., Bhagoji, A.N., et al.: Advances and open problems in federated learning. Found. Trends® Mach. Learn. **14**(1-2), 1–210 (2021)
7. Khanam, T., Siuly, S., Wang, K., Wang, H.: Based-bci technology. In: Health Information Science: 13th International Conference, HIS 2024, Hong Kong, China, December 8–10, 2024, Proceedings. Springer Nature (2025)
8. Khanam, T., Siuly, S., Wang, H.: Analysing big brain signal data for advanced brain computer interface system. In: Australasian Database Conference, pp. 103–114. Springer (2022)
9. Khanam, T., Siuly, S., Wang, H.: An optimized artificial intelligence based technique for identifying motor imagery from EEGS for advanced brain computer interface technology. Neural Comput. Appl. **35**(9), 6623–6634 (2023)
10. Khanam, T., Siuly, S., Wang, K., Wang, H.: An AI driven framework for EEG based-BCI technology. In: International Conference on Health Information Science, pp. 209–220. Springer (2025)
11. Khanam, T., Siuly, S., Wang, K., Zheng, Z.: A privacy-preserving encryption framework for big data analysis. In: International Conference on Web Information Systems Engineering, pp. 84–94. Springer (2024)
12. Khanam, T., Siuly[1], S., Wang, K., Wang, H.: Based-BCI technology. In: Health Information Science: 13th International Conference, HIS 2024, Hong Kong, China, December 8–10, 2024, Proceedings. vol. 15336, p. 209. Springer Nature (2025)
13. Lawhern, V.J., Solon, A.J., Waytowich, N.R., Gordon, S.M., Hung, C.P., Lance, B.J.: Eegnet: A compact convolutional neural network for EEG-based brain–computer interfaces. J. Neural Eng. **15**(5), 056013 (2018)
14. Li, X., Jiang, M., Zhang, X., Kamp, M., Dou, Q.: Fedbn: Federated learning on non-iid features via local batch normalization. arXiv preprint arXiv:2102.07623 (2021)
15. Liu, X.H., Lu, B.L., Zheng, W.L.: mixeeg: Enhancing eeg federated learning for cross-subject eeg classification with tailored mixup. arXiv preprint arXiv:2504.07987 (2025)
16. Sadiq, M.T., Siuly, S., Li, Y., Wen, P.: A comprehensive approach for enhancing motor imagery eeg classification in bci's. In: International Conference on Health Information Science, pp. 247–260. Springer (2023)
17. Santamaria-Vazquez, E., Martinez-Cagigal, V., Vaquerizo-Villar, F., Hornero, R.: Eeg-inception: a novel deep convolutional neural network for assistive erp-based brain-computer interfaces. IEEE Trans. Neural Syst. Rehabil. Eng. **28**(12), 2773–2782 (2020)
18. Schirrmeister, R.T., et al.: Deep learning with convolutional neural networks for EEG decoding and visualization. Hum. Brain Mapp. **38**(11), 5391–5420 (2017)
19. Shahid, J., Ahmad, R., Kiani, A.K., Ahmad, T., Saeed, S., Almuhaideb, A.M.: Data protection and privacy of the internet of healthcare things (iohts). Appl. Sci. **12**(4), 1927 (2022)
20. Siuly, Li, Y., Wen, P.: Identification of motor imagery tasks through cc–lr algorithm in brain computer interface. Int. J. Bioinform. Res. Appl. **9**(2), 156–172 (2013)
21. Siuly, S., Li, Y.: Discriminating the brain activities for brain-computer interface applications through the optimal allocation-based approach. Neural Comput. Appl. **26**(4), 799–811 (2015)
22. Siuly, S., Li, Y., Zhang, Y.: Eeg signal analysis and classification. IEEE Trans Neural Syst Rehabilit Eng **11**, 141–144 (2016)

23. Siuly, S., Li, Y., Zhang, Y.: Improving prospective performance in mi recognition: Ls-svm with tuning hyper parameters. In: EEG Signal Analysis and Classification: Techniques and Applications, pp. 189–209. Springer (2017)
24. Sun, T., Li, D., Wang, B.: Decentralized federated averaging. IEEE Trans. Pattern Anal. Mach. Intell. **45**(4), 4289–4301 (2022)
25. Tawhid, M.N.A., Siuly, S., Kabir, E., Li, Y.: Exploring frequency band-based biomarkers of EEG signals for mild cognitive impairment detection. IEEE Trans. Neural Syst. Rehabil. Eng. **32**, 189–199 (2023)
26. Tawhid, M.N.A., Siuly, S., Li, T.: A convolutional long short-term memory-based neural network for epilepsy detection from EEG. IEEE Trans. Instrum. Meas. **71**, 1–11 (2022)
27. Wu, H., et al.: Online privacy-preserving EEG classification by source-free transfer learning. IEEE Trans. Neural Syst. Rehabil. Eng. (2024)

AI-Powered Ergonomic Innovation to Improve Workplace Wellbeing and Productivity

Eka Prita Yuliatin[1(✉)] and Rienna Oktarina[2]

[1] Industrial Engineering Department, Binus Graduate Program-Master of Industrial Engineering, Bina Nusantara University, Jakarta 11480, Indonesia
eka.yuliatin@binus.ac.id

[2] Industrial Engineering Department, Faculty of Engineering, Bina Nusantara University, Jakarta, Indonesia

Abstract. Workplace ergonomics plays a crucial role in maintaining productivity and preventing musculoskeletal disorders (MSDs), which remain among the most common occupational health issues in manufacturing environments. At PT. X, a large-scale automotive manufacturing company in Indonesia, clinic data indicated that prior to 2022, the monthly average of visits related to fatigue and posture related complaints reached 434 cases. Following the implementation of an AI-powered ergonomic evaluation system in 2023, this number decreased significantly to 91 cases per month. The system was developed to automate posture assessment using computer-vision techniques, integrating Open Pose for human-pose estimation and a proprietary classification algorithm derived from the internal TEBA (T-Ergonomic Burden Assessment) framework, which references RULA and REBA standards. A pilot study was carried out at a standing assembly workstation using fixed and movable webcams to capture operator movements in real time without interrupting production. The AI model classified postures into ergonomic risk categories and automatically generated summary reports after each observation. Implementation results demonstrated measurable improvements: average evaluation time per operator decreased from 30 to 6 min (a 60% productivity increase), and indirect ergonomic related costs were reduced by 83%. The notable decline in MSD-related clinic visits also reflected tangible improvements in workplace well-being. These findings confirm that integrating AI into ergonomic evaluation not only increases operational efficiency but also advances human-centered digital transformation aligned with Industry 4.0 principles.

Keywords: Artificial Intelligence · Ergonomic Assessment · Manufacturing Innovation

1 Introduction

The Fourth Industrial Revolution (Industry 4.0) integrates Artificial Intelligence (AI), cyber-physical systems, and the Internet of Things (IoT) to enable intelligent automation and flexible, data driven production [1, 2]. Among these technologies, AI has become a key enabler of predictive maintenance, process optimization, and real-time decision

E. R. Kaburuan and S. Goundar (Eds.): HIS 2025, LNCS 16392, pp. 191–202, 2026.
https://doi.org/10.1007/978-981-95-6304-3_17

support [3, 4]. As automation advances, the human centered aspect of Industry 4.0 particularly occupational safety and ergonomics remains critical. Musculoskeletal disorders (MSDs) are among the most common causes of work related illness and absenteeism in labor-intensive industries [5, 6]. Effective ergonomic design helps prevent injuries and enhances worker satisfaction and productivity [7, 8].

At PT. X, internal clinic data showed increasing visits related to muscle pain and fatigue, often caused by repetitive motions and awkward standing postures. Figure 1 illustrates that in 2022, muscle pain ranked third with 252 cases (5.6%) and low back pain ranked thirteenth with 91 cases (2.1%). This trend highlighted the need for proactive ergonomic risk management. Recent advances in AI-based computer vision, such as Open Pose and YOLOv8, enable real-time posture detection from video input without wearable sensors [9, 10]. This study explores how AI can automate posture assessment aligned with PT. X's internal framework to promote human-centered and sustainable manufacturing.

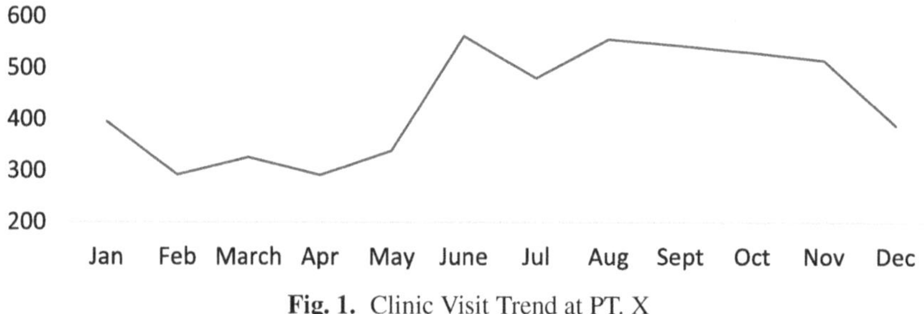

Fig. 1. Clinic Visit Trend at PT. X

According to OSH (Occupational Safety and Health) Academy, five major ergonomic risk factors: repetition, awkward posture, vibration, force, and contact stress are key contributors to MSD development [5]. To manage these risks, PT. X has established a structured shop floor management system that integrates safety and ergonomic observations into daily operations. For ergonomic evaluation, the company applies two standardized tools: TEBA (T-Ergonomic Burden Assessment), focusing on posture related risks, and MEBA (Material Handling Burden Assessment), assessing risks related to manual load handling. These tools were developed through internal ergonomic training and benchmarking against international standards such as RULA (Rapid Upper Limb Assessment) and REBA (Rapid Entire Body Assessment) [9, 10]. Figure 2 illustrates posture categories and risk levels within the TEBA framework.

The structured TEBA approach ensures that ergonomic risks are consistently identified and quantified. Figure 3 presents the TEBA ergonomic assessment sheet used by line supervisors to document posture observations. However, this method is resource intensive and time consuming. A time study showed that a single workstation evaluation could take more than 30 min, resulting in an estimated 392.5 h of manual assessment per month.

To overcome these challenges, PT. X explored AI as an enabler for automation in ergonomic risk evaluation. Computer vision techniques, such as Open Pose and YOLOv8, allow accurate human pose estimation and object detection using standard

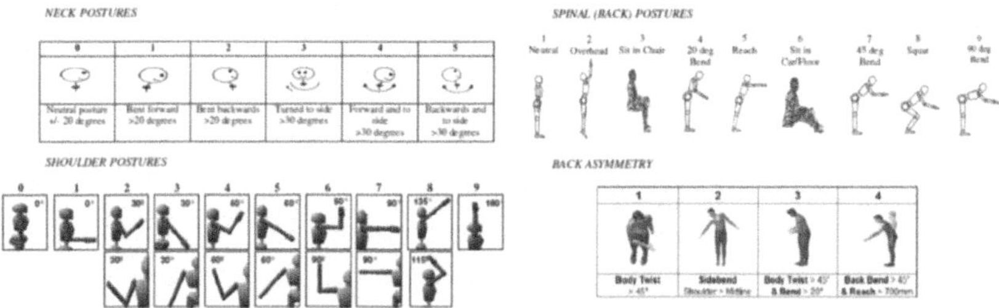

Fig. 2. TEBA Posture Chart

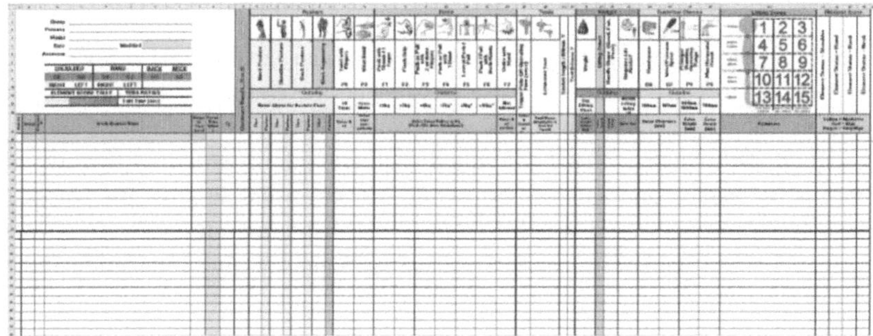

Fig. 3. TEBA ergonomic assessment sheet

video input without wearable sensors [11, 12]. The purpose of this study is to investigate how AI can be utilized to automate posture assessment while maintaining compliance with the internal TEBA framework. This research contributes to the growing field of human centered AI by demonstrating how digital tools can enhance worker safety and well-being while improving efficiency [13, 14]. The study aims to bridge the gap between technology and ergonomics in the journey toward sustainable, data driven manufacturing.

2 Literature Review

2.1 Industry 4.0 and Manufacturing Transformation

The concept of Industry 4.0 represents the integration of digital and physical systems through technologies such as the Internet of Things (IoT), cyber-physical systems, big data analytics, and Artificial Intelligence (AI). These technologies enable smart factories that are interconnected, flexible, and data-driven [1, 2]. Research has shown that Industry 4.0 enhances operational efficiency while promoting sustainability and adaptability in dynamic industrial contexts [3, 10]. In manufacturing, it serves as a key driver of competitive advantage, improving productivity, reducing downtime, and enhancing decision making through predictive insights [11]. However, successful implementation requires balancing technological innovation with human adaptability [12]. Beyond operational improvements, the digital transformation of manufacturing is also linked to the broader phenomenon of digital globalization, where data flows and interconnected systems redefine competitiveness and innovation dynamics across industries [19].

2.2 Artificial Intelligence and Industrial Performance

Artificial Intelligence (AI) plays a pivotal role within Industry 4.0 by enabling intelligent automation, predictive maintenance, and process optimization. AI-driven systems support data driven decision making and improve industrial performance when strategically aligned with organizational goals [4]. Kamble et al. [3] highlight that AI integration complements lean manufacturing practices, promoting sustainable performance. However, human involvement remains crucial technology serves as an enabler, not a replacement, for human judgment and experience in industrial operations [12].

2.3 Ergonomics and Occupational Health

Ergonomics focuses on aligning work systems with human capabilities to prevent injuries and improve performance. Studies consistently link poor ergonomics with musculoskeletal disorders (MSDs), which remain a leading cause of work-related illness and absenteeism [5, 6]. Koirala and Nepal [5] noted that ergonomic practices directly affect employee performance and satisfaction, while Marková and Prajová [6] emphasized that quantifying physical burden helps identify high risk tasks in production. Despite advancements, traditional observation-based assessments are time consuming and often subjective [7].

2.4 Ergonomic Risk Assessment Standards (RULA, REBA, and Internal Frameworks)

Standardized ergonomic evaluation methods such as RULA (Rapid Upper Limb Assessment) and REBA (Rapid Entire Body Assessment) are widely adopted to assess posture-related risks [8, 9]. Many manufacturing companies, including PT. X, have developed internal frameworks referencing these standards. PT. X's TEBA (T-Ergonomic Burden Assessment) and MEBA (Material Handling Burden Assessment) frameworks ensure consistent evaluation of posture and material-handling risks through structured, quantitative scoring aligned with international best practices.

2.5 Digital Ergonomics and AI-Based Assessment

Recent studies highlight a shift toward digital ergonomics, where AI and computer vision enhance the precision and scalability of ergonomic evaluations. Tirupachuri et al. [8] developed a real-time ergonomics assessment system using stress and payload data, while Ahmad and Kim [9] implemented an AI-based posture recognition system combining Open Pose with RULA scoring. Li et al. [12] and Kang and Park [13] demonstrated that AI can perform accurate, contactless posture evaluations in real industrial settings. However, challenges remain in ensuring data privacy, adaptability, and user acceptance [10, 11]. Recent works also underline that the adoption of data-driven ergonomics enables continuous workplace monitoring and safety improvement through AI-assisted analytics, reinforcing a proactive safety culture [20].

2.6 Research Gap and Contribution

Previous research has explored AI applications in manufacturing and ergonomics separately, yet few studies have integrated AI-based posture assessment within company specific ergonomic frameworks grounded in real industrial practice. Most rely solely on RULA or REBA without customization to local standards or operational constraints. This study addresses that gap by developing and testing an AI-driven ergonomic evaluation system aligned with PT. X's internal TEBA framework, combining AI based pose estimation with standardized ergonomic scoring. This approach transforms ergonomic risk evaluation from a subjective, periodic process into a data-driven, real-time assessment supporting both safety performance and workforce sustainability.

3 Methodology

This study adopts a Design Science Research (DSR) approach to develop and validate an AI-based ergonomic posture assessment system. The DSR framework was chosen because it emphasizes problem solving through the creation and evaluation of an artifact in this case, an intelligent ergonomic monitoring tool applied in a real manufacturing environment [1, 2]. Unlike conventional methods relying on manual observation or wearable sensors, the proposed system integrates pose estimation and object detection using standard cameras, providing a lightweight and scalable solution while preserving data confidentiality and operational efficiency.

3.1 Problem Identification and Context

The study was conducted at PT. X, a large scale automotive manufacturing company engaged in casting, machining, and assembly processes. Operators perform standing tasks involving repetitive actions such as component fitting, tightening, and part handling. Internal clinic data revealed increasing musculoskeletal complaints, particularly in the shoulder and lower back, typical of static or awkward postures. Manual assessments using the T-Ergonomic Burden Assessment (TEBA) adapted from RULA and REBA, required approximately 30 min per workstation, accumulating around 392.5 h monthly across all lines. The process was labor intensive and prone to observer bias, reinforcing the need for an objective, efficient, and data-driven approach.

3.2 System Design and Development

The AI-based ergonomic system automates posture evaluation through three core modules:

Pose Detection Module: Built on the Open Pose framework, it extracts 18 skeletal key points from live video input. To maintain confidentiality, fixed webcams were used instead of mobile devices to prevent unauthorized data transfer.

Posture Classification Algorithm: A custom algorithm classifies postures into low, moderate, or high risk levels using thresholds derived from internal TEBA scoring.

Visualization Dashboard: Developed in Python and integrated with Open Pose and YOLOv8, the web based dashboard visualizes posture status and generates automated reports for supervisors. The system operates locally without wearable sensors, minimizing disruption to production. The overall architecture is presented in Fig. 4.

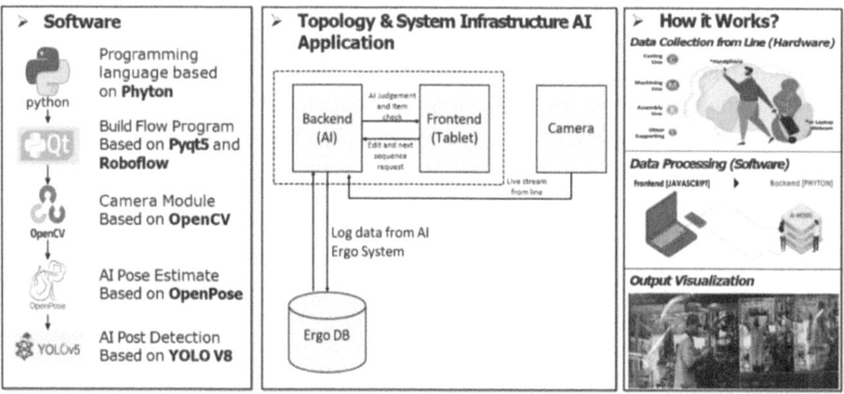

Fig. 4. AI Ergonomic System Architecture

3.3 Pilot Implementation

A pilot was conducted at a standing assembly workstation characterized by repetitive bending and twisting. Movable camera equipment allowed flexible setup without halting production. The system processed live video to identify operator postures, providing real time color coded visualization: green for acceptable, yellow for moderate, and red for high risk postures. After each session, the system automatically generated a summary highlighting unsafe positions, supporting immediate feedback and corrective action discussions. The user interface output is shown in Fig. 5.

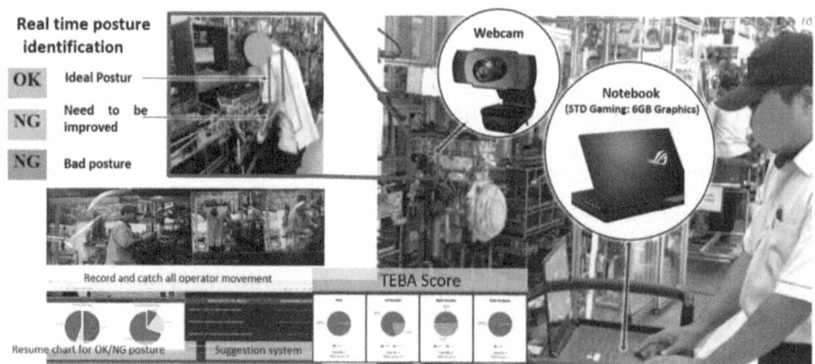

Fig. 5. AI Ergonomic user interface

The pilot demonstrated efficiency gains: average assessment time was reduced from 30 to 6 min per operator, improving productivity by 60%. Additionally, indirect ergonomic related costs including medical treatment, absenteeism, and overtime coverage declined by approximately 83% over a three-month observation period.

3.4 User Acceptance and Ethical Consideration

User feedback indicated strong acceptance among both operators and supervisors. Supervisors appreciated the consistent and objective analysis, while operators favored the non-intrusive setup without wearable sensors. To address privacy concerns, all data collection was limited to scheduled observation sessions using movable webcams. Video processing occurred entirely within the company's internal network, with anonymized posture data retained solely for ergonomic improvement purposes. No cloud storage or external data transmission was involved, ensuring ethical compliance and worker trust.

3.5 Evaluation and Scalability

Performance testing using Apache JMeter simulated 100 concurrent dashboard users, confirming system stability and responsiveness (Fig. 6). The system achieved an average response time of 1.35 s, well within the 3-s threshold.

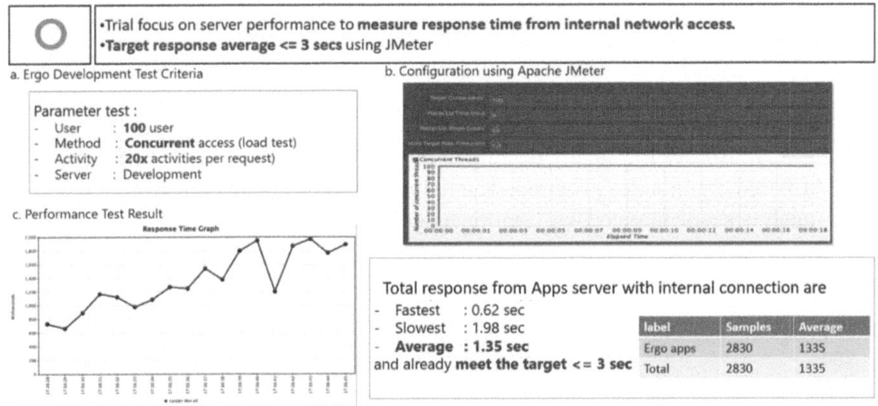

Fig. 6. System Test

Although piloted at a single workstation, the modular design supports future scalability across production areas and integration with broader digital safety dashboards for predictive ergonomic monitoring.

4 Result and Discussion

4.1 Operational Performance Improvement

The implementation of the AI-based ergonomic posture assessment system significantly improved efficiency and data consistency. Before deployment, each TEBA-based ergonomic evaluation required around 30 min per operator. After automation, the same task was completed in under 6 min, representing a 60–80% reduction in evaluation time. This gain resulted from automatic posture detection, risk classification, and digital reporting, eliminating manual form filling and assessor variation. Table 1 summarizes the improvement across operational and health indicators.

Table 1. Operational and Health Impact of AI-based Ergonomic System

Indicator	Before	After	Improvement
Average time per ergonomic assessment	30 min	6 min	↓ 80%
Workstations evaluated per month	40	120	↑ 200%
Clinic visits related to MSD cases (average/month)	434	91	↓ 63,9%
MSD rank among top 10 clinic cases	Ranked #3	Ranked#13	Eliminated
Indirect ergonomic-related costs (absenteeism, overtime, treatment)	Baseline 100%	17% of baseline	↓ 83%

Figure 7 illustrates the steady decline in monthly clinic visits after the introduction of the AI-based ergonomics program. The reduction confirms that integrating real-time posture analytics with targeted workstation redesign effectively enhances employee well-being and lowers work-related health incidents.

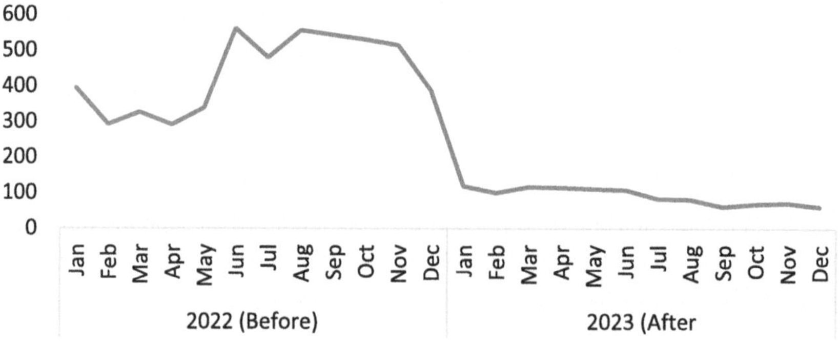

Fig. 7. Clinic Visit Trend at PT. X after Ergonomy Improvement

4.2 Ergonomic Risk Detection and Corrective Action

The AI-based ergonomic system provides real-time visual feedback through a color-coded skeletal overlay on the operator's body. Green indicates an acceptable posture (OK), yellow signals a moderate risk posture requiring improvement, and red highlights a high risk or poor posture. Throughout the observation, these visual cues allow both operators and supervisors to instantly recognize postural deviations during work activities. At the end of each session, the system automatically generates a summary report and stores the analyzed video data within the internal network. This summary highlights the frequency and type of postures observed, serving as a trigger for workplace improvement actions. Operators and team leaders can review these results together to evaluate workstation conditions and identify ergonomic improvement needs. For instance, equipment adjustments were made to match operator anthropometry, such as height, reach distance, and working angles, resulting in the design of adjustable jigs and fixtures that better accommodate diverse body dimensions. This data driven approach enabled multiple local improvements across different posts, fostering a massive ergonomic enhancement initiative that improved comfort, safety, and overall workplace wellbeing.

4.3 Health and Safety Impact

Beyond efficiency, the system delivered measurable health benefits. Average monthly clinic visits related to MSDs dropped from 434 to 91, and MSD-related complaints were no longer among the top 10 causes of medical visits. Supervisors reported greater awareness of ergonomic hazards, while operators demonstrated improved posture habits after repeated AI-based feedback. These findings echo Wamba-Taguimdje et al. [12] and Kamble et al. [3], who emphasize that successful Industry 4.0 initiatives align technological innovation with human sustainability and safety.

4.4 Discussion

This study confirms that AI-enabled ergonomics transforms evaluation from a subjective, periodic task into a real-time, data-driven process. Automation ensures objectivity, reduces assessor bias, and maintains compliance with internal TEBA standards, ensuring compatibility with existing factory routines. The intuitive visualization also encourages collaboration between supervisors and operators, fostering a culture of shared responsibility for safety. Although the pilot covered only one standing assembly line, the system's modular architecture supports scaling to other production areas and integration into broader digital safety dashboards. Future development will extend analytics to predict posture risk trends and link AI results with productivity metrics, reinforcing the company's progress toward Industry 4.0 maturity and sustainable human-centered manufacturing.

5 Conclusion and Recommendation

This study developed and validated an AI-powered ergonomic assessment system to improve posture evaluation efficiency and workplace wellbeing in a real manufacturing environment. The system integrates Open Pose based pose estimation and custom classification logic derived from the internal TEBA framework, enabling real time, objective, and non-intrusive ergonomic assessments using standard cameras. The implementation at PT. X, a large-scale automotive manufacturer in Indonesia, demonstrated measurable improvements. The average assessment time decreased from 30 to 6 min per operator, while clinic visits related to musculoskeletal disorders dropped from an average of 434 to 91 cases per month, effectively removing MSDs from the company's top-ten health issues. In addition, indirect ergonomic-related costs decreased by 83%, and 72% of previously high-risk postures were reclassified as acceptable after targeted workplace adjustments. Beyond operational gains, this research highlights how AI-based ergonomics can strengthen human centered manufacturing by turning subjective evaluations into data driven insights. The system empowered operators and supervisors to visualize posture risks, initiate real-time corrective actions, and collaborate on equipment design improvements such as adjustable jigs and workstation layouts. In essence, this study demonstrates that integrating AI into ergonomic management not only enhances productivity and safety but also promotes a culture of continuous improvement aligned with Industry 4.0 maturity goals. Future work will focus on expanding the model to multi-station monitoring, dynamic load analysis, and integration with predictive analytics dashboards to support sustainable, data-driven occupational health management.

Acknowledgments. The authors would like to express their gratitude to the industrial partner for providing access to workplace data and valuable insights during the development of the AI-based ergonomic evaluation model. The authors also appreciate the constructive feedback from academic advisors that helped refine this research.

Authors' Contributions. Eka Prita Yuliatin contributed to data collection, preprocessing, and initial manuscript drafting. Rienna Oktarina contributed to the research methodology design and manuscript review. Both authors approved the final version of the paper.

Data Availability Statement. The data supporting the findings of this study are available within this article. Additional information may be provided upon reasonable request to the corresponding author, subject to confidentiality constraints and data protection policies.

Declaration of Generative AI Use in Scientific Writing. During the preparation of this work, the authors used ChatGPT to improve the clarity and flow of the writing. After using the tool, the authors carefully reviewed, edited, and validated all content, and take full responsibility for the final version of the manuscript.

Disclosure of Interest. The authors declare that they have no conflict of interest related to the content or outcomes of this research.

References

1. Sordan, J., Oprime, P., Pimenta, M., Chiabert, P., Lombardi, F.: Industry 4.0: a bibliometric analysis in the perspective of operations management. Oper. Supply Chain Manag. **15**(2), 93–104 (2022). https://doi.org/10.31387/oscm0480333
2. Dalenogare, L.S., Benitez, G.B., Ayala, N.F., Frank, A.G.: The expected contribution of industry 4.0 technologies for industrial performance. Int. J. Prod. Econ. **204**, 383–394 (2018). https://doi.org/10.1016/j.ijpe.2018.08.019
3. Kamble, S.S., Gunasekaran, A., Dhone, N.C.: Industry 4.0 and lean manufacturing practices for sustainable organizational performance in Indian manufacturing companies. Int. J. Prod. Res. **58**(5), 1319–1337 (2019). https://doi.org/10.1080/00207543.2019.1630772
4. Wamba-Taguimdje, S.L., Wamba, S.F., Kamdjoug, J.R.K., Wanko, C.E.T.: Influence of artificial intelligence (AI) on firm performance: the business value of AI-based transformation projects. Bus. Process. Manag. J. **26**(7), 1663–1690 (2020). https://doi.org/10.1108/BPMJ-10-2019-0411
5. Koirala, R., Nepal, A.: A literature review on ergonomics, ergonomic practices, and employee performance. Quest J. Manag. Soc. Sci. **4**(2), 273–288 (2022)
6. Marková, P., Prajová, V.: Evaluation of physical burdens of operators using ergonomics. MM Sci. J., 4872–4875 (2021). https://doi.org/10.17973/MMSJ.2021_10_2021016
7. Ahmad, T., Kim, Y.G.: Vision-based ergonomic risk assessment using OpenPose and RULA. Sci. Total. Environ. **737**, 139878 (2020). https://doi.org/10.1016/j.scitotenv.2020.139878
8. Tirupachuri, Y., et al.: Online non-collocated estimation of payload and articular stress for real-time human ergonomy assessment. IEEE Access **9**, 123260–123275 (2021). https://doi.org/10.1109/ACCESS.2021.3109238
9. Otten, L., Zhang, Z., Langer, D.: Deep learning-based posture recognition for ergonomic risk assessment in industrial workplaces. Appl. Ergon. **108**, 103941 (2023). https://doi.org/10.1016/j.apergo.2023.103941
10. Kim, H., Lee, W.: AI-powered ergonomic evaluation system using pose estimation and biomechanical metrics. Sensors **24**(3), 1152 (2024). https://doi.org/10.3390/s24031152
11. Rahman, M., Hossain, M.: Integration of computer vision and IoT for ergonomic risk detection in smart manufacturing. IEEE Access **12**, 56789–56801 (2024). https://doi.org/10.1109/ACCESS.2024.3456710
12. Li, H., Chen, Y., Zhang, Q.: AI-based real-time ergonomic risk evaluation in industrial assembly lines. Appl. Ergon. **121**, 104205 (2024). https://doi.org/10.1016/j.apergo.2024.104205
13. Kang, J., Park, S.: Human–AI collaboration for safe and smart workplaces: a review of computer vision applications. Saf. Sci. **167**, 106246 (2023). https://doi.org/10.1016/j.ssci.2023.106246
14. Ghosh, A., Sarkar, S.: A review of AI applications in occupational health and safety management. Saf. Sci. **168**, 106966 (2023). https://doi.org/10.1016/j.ssci.2023.106966
15. Nguyen, T., et al.: Human pose estimation and action recognition for real-time ergonomic monitoring in industrial environments. Rob. Comput.-Integr. Manuf. **79**, 102512 (2025). https://doi.org/10.1016/j.rcim.2025.102512
16. Binias, B., Czapla, P.: Explainable AI in ergonomic risk classification based on pose estimation. J. Manuf. Syst. **69**, 142–156 (2023). https://doi.org/10.1016/j.jmsy.2023.02.007
17. Rojas, R., Frank, A.G.: Industry 4.0 technologies for sustainable human–machine collaboration. Comput. Ind. Eng. **171**, 108397 (2022). https://doi.org/10.1016/j.cie.2022.108397
18. Park, S., Lee, J.: Digital transformation of human factors and ergonomic systems. Hum. Fact. Ergon. Manuf. **33**(2), 111–128 (2023)

19. Baldwin, R., Forslid, R.: The new globalization: going digital. Rev. World Econ. **157**, 3–28 (2021). https://doi.org/10.1007/s10290-020-00395-2
20. Maynard, A., et al.: Data-driven ergonomics: leveraging artificial intelligence for safer workplaces. Procedia Manuf. **55**, 1145–1152 (2021)

Heart Attack Prediction Using Deep Learning Methods

Ivo Herid Lesmana[1], Syarifah Diana Permai[1](✉), Jeklin Harefa[2], and Gredion Prajena[2]

[1] Statistics Department, School of Computer Science, Bina Nusantara University, Jakarta 11480, Indonesia
syarifah.permai@binus.ac.id

[2] Computer Science Department, School of Computer Science, Bina Nusantara University, Jakarta 11480, Indonesia

Abstract. Heart disease is one of the diseases known to have highest mortality rate, with estimated that one in third of death per year is caused by heart disease. Heart disease comes randomly and can't be predicted on whether a patient has a heart attack. Potential of heart attack can be predicted with analysing the health situation of the patient. This research is used to predict the heart disease potential in a patient. This research uses statistical methods, namely Logistic Regression and uses deep learning, namely Neural Network. Comparison between the two models is expected to produce the best model for predicting heart disease. In this experiment the neural network has a very high accuracy reaching from 80% to 94% with minimal loss and based on the curve of the model it does not seems to have an overfitting.

Keywords: Heart Attack · Logistic Regression · Neural Network · Deep Learning

1 Introduction

Heart disease is one of the diseases known to have highest mortality rate, with estimated that one in third of death per year is caused by heart disease. Heart Disease also known as cardiovascular disease is not an infectious disease rather, it's a chronic disease and mostly is a product of unhealthy lifestyle. Most of heart disease are caused by clogged artery caused by cholesterol, high blood sugar, and obesity. This can be prevented by having a healthier life, like exercising and eating clean and healthy [1]. However, most people are ignorant towards their potential of heart disease even if heart disease are caused by unhealthy lifestyle, heart attack can also be triggered by panic attacks and such other things, thus its attack is random and can't be predicted in the exact time. The potential of heart attack however could be predicted in a way so that it could be prevented before it even happens.

E. R. Kaburuan and S. Goundar (Eds.): HIS 2025, LNCS 16392, pp. 203–213, 2026.
https://doi.org/10.1007/978-981-95-6304-3_18

As stated before, Heart disease is one of the deadliest disease known to mankind, it is however cannot be comprehended as a commonly known disease, it is most presumably known as a medical condition or emergency in which happens when an artery is clogged overtime, resulting in the blood circulation being blocked completely, thus causing heart attack this heart disease is called Coronary Artery Disease [2]. Heart attack however while deadly, isn't always known to have a symptom. Though there are some symptoms namely: Chest Pain, Fatigue, Cold Sweat, etc. It is not guaranteed to have a symptom, or whether the symptom is caused by heart disease.

Heart Disease itself has different types, which indicates different case of disease, this type could be discovered as a result of different situations, such as coronary artery disease, which is as described before, caused by clogged artery vein, which causes malfunction in the heart and the blood circulation. There is also Congenital Heart Defects, which is a type of defect rather than a heart disease, where in this case, the patient is born with a defects in heart, this situation, means that the patient is at risk of heart attack from birth, and not caused by lifestyle [3], but is recommended to have a healthier lifestyle as to prevent from worsening the effect. The proposed Model is based of Artificial Neural Network, where it is inspired by neuron in human brains. Similar to human brain, the neurons of ANN are interconnected to one another, and the connections are similar to synapses in brains. ANN can learn representative feature automatically, this means compared to simple machine learning models such as Logistic Regression, ANN can learn important features without manual feature engineering, this advantage is caused by the neuron adjusted the weight and biases to learn the most of relevant features from the data, thus making it more non-linear [4].

There have been several research done to predict heart disease using various machine learning algorithms. This research provided results with high accuracy ranging from 70% to 90%, which even 85% should be enough for a classification. One of these results having 99% which might be a result of overfitting but might also mean a near perfect classification and are possible to be developed further [5]. Other having accuracy as low as 70% to 85% this however is caused by having tested different methods of algorithm and comparing their results [6]. Most of these research differs from the current research however as most of it is a comparison on how well an algorithm model against the particular dataset, although there are some which creates an application to diagnose heart disease, such as Heart Diseases Diagnose via Mobile Application [7] which uses heart sound as data. Which uses a different type of data altogether. The objectives of this study include: (1) to create a prediction of heart attack using neural network, (2) compare the result of Logistic Regression and Neural Network model, (3) find the most influential feature using feature importance.

2 Logistic Regression

Logistic Regression is one of the statistical methods to predict categorical variable, logistic regression is commonly used for binary classification tasks but can also be extended to multi-class classification. Unlike linear regression, which predicts continuous values, logistic regression predicts categorical outcomes. The output is a probability between 0 and 1, which can be thresholder to assign class labels (e.g., 0 or 1). Logistic regression uses the logit function (logistic function or sigmoid function) to map any real-valued input to a probability:

$$P(y = 1|X) = \frac{1}{1 + e(\beta 0 + \beta 1 * X1 + \ldots \beta \mathrm{n} * \mathrm{Xn})} \tag{1}$$

where:

- $P(y = 1|X)$ is Probability that the dependent variable y equals 1 given the input X.
- $\beta 0 \ldots \beta n$ are the coefficient during training.

Logistic Regression has a threshold for probability where if the probability is bigger than the threshold then it is considered category/class 1 [8], however there are some test needed to make sure the logistic regression model is significant and fit to the data. These tests are:

1. Simultaneous Test

This test assesses the independence of all variables in a model taken together, have a significant effect on the dependent variable. In other words, it assesses whether the entire model is statistically significant.

2. Partial Test

The tests assess the statistical significance of individual variables, this test is calculated based on the estimated coefficient, and it's standard deviation. The Partial Test essentially measures how many standard deviations the estimated parameter value (^θ) is away from the hypothesized value (θ_0). A larger value of Z indicates that the estimated value is further from the hypothesized value, suggesting stronger evidence against the null hypothesis.

3. Hosmer-Lemenshow Test

The hosmer-Lemenshow test is a statistical test used to assess the overall goodness of fit for logistic regression model. It essentially does an assessment of how well the predicted probability from LR model aligns with the actual observed outcome, in different subgroup of data [9]. It uses Chi-Square statistic to compare the observed probabilities and expected probabilities, which uses formula as

$$HLstatistics = \sum \left(\frac{(observed - expected)^2}{expected} \right) \tag{2}$$

where:

- *observed* : observed number of events
- *expected* : expected number of events (based on the logistic regression model predictions)

A significant test result indicates that the model is not a good fit, while a non-significant test result indicates a good fit. A model is considered to fit well if its value is greater than 0.05, as this means the null hypothesis is not rejected. The null hypothesis states that there is no difference between the observed and model- predicted values.

3 Artificial Neural Network

Artificial Neural Network is a method of Deep Learning which are inspired by biological neural networks or brain, where they process information through interconnected nodes, called neurons, which are inspired by neurons in brain [10]. Artificial Neural Networks is not defined by one single formula as different codes might change the Neuron Architecture in a model, thus it is highly customizable and are possible to change depending on the different parameters. As it was with a brain of different person having different sum of nodes, neurons and brain parts that might be unique on one person. The architecture of Artificial Neural networks consists of Neurons as it's main computational unit, where each Neuron receives input signals and applies transformation and produces an output, with formula of

$$y = f(\sum\nolimits_{i=1}^{n} w_i * x_i + b) \tag{3}$$

where :

- wi : weight of the connections from the input neurons
- xi : input to the neurons
- b : bias
- $f()$: activation function

ANN has 4 different Activation Function each with different formula, these Activation function are

- Sigmoid: $f(Z)\frac{1}{1+e^{z}}$
- ReLU (Rectified Linear Unit): $f(z) = \max(0, z)$
- Tanh (Hyperbolic Tangent): f$f(z) = \tanh(z)$
- Softmax : $f(z)_i = \frac{e^{z_i}}{\sum e^{z_j}}$ for I = 1, 2, … K number of classes

Ann's architecture has 3 type of neuron layers : input layer, Hidden layer, and output layer. Except for input layer, each layer has an associated weight matrix W and bias vector b, with the output layer is calculated as

$$Z = W * X + b \tag{4}$$

where:

- X is the input to the layer.
- W is weight
- b is the bias

Output layer for binary classification uses Sigmoid function, as Sigmoid function effectively maps the output of neural networks to a probability value between 0 and 1.

Ann layers follow Forward Propagation where each output of neuron in a layer is used as the input of neuron in the subsequent layer (Fig. 1).

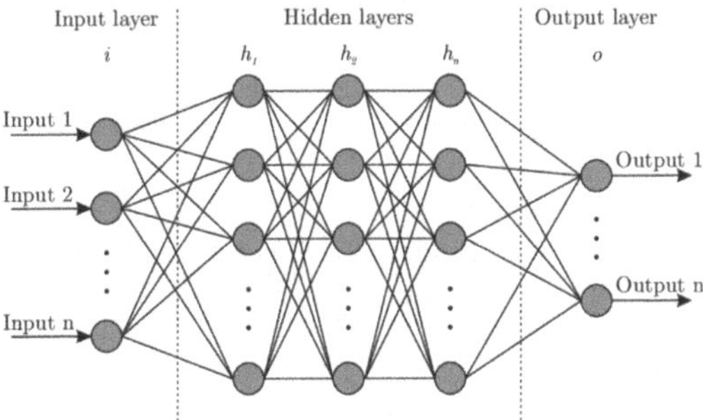

Fig. 1. ANN Architecture [11]

3.1 Loss Function

ANN has a lost function to measure between the predicted outputs and the actual outputs [12], for binary classification such that is used for this research, it uses cross-entropy loss, where it essentially measures the difference between the discovered probability distribution of a classification model and the predicted values [13].

$$L = \frac{1}{N}\sum\nolimits_{i=1}^{N} (y_i \log(\hat{y}i) + (1 - yi) * \log(1 - \hat{y}i)) \tag{5}$$

where N is the number of samples, $\boldsymbol{yi}$ is the true label and $\boldsymbol{\hat{y}i}$ is the predicted output

3.2 Model Evaluation

For the model to be validated in performance, the model needs to be evaluated in such ways that it might prove its results. The evaluation metrics used to assess the performance of model in this research are as follows: F1-Score, Precision, Recall and Accuracy, which is calculated using Confusion matrix of True Positive and True Negative.

4 Methodology

The Dataset used would be derived from the UCI Machine Learning dataset Heart disease dataset. The dataset contains 1025 data with 13 independent features and 1 dependent variables being the heart attack binary value [14]. the medical dataset classifies either heart attack or none. The gender column in the data is normalized: the male is set to 1 and the female to 0. The rest of the variables are comprised as Age as age, Chest Pain Type (angina, non-angina, atypical angina, asymptomatic) as cp, Resting Blood Pressure in mm/hg as trestbps, Cholesterol in mg/dl as chol, Fasting blood sugar (0 : $<$120 mg/dl, 1 : $>$120 mg/dl) as fbs, Rest ecg result as rest_ecg, Maximum heart rate in bpm as Thalach, Exercise induced angina (1 : anginas caused by exercise, 0: not caused by exercise) as exang, Oldpeak as oldpeak, Slope as slp, Number of Major Vessel colored by Fluoroscopy as ca, and Heart attack output as output.

The flow of the research is designed in a flowchart to showcase the steps done in this research, this would hopefully 1made it easier to know the steps necessary

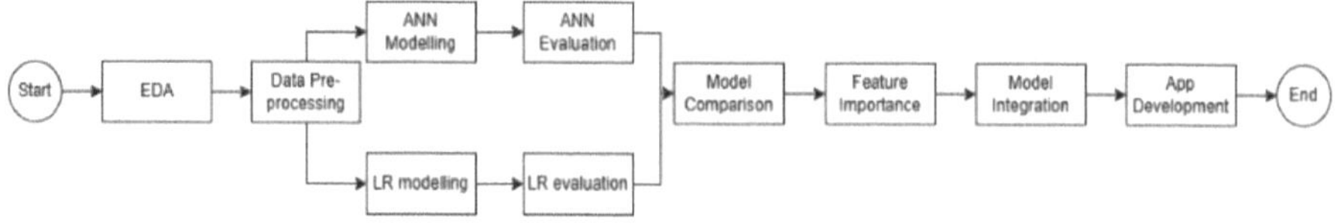

Fig. 2. Research Flowchart

Figure 2 showed that the first step is the EDA where it explores the dataset through chart and plots, then Data Pre- processing include cleaning null data, outlier and tests of independence for each variable. The next step is modelling, where it is split into 2 ANN and LR, this step is similar but not the same, as ANN modelling and LR is 2 different thing, ANN would test different layer, while LR would tests different variables significance, next the evaluation process where in ANN uses only classification report while LR uses both classification report and Summary of model. The next step is compare all models, where LR and ANN are compared, then the best method is used for feature importance. The 2 final steps are model integration and application development.

5 Results and Discussion

This section would explore the result for this research, first there needs to be done is the EDA, where it uses chart and plots. First, pie chart was done for categorical variables, this include predicted and predictor (Fig. 3).

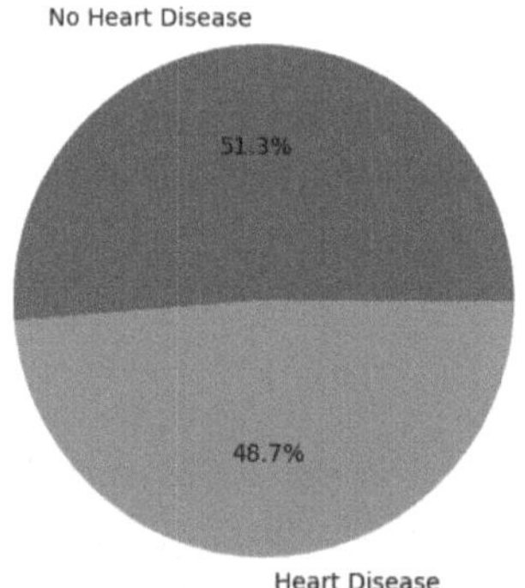

Fig. 3. Pie chart of heart disease variable

Above are the pie chart for predicted variables, see that the percentage of non-heart disease patients and heart disease patients are close, this means the dataset is equally distributed for heart disease and non-heart disease. Then the next step for EDA is to plot, first the plot is boxplot used to find outliers (Fig. 4).

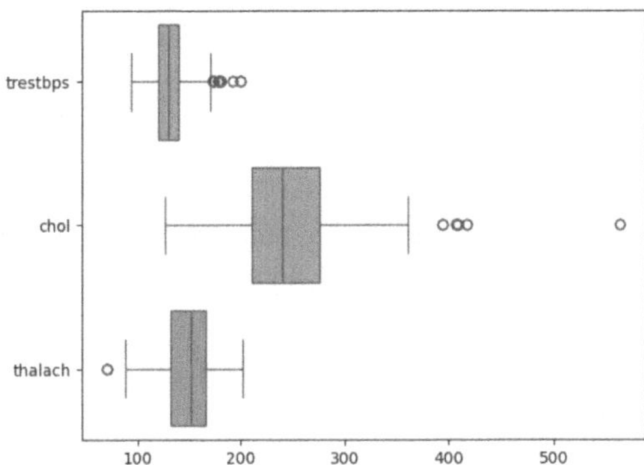

Fig. 4. Boxplot Continuous variable

See that there are some outliers, in this dataset even the cholesterol has some extreme values, reaching to 500+, however outliers are possible to exist in real life, thus the researchers decided not to erase or impute the outlier as this might cause miscalculation in modelling phase. The Chi-Square test would allow for only the independent variables that shows no association to the predicted variable to be used, thus allowing a less bias model later on. This test would create a contingency table between each variable and the target variable.

H0 : The variables are independent to each other.

H1 : The variables are strongly associated (Table 1).

Table 1. Chi-Square test

Variables	χ^2 value	P-value	df
Gender	78.86	6.5×10^{-19}	1
fbs	1.51	0.218	1
cp	280.98	1.2×10^{-60}	3
exang	194.815	2.82×10^{-44}	1

From the result of chi square tests, see that only fbs is above 0.05. Thus, only fbs is considered independent or has no relation with the target variable. While other categorical independent variables have a relationship with the heart disease variable. The first model implemented to predict heart disease was logistic regression. Table 2 would explore the final model for Logistic Regression, here the model has already been done on assumption tests, such as partial and full parameter significance test, and hoslem goodness of fit test. There are a few variables being removed as it is tested to be not significant, the model has also been tested for hoslem and that the final LR model has a good fit for the dataset.

The equation of Logistic Regression based on the Estimate in the Table 2 are as follows:

$$
\begin{aligned}
logit(p) = 2.4821 - 1.6826 \times sex - 0.0190 \times trestbps \\
-0.0059 \times chol + 0.0264 \times thalach - 0.8365 \\
\times exang - 0.6710 \times oldpeak + 1.1277 \times cp_1 \\
+ 1.7372 \times cp_2 + 1.8696 \times cp_3 + 0.0297 \\
\times thal_2 - 1.55 \times thal_3 - 2.0769 \times ca_1 \\
- 3.0676 \times ca_2 - 1.8998 \times ca_3
\end{aligned}
$$

Table 2. Logistic Regression Model

Variables	Estimate	P-value
Intercept	1.0396	0.075
gender	−1.6826	0
trestbps	−0.019	0.004
chol	−0.0059	0.012
thalach	0.0264	0
exang	−0.8365	0.002
oldpeak	−0.671	0
cp_1	1.1277	0.001
cp_2	1.7372	0
cp_3	1.8696	0
thal_2	0.029	0.95
thal_3	−1.475	0.002
ca_1	−2.0769	0
ca_2	−3.067	0
ca_3	−1.899	0.001

Based on Table 2 and the equation above, most of the continuous variables give negative and small outcome. While most category variables and its dummies gives positive outcome, which means increasing the likelihood of heart disease. The ANN model was tested using 2 type, 5 layer model and 4 layer model, and as the 5-layer works evaluated better than 4-layer, only 5-layer model is shown in Table 3.

Based on the Table 3, the best result is achieved at model 3, where all activation function except output layer uses reLU and using the neuron combination of 64, 32, 16, 8, 4. All the model of ANN achieved an accuracy higher than LR, this include 4 layer and 5 layer model, thus the comparison table is shown below

Table 3. The ANN Model with 5 layers

H1	H2	H3	H4	H5	Dropout	Accuracy	Precision	Recall
32 (reLU)	16 (reLU)	8 (reLU)	4 (tanh)	2 (tanh)	after H5	0.85	0.85	0.85
64 (reLU)	32 (reLU)	16 (reLU)	8 (tanh)	4 (tanh)	after H2	0.90	0.90	0.89
64 (reLU)	**32 (reLU)**	**16 (reLU)**	**8(reLU)**	**4 (reLU)**	**none**	**0.94**	**0.94**	**0.95**
50 (reLU)	40 (reLU)	20 (reLU)	10(tanh)	5 (reLU)	none	0.92	0.92	0.92

Table 4. Model Comparison

Model	Accuracy	Precision	Recall
ANN Model with 4-Layers	0.94	0.94	0.93
ANN Model with 5-Layers	**0.94**	**0.94**	**0.95**
Logistic Regression	0.83	0.83	0.83

Based on Table 4, the ANN 4-layers and 5-layers comes close in performance, while LR model is below them. Although 0.83 is considered a good result, a better result would supposedly achieve better predictions. Feature Importance is a machine learning technique that calculates a score for each input feature in a model to indicate how important it is in predicting a target variable [15]. In this feature importance, the model used is the best model which is 5-layer ANN (Fig. 5).

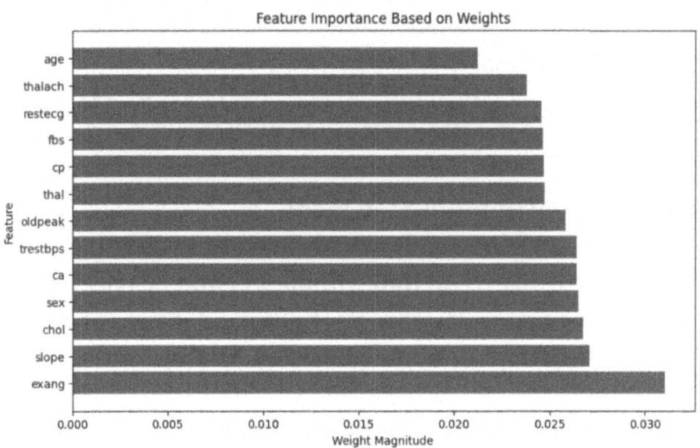

Fig. 5. Feature Importance

Based on the feature importance above, the most influential feature is exang (Exercise induced angina), with the highest weight magnitude, also the weight of all variable does not differs that much and there are no extremely low or extremely high weight magnitudes, meaning that according to ANN model all variables are needed.

6 Conclusion

This research explores the relationship between Machine Learning and Medical Fields, focusing on the use of Neural Network models for early heart disease prediction. The study found that neural networks have high performance in classifying early cases and predicting heart disease risk, with a high performance of 80-94%. However, the model had flaws, the model primarily focused on structured clinical data, and it did not include other important factors such as lifestyle behaviors, genetic history, or imaging data, which could enhance predictive accuracy. A more spread-out dataset could improve the model's results, as the normal range should be less than 200 mg/dl. The most influential features were Exercise Induced Angina, which has the highest weight.

7 Future Work

Future research should focus on expanding datasets with larger and more diverse populations to improve generalizability. Incorporating additional health indicators—such as genetics, lifestyle, and imaging data—could further enhance predictive accuracy. Improving model explainability will be essential for clinical adoption, while real-world clinical evaluations over time can validate its practical utility for early detection and prevention of heart disease.

8 Data Availability Statement

The dataset used in this study is publicly available on the UCI Machine Learning Heart disease dataset and has been cited in this paper as follows:

Janosi, A., Steinbrunn, W., Pfisterer, M., & Detrano, R. (1989). Heart Disease [Dataset]. UCI Machine Learning Repository. https://doi.org/https://doi.org/10.24432/C52P4X.

Credit Authorship Contribution Statement

Ivo Herid Lesmana: Data Curation, Visualization, Writing - Original Draft, Methodology, Formal analysis. **Syarifah Diana Permai**: Conceptualization, Supervision, Methodology, Writing - Review & Editing. **Jeklin Harefa**: Methodology, Supervision. **Gredion Prajena**: Writing - Review & Editing.

Acknowledgment. This research paper is part of the project initiative under Binus University in 2024 titled "Certified Specific Independent Study in Health Informatics." The authors gratefully acknowledge Binus University for funding and supporting this project. This support has been essential in enabling the research to be conducted and completed successfully.

References

1. Gielen, S., Laughlin, M.H., O'Conner, C., Duncher, D.J.: Exercise training in patients with heart disease: review of beneficial effects and clinical recommendations (2014)
2. Angelantonio, E.D., Thompson, A., Wensley, F., Danesh, J.: Coronary heart disease (2011)
3. Sun, R.R., Liu, M., Lu, L., Zheng, Y., Zhang, P.: Congenital Heart Disease: Causes, Diagnosis, Symptoms, and Treatments (2015)
4. Gawlikowski, J., et al.: A survey of uncertainty in deep neural networks. Artif. Intell. Rev. (2023)
5. Amin, A.H., Ahmed, B.K., Maroof, B.B., Rashid, T.A.: Heart attack classification system using neural network trained with particle swarm optimization (2022)
6. William Tchin, A.J.A.R., Putro, P.H., Darmawan, Y.P., Gunawan, A.A.S.: Prediction of heart disease UCI dataset using machine learning algorithms (2022)
7. Hemanth, J.D., Kose, U.: Heart Diseases Diagnose via Mobile Application (2018)
8. Schober, P., Vetter, T.: Logistic regression in medical research (2021)
9. Surjanovic, N., Lockhart, R.A., Loughin, M.T.: A generalized Hosmer–Lemeshow goodness-of-fit test for a family of generalized linear models. Official J. Spanish Soc. Stat. Oper. Res. (2023)
10. Shihuru, K.: An introduction to artificial neural network (2016)
11. Bre, F., GImінez, J.M.: Prediction of wind pressure coefficients on building surfaces using artificial neural networks (2017)
12. Tian, Y., Su, D., Lauria, S., Liu, X.: Recent advances on loss functions in deep learning for computer vision. Neurocomputing, 129–158 (2022)
13. Mao, A., Mohri, M., Zhong, Y.: Cross-entropy loss functions: theoretical analysis and applications. In: Proceedings of the 40th International Conference on Machine Learning (2023)
14. Janosi, A., Steinbrum, W., Pfiesfer, M., Detrano, R.: International application of a new probability algorithm for the diagnosis of coronary artery disease. UCI Mach. Learn. Repository (1989)
15. Wojitas, M.A., Chen, K.: Feature importance ranking for deep learning. In: Advances in Neural Information Processing Systems, NeurIPS 2020, vol. 33 (2020)

Can Machine Learning be Effective with Small Datasets? Insights from Modeling in Neuroscience

Maria Cristina De Cola, Fabiana Pia Vitiello(✉), Angelo Quartarone, and Maria Lui

IRCCS Centro Neurolesi Bonino-Pulejo, Messina 98155, Italy
fabiana.vitiello@irccsme.it

Abstract. Recent advances in neuroimaging, genomics, and other technology driven data acquisition methods have greatly increased the complexity and volume of medical data. Traditional machine learning (ML) approaches are becoming increasingly difficult to apply in this context, particularly in neuroscience, where datasets are often high-dimensional but contain a limited number of samples because of the difficulty of collecting data from human participants. Although ML techniques are powerful tools for analyzing large datasets, they typically require substantial training sets containing balanced data and accurate labels. In real-world medical research, such data is rather rare. Consequently, small sample sizes can introduce bias in model performance estimates, thereby limiting the feasibility of predictive modeling. Nevertheless, such datasets are essential for identifying potential biomarkers and for conducting pilot or feasibility studies within the framework of personalized medicine. However, the limited sample size can lead to biased machine learning performance estimates, which makes it impossible to apply ML methods to predictive modeling. Therefore, artificial intelligence-based data mining tools are being developed to process large volumes of data and explore hidden features and correlations.

This narrative review provides an overview of ML strategies tailored to neurological datasets with limited sample sizes, to better understand recent trends in this area and identify opportunities for future research. Particular attention is given to dimensionality reduction in complex data with few instances, as well as the integration of data mining and statistical learning techniques to improve the analysis and interpretation of small-scale but information-rich datasets.

Keywords: artificial intelligence · data mining · machine learning · neurological data · small datasets

1 Introduction

Machine learning (ML) and deep learning (DL) rely on large amounts of data to learn patterns and make decisions about new input. The key difference is that

E. R. Kaburuan and S. Goundar (Eds.): HIS 2025, LNCS 16392, pp. 214–225, 2026.
https://doi.org/10.1007/978-981-95-6304-3_19

DL processes data through multi-layered neural networks to automatically learn complex features from data. Convolutional-Neural Network (CNN) is the most popular type of neural network used in DL [8]. A CNN does not require manual feature extraction. It can extract features directly from a set of data and perform classification without user interpretation. On the contrary, ML approaches manually extract features and classify objects using separate algorithms. For this reason, deep learning has gained popularity in many real-time applications.

Over the past decade, researchers have been working to apply ML and DL to a variety of fields, becoming a major data-driven discovery tool. Their popularity stems from their ability to accurately estimate behavior in unknown domains by learning patterns from large scales of training data, which always require millions of training data to help the model achieve satisfactory performance.

In contrast to fields such as text mining [39], language translation [47], and gaming [51], where datasets containing billions or even trillions of instances are common, medical research rarely has access to data of this magnitude due to the time and expense involved, as well as challenges with data quality [14]. Thus, researchers often have to handle large and varied volumes of data that are not always accurate. For instance, the data may contain errors, inconsistencies, or missing information. The analysis stages significantly reduce the sample size, resulting in a smaller dataset for subsequent modeling. In addition, a vast array of features is often collected, resulting in high-dimensional data with small sample size. In these cases, the performance of the ML and DL-based models decreases, leading to poor prediction accuracy and generalized capability for the new scenario in addition to rapid overfitting of the training model. This significant challenge has prompted the development of various approaches to promote the growth of ML and DL methods [9].

This paper is not a systematic or quantitative meta-analysis of machine learning methods applied in neuroscience, as extensive literature on the topic already exists [1–3,7,10,11,13,26,62]. Instead, this paper aims to provide a narrative review that aims to map and synthesize methodological strategies for small-scale ML to improve the robustness of classification performance when applied to neuroscience datasets.

In their work [70], Zhang and Ling wrote: "a good classifier should have a small prediction error (predictability); converge to the Bayes-rule classifier asymptotically (consistency); be stable when adding/ removing an observation (generality); be stable for different data sets of the same kind (stochastic stability); be stable when there are a small number of contaminated observations (robustness); and have a small number of variables in the classifier (interpretability or sparsity)". We will refer to these definitions throughout the rest of the paper, which is structured as follows: Sect. 2 examines the limitations of small datasets. Section 3 reviews strategies for increasing the number of instances. These methods include Data Augmentation, Transfer Learning, Self-supervised learning, Semi-supervised learning, and Active learning. Section 4 focuses on methods for reducing the number of features, such as feature extraction and feature selection. Finally, the paper outlines future directions for applying machine learning with small data in neuroscience.

2 Model Accuracy When Working with Small Datasets

Results showing very high performance in small cohorts should be interpreted with caution, as overfitting and lack of external validation can inflate apparent precision. High-accuracy estimates reported in some studies conducted on small cohorts may not be a true reflection of generality, but may reflect sampling variability rather than model robustness [68]. Vabalas et al. [67] hypothesized that some of the bias is due to validation methods, which did not sufficiently control overfitting. Particularly when feature selection is performed before data splitting or when cross-validation folds are not properly nested. This highlights the need for specific strategies to overcome biases in classifier performance estimates produced by the intrinsic structure and variance of smaller datasets [58]. Therefore, appropriate validation design is essential to ensure reproducible and unbiased model performance.

2.1 Validation Strategies for Small Samples

Several validation techniques have been proposed for small datasets to reduce bias in model evaluation. Leave-one-out cross-validation (LOO-CV) and bootstrap resampling are effective alternatives, providing stable estimates with minimal data loss. LOO-CV is particularly suitable for very small datasets because each training set differs from the full dataset by only one sample, making it approximately unbiased. However, this approach tends to exhibit high variance, as the strong overlap among training sets produces highly correlated error estimates. In contrast, k-fold cross-validation (k-fold CV) reduces this correlation by using less overlapping partitions, thus yielding lower variance but more biased performance estimates when sample sizes are small. Consequently, there is always a biasâĂŞvariance trade-off between LOO-CV and k-fold CV. When sample sizes are extremely limited, repeated stratified k-fold CV represents a good compromise between bias and variance. Steinert et al. [58] recommend the use of repeated nested cross-validation, which provides more stable and reliable estimates than a single cross-validation run. Nested cross-validation is widely regarded as the most robust technique for preventing data leakage between feature selection and testing stages, producing unbiased performance estimates regardless of sample size. Repeated evaluations should be performed with different random splits, changing the random seed between repetitions to reduce the bias introduced by a unique data partition. Moreover, the integration of repetitions should not be limited to a simple averaging after testing, but rather incorporated directly into the permutation test, ensuring that the resulting probabilities adequately capture the variability arising from different splits.

3 Managing Small Datasets: Different Approaches

There are several viable strategies to improve the predictive power of ML or DL models when dealing with small datasets. In this section, we explore the most common. We also report some applications in neuroscience.

3.1 Data Augmentation

Data augmentation (DA) allows to generate synthetic data, providing meaningful guidance during training. The purpose was to generate additional samples of the class while keeping the underlying category unchanged. By applying transformations such as rotation, flipping, cropping, scaling, etc. of existing data, it is able to generate additional data samples, thereby expanding the dataset [43].

In neuroscience, DA can be used to improve the accuracy of multiple sclerosis classifications, even if classes are unbalanced [15]. We found that most applications of data augmentation methods focus on generating new functional magnetic resonance imaging (fMRI) scans that resemble realistic brain structures. In fact, DA produces new samples by displaying various spatial differences and remaining consistent with the original maps [44]. DA was also used to improve the classification performance of Alzheimer's disease [4,19,25], Schizophrenia [53], as well as in Parkinson's disease classification through gait data [66], where rotation was found to produce the highest level of accuracy.

3.2 Transfer Learning

Recently, transfer learning (TL) emerged as a key technique in deep learning, allowing models trained on large datasets to be adapted for tasks with limited labeled data. TL applies knowledge learned in one domain to another domain for which no data exists [40]. TL has gained considerable importance because it can work with little or no information during the training phase. Therefore, there is considerable interest among researchers in using transfer learning to efficiently train models in situations where data is scarce [36]. The model is trained on a large volume of data, learning the weights and biases during the training process. These learned weights can then be transferred to other network models, which starts with these pre-trained values [38]. The use of related but different available datasets makes this learning approach a viable method in many different contexts [29]. Thus, TL is applied in several fields, including neuroscience, where it has become the standard method for deep learning applications in neuroimaging [71]. For example, Altwijiri et al. [5] used TL as image processing module before of the training phase through a pre-trained CNN, reaching 99.3% accuracy in detecting the severity levels of Alzheimer's disease. There are applications of TL in classification problems related to the diagnosis of epilepsy [57], attention deficit hyperactivity disorder [30], as well as schizophrenia [52]. There are models pre-trained on large data sets before applying CNNs and transformers for the diagnosis of Parkinson's disease from voice data [61]. Regarding regression problems, TL was used in applications related to the severity of autism [42] and Alzheimer's disease [21,32].

Empirical evidence shows that transfer learning approaches are effective in counteracting overfitting, accelerating training times, and significantly reducing the amount of data required for retraining [71].

3.3 Self-supervised Learning

Self-supervised learning (SSL) is another new pre-training method similar to TL. It extracts reusable features from source data and uses them to improve the training of new models. In contrast to other pre-training methods, SSL creates pseudo-labels from unlabeled data through pretext tasks, and is often viewed as a bridge between supervised and unsupervised learning [71].

To date, SSL research has shown promising performance in addressing data scarcity issues in a wide range of application domains [63]. In particular, it outperformed other methods when dealing with extremely small datasets, making it a compelling option for developing deep learning models. For instance, Banville et al. proved the benefit of SSL approaches in EEG data [12]. They demonstrated that linear classifiers trained using SSL-learned features outperformed supervised deep neural networks in a regime with limited labeled data, achieving competitive performance when all available labels were used. In addition to the classification of EEG signals, which has yielded several results [35], SSL is also applied in the context of neuroimaging [22,31]. However, unlike other types of signals, neurological signals contain less information, which complicates the generalization for self-supervised training. This issue is addressed by several models, including Neuro-BERT [64]. This model predicts the frequency of masked segments of the neurological signal through the reconstruction of the original signal. In contrast, the recent work of Zhou et al. [72] describes a transformer-based self-supervised framework that directly analyzes time-series fMRI data without computing functional connectivity. This method includes a self-supervised pre-training tasks to reconstruct the randomly masked fMRI time-series data, investigating the effects of various masking strategies.

3.4 Semi-supervised Learning

Semi-supervised learning is a machine learning technique that allows a model to be trained using a small amount of labeled data alongside a large amount of unlabeled data. Therefore, the user provides a small set of labels to guide the model, and the remaining unlabeled data is exploited to improve generalization.

This makes it particularly useful for labeling data such as magnetic resonance imaging, electrophysiological signals, and microscope images. Various studies have applied this technique for tumor classification [23], brain tissue segmentation [34], and to improve robustness and noise reconstruction [45]. In addition, several studies have applied semi-supervised learning pipelines to extract EEG representations for emotion recognition. Zhang et al. [69] showed strong performance even with extremely limited labels, and Sha et al. [50] presented a semi-supervised regression model with adaptive graph learning.

3.5 Active Learning

When large amounts of unlabeled data is available but manual labeling is expensive, active learning (AL) can be applied. AL is a form of supervised machine learning in which the system actively queries the user for labels, thereby training a classification model more efficiently. Specifically, the model iteratively requests expert labels, also known as gold-standard annotations, and selects the most informative data points [49]. This strategy improves the overall classification performance and ensures high generalizability across the space [60].

Applications of AL in the field of neuroscience cover neuroimaging, addressing tasks as MRI tumor segmentation [18] and hippocampus segmentation [65], as well as connectivity inference [17], and knowledge base creation [6]. Furthermore, combining AL with transfer learning can reduce annotation costs while maintaining the stability and robustness of model performance in brain tumor classification [27].

4 Data Reduction

High-dimensional and low-sample-size (HDLSS) datasets present significant challenges for many machine learning methods. This occurs when the number of variables (features) in a dataset is significantly greater than the number of instances (samples). The sparsity of data makes traditional statistical methods unreliable, which represents a challenge in data analysis [54]. In neuroscience, for example, datasets are often characterized by very high feature dimensionality (e.g., voxel-wise neuroimaging, multi-site electrophysiological recordings, gene expression per cell), coupled with limited sample sizes (e.g., tens of subjects or trials). Thus, it is often necessary to determine a subset of features that are relevant for the outcome of interest.

Reduction methods can be supervised or unsupervised, and are often classified as feature extraction (FE) or feature selection (FS) methods. Feature extraction identifies a smaller set of representative data that accurately describes the original ones. This helps to build a robust and efficient pattern classifier system [37]. In contrast, feature selection chooses a subset of existing features that are most predictive or stable. Therefore, FE and FS answer related but distinct needs: extraction compresses and denoises, selection preserves interpretability and task relevance.

Feature reduction methods are widely used in neuroscience, particularly in neuroimaging and biosignal processing [16]. Palmar et al. applied a CNN directly to the fMRI of the resting state to extract spatio-temporal characteristics and improve accuracy in the classification of Alzheimer's disease and mild cognitive impairment [46]. Similarly, new algorithms for computerized voice analysis showed very accurate results [28,59]. However, these algorithms were developed using limited datasets with subjects with similar demographics. Hireš et al. analyzed four datasets demonstrating that even if the algorithms yielded excellent performance on a single dataset, the results obtained on new data or even a mix of datasets were very unsatisfactory [28].

Recent studies suggest that unsupervised methods are essential when labels are unavailable or unreliable. These methods offer general-purpose feature compression and representation learning [20,55]. Unsupervised approaches, such as principal component analysis (PCA), independent component analysis (ICA), and autoencoders, aim to compress data without requiring labeled samples. However, a key limitation of these methods is that they often retain dimensions with high variance that are not necessarily discriminative for the task at hand. In contrast, supervised methods yield superior performance in predictive tasks when even a modest number of labels are available because they prioritize task-relevant discriminability [24].

Hybrid strategies in HDLSS neuroscience, which combine unsupervised pre-training (e.g., autoencoders or self-supervised embeddings) with supervised fine-tuning and stability-aware selection, have emerged as the most robust approach, balancing data efficiency, task specificity, generalization, interpretability, and statistical reliability when samples are very limited [48,56]. Similarly, hybrid approaches that use an unsupervised reduction method as a preprocessing step before applying CNNs are showing promising results [33].

5 Conclusion

Generally, the availability of larger datasets allows machine learning algorithms to capture more complex patterns, thereby enhancing predictive performance. The right threshold at which a dataset is considered "too small" depends on the specific task and model architecture, although to achieve reliable and satisfactory results, it is often necessary to have hundreds or thousands of samples. However, neuroscience researchers often have to analyze datasets that are limited to less than one hundred samples. Therefore, it is crucial to adopt strategies that address this challenge and enable machine learning and deep learning models to learn effective patterns from limited data trying to avoid overfitting.

Through this review, we established two primary approaches for dealing with the difficulties presented by limited datasets. From a data perspective, the rows of the dataset can be increased using approaches such as data augmentation, which synthetically expands the dataset, whereas the columns can be decreased by extracting the most informative features. Another approach is to collect additional instances, although this is often difficult to achieve in practice. From a machine learning perspective, it is possible to adopt strategies that help algorithms to learn effective patterns from the limited dataset. Some approaches require initial user labeling, such as transfer learning and semi-supervised learning, while others operate independently, including self-supervised learning and active learning (see Table 1).

Table 1. Strategies to handle small datasets: advantages and disadvantages.

Strategy	Advantages	Disadvantages
Data Augmentation	- Reduces overfitting by increasing data variety - Techniques such as rotation, flipping, and image enlargement are straightforward and well supported - Can improve model generalization without collecting new data	- Creates only variations and not new instances - Inappropriate alterations may be introduced, potentially affecting model performance - Less effective for non-image or non-structured data
Transfer Learning	- Leverages knowledge from pre-trained models - Requires less time and resources, speeding up learning - Uses proven models	- Some pre-trained models require a lot of memory - Possible transfer of bias from source data - Reliance on the original task
Self-Supervised Learning	- Reduces labeling costs - Versatile; can be adapted to different types of data - Works well with large raw datasets	- Requires more computational resources - Difficult to interpret what the model is learning - May perform poorly with very small datasets
Semi-Supervised Learning	- Useful when unlabeled data is available - Achieves good results even with limited labels - Excellent for pre-training	- Performance depends on quality of labeled subset - Potential errors in the generation of pseudo labels - May propagate labeling biases if initial labels are poor
Active Learning	- Reduces labeling effort by selecting informative samples - Suitable for small datasets - Can improve model performance with fewer labels	- Computational expensive - Requires new labels during training - Biases may occur if starting from unrepresentative data

Future research should focus on integrating multiple strategies, such as the combination of self-supervised and semi-supervised learning or the use of SSL for feature extraction. In addition, neuroscience-specific data augmentation techniques should be developed. Meta-learning could help models generalize from very few samples, while explainable AI could ensure neurobiologically meaningful patterns. Standardized small-scale datasets and cross-modality transfer learning could further improve reproducibility and maximize the utility of limited data.

Acknowledgments. This study was funded by the European Union - Next Generation EU (project code PNRR-MCNT1-2023-12378447).

Disclosure of Interests. Authors have no competing interests.

References

1. Abdaltawab, A.: How accurate are machine learning models in predicting anti-seizure medication responses: a systematic review. Epilepsy Behav. **163**, 110212 (2025)
2. Abdi-Sargezeh, B.: A review of signal processing and machine learning techniques for interictal epileptiform discharge detection. Comput. Biol. Med. **168**, 107782 (2024)
3. Aberathne, I.: Detection of Alzheimer's disease onset using MRI and PET neuroimaging: longitudinal data analysis and machine learning. Neural Regen. Res. **18**(10), 2134–2140 (2023)
4. Ahamed, M.K.U.: A hybrid filtering and deep learning approach for early Alzheimer's disease identification. Sci. Rep. **15**(1), 27694 (2025)
5. Altwijri, O.: Novel deep-learning approach for automatic diagnosis of Alzheimer's disease from MRI. Appl. Sci. **13**(24), 13051 (2023)
6. Ambert, K.H.: Virk: an active learning-based system for bootstrapping knowledge base development in the neurosciences. Front. Neuroinform. **7**, 38 (2023)
7. Abualnaja, S.Y.: Machine learning for predicting post-operative outcomes in meningiomas: a systematic review and meta-analysis. Acta Neurochir. **166**(1), 505 (2024)
8. Alzubaidi, L.: Review of deep learning: concepts, CNN architectures, challenges, applications, future directions. J. Big Data **8**(1), 53 (2021)
9. Alzubaidi, L.: A survey on deep learning tools dealing with data scarcity: definitions, challenges, solutions, tips, and applications. J. Big Data **10**(1), 46 (2023)
10. Amanollahi, M.: Machine learning applied to the prediction of relapse, hospitalization, and suicide in bipolar disorder using neuroimaging and clinical data: a systematic review. J. Affect. Disord. **361**, 778–797 (2024)
11. Arya, A.D.: A systematic review on machine learning and deep learning techniques in the effective diagnosis of Alzheimer's disease. Brain Inform. **10**(1), 17 (2023)
12. Banville, H.: Uncovering the structure of clinical EEG signals with self-supervised learning. J. Neural Eng. **18**(4), 046020 (2021)
13. Badrulhisham, F.: Machine learning and artificial intelligence in neuroscience: a primer for researchers. Brain Behav. Immun. **115**, 470–479 (2024)
14. Bansal, M.A.: A systematic review on data scarcity problem in deep learning: solution and applications. ACM Comput. Surv. (Csur) **54**(10s), 1–29 (2022)
15. Barile, B.: Data augmentation using generative adversarial neural networks on brain structural connectivity in multiple sclerosis. Comput. Methods Programs Biomed. **206**, 106113 (2021)
16. Beaulac, C.: Neuroimaging feature extraction using a neural network classifier for imaging genetics. BMC Bioinform. **24**(1), 271 (2023)
17. Bertrán, M.A.: Active learning of cortical connectivity from two-photon imaging data. PLoS ONE **13**(5), e0196527 (2018)
18. Boehringer, A.S.: An active learning approach to train a deep learning algorithm for tumor segmentation from brain MR images. Insights Imaging **14**, 141 (2023)
19. Chen, X.: A deep learning approach for non-invasive Alzheimer's monitoring using microwave radar data. Neural Netw. **181**, 106778 (2025)
20. Dattola, S.: Integrating wearable sensor signal processing with unsupervised learning methods for tremor classification in Parkinson's disease. Bioengineering **12**(1), 37 (2025)

21. Dong, Q.: Integrating convolutional neural networks and multi-task dictionary learning for cognitive decline prediction with longitudinal images. J. Alzheimers Dis. **75**(3), 971–992 (2020)
22. edForov, A.: Self-supervised multimodal learning for group inferences from MRI data: discovering disorder-relevant brain regions and multimodal links. NeuroImage **285**, 120485 (2024)
23. Ge, C.: Deep semi-supervised learning for brain tumor classification. BMC Med. Imaging **20**(1), 87 (2020)
24. Glaser, J.I.: The roles of supervised machine learning in systems neuroscience. Prog. Neurobiol. **175**, 126–137 (2019)
25. Goenka, N.: A regularized volumetric ConvNet based Alzheimer detection using T1-weighted MRI images. Cogent Eng. **11**(1), 2314872 (2024)
26. Gupta, A.: Advancing rare neurological disorder diagnosis: addressing challenges with systematic reviews and AI-driven MRI meta-trans learning framework for neurodegenerative disorders. Ageing Res. Rev. 102831 (2025)
27. Hao, R.: A transfer learning–based active learning framework for brain tumor classification. Front. Artif. Intell. **4**, 635766 (2021)
28. Hireš, M.: On the inter-dataset generalization of machine learning approaches to Parkinson's disease detection from voice. Int. J. Med. Inform. **179**, 105237 (2023)
29. Hosna, A.: Transfer learning: a friendly introduction. J. Big Data **9**(1), 102 (2022)
30. Huang, Y. : Conditional domain adversarial transfer for robust cross-site ADHD classification using functional MRI. In ICASSP 2020-2020 IEEE International Conference on Acoustics, Speech and Signal Processing (ICASSP), pp. 1190–1194. IEEE (2020)
31. Huang, S.C.: Self-supervised learning for medical image classification: a systematic review and implementation guidelines. NPJ Digit. Med. **6**(1), 74 (2023)
32. Huang, S.: A transfer learning approach for network modeling. IIE Trans. **44**(11), 915–931 (2012)
33. Ielo, A.: A convolutional neural network model for classifying resting tremor amplitude in Parkinson's disease. IEEE Trans. Neural Syst. Rehab. Eng. Publication IEEE Eng. Med. Biol. Soc. **33**, 2034–2043 (2025)
34. Ito, R.: Semi-supervised deep learning of brain tissue segmentation. Neural Netw. **116**, 25–34 (2019)
35. Jiang, X.: Self-supervised contrastive learning for EEG-based sleep staging. In: 2021 International Joint Conference on Neural Networks (IJCNN), pp. 1–8. IEEE (2021)
36. Khuat, T.T.: Applications of machine learning in antibody discovery, process development, manufacturing and formulation: current trends, challenges, and opportunities. Comput. Chem. Eng. **182**, 108585 (2024)
37. Krishnan, S.: Trends in biomedical signal feature extraction. Biomed. Sig. Process. Control **43**, 41–63 (2018)
38. Krishna, S.T.: Deep learning and transfer learning approaches for image classification. Int. J. Recent Technol. Eng. (IJRTE) **7**(5S4), 427–432 (2019)
39. Li, J.: A local discrete text data mining method in high-dimensional data space. Int. J. Comput. Intell. Syst. **15**, 53 (2022)
40. Lu, J.: Transfer learning using computational intelligence: a survey. Knowl.-Based Syst. **80**, 14–23 (2015)
41. Marques, J.A.L.: Artificial neural network-based approaches for computer-aided disease diagnosis and treatment. In: Cognitive and Soft Computing Techniques for the Analysis of Healthcare Data, pp. 79–99. Academic Press (2022)

42. Moradi, E.: Predicting symptom severity in autism spectrum disorder based on cortical thickness measures in agglomerative data. Neuroimage **144**, 128–141 (2017)
43. Nanthini, K.: A survey on data augmentation techniques. In: 2023 7th International Conference on Computing Methodologies and Communication (ICCMC), pp. 913–920. IEEE (2023)
44. Nguyen, K.P.: Anatomically informed data augmentation for functional MRI with applications to deep learning. In: Medical Imaging 2020: Image Processing, vol. 11313, pp. 172–177 (2020)
45. Nguyen, H., Luo, S., Ramos, F.: Semi-supervised learning approach to generate neuroimaging modalities with adversarial training. In: Lauw, H.W., Wong, R.C.-W., Ntoulas, A., Lim, E.-P., Ng, S.-K., Pan, S.J. (eds.) PAKDD 2020. LNCS (LNAI), vol. 12085, pp. 409–421. Springer, Cham (2020). https://doi.org/10.1007/978-3-030-47436-2_31
46. Parmar, H.: Spatiotemporal feature extraction and classification of Alzheimer's disease using deep learning 3D-CNN for fMRI data. J. Med. Imaging **7**(5), 056001–056001 (2020)
47. Popel, M.: Transforming machine translation: a deep learning system reaches news translation quality comparable to human professionals. Nat. Commun. **11**, 4381 (2020)
48. Sauvalle, B.: Hybrid diffusion models: combining supervised and generative pretraining for label-efficient fine-tuning of segmentation models. arXiv preprint arXiv:2408.03433 (2024)
49. Settles, B: Active learning literature survey (2009)
50. Sha, T.: Semi-supervised regression with adaptive graph learning for EEG-based emotion recognition. Math. Biosci. Eng. **20**(6), 11379–11402 (2023)
51. Shah, M.: Predictive analytics, strategic game analysis, and injury prevention in sports: the role of big data and artificial intelligence. Mach. Learn. Comput. Sci. Eng **1**, 17 (2025)
52. Shalbaf, A.: Transfer learning with deep convolutional neural network for automated detection of schizophrenia from EEG signals. Phys. Eng. Sci. Med. **43**(4), 1229–1239 (2020)
53. Shams, A.: A deep learning approach for diagnosis of schizophrenia disorder via data augmentation based on convolutional neural network and long short-term memory. Biomed. Eng. Lett. **14**(4), 663–675 (2024)
54. Shen, L.: Classification for high-dimension low-sample size data. Pattern Recogn. **130** (2022)
55. Shi, Y.: Robust representation learning for unreliable partial label learning. arXiv preprint arXiv:2308.16718 (2023)
56. Shin, H.: An effective heuristic for developing hybrid feature selection in high dimensional and low sample size datasets. BMC Bioinform. **25**(1), 390 (2024)
57. Si, X.: Automated detection of juvenile myoclonic epilepsy using CNN based transfer learning in diffusion MRI. In: 2020 42nd Annual International Conference of the IEEE Engineering in Medicine and Biology Society (EMBC), pp. 1679–1682. IEEE (2020)
58. Steinert, S.: A refined approach for evaluating small datasets via binary classification using machine learning. PLoS ONE **21**; **19**(5), e0301276 (2024)
59. Sugiharti, E.: Optimizing support vector machine performance for Parkinson's disease diagnosis using GridSearchCV and PCA-based feature extraction. J. Inf. Syst. Eng. Bus. Intell. **10**(1) (2024)
60. Tharwat, A.: A survey on active learning: state-of-the-art, practical challenges and research directions. Mathematics **11**(4), 820 (2023)

61. Tougui, I.: Transformer-based transfer learning on self-reported voice recordings for Parkinson's disease diagnosis. Sci. Rep. **14**(1), 30131 (2024)
62. Yeung, J.A.: Artificial intelligence (AI) for neurologists: do digital neurones dream of electric sheep? Pract. Neurol. **23**(6), 476–488 (2023)
63. Yu, J.: Self-supervised learning for recommender systems: a survey. IEEE Trans. Knowl. Data Eng. **36**(1), 335–355 (2023)
64. Wu, D.: Neuro-BERT: rethinking masked autoencoding for self-supervised neurological pretraining. arXiv preprint arXiv:2204.12440 (2022)
65. Wu, J.: Active transfer learning for 3D hippocampus segmentation. In: Xue, Z., et al. (eds.) MILLanD 2023. LNCS, vol. 14307, pp. 224–234. Springer, Cham (2023). https://doi.org/10.1007/978-3-031-44917-8_22
66. Uchitomi, H.: Classification of mild Parkinson's disease: data augmentation of time-series gait data obtained via inertial measurement units. Sci. Rep. **13**(1), 12638 (2023)
67. Vabalas, A.: Machine learning algorithm validation with a limited sample size. PLoS ONE **14**(11), e0224365 (2019)
68. Varoquaux, G.: Cross-validation failure: small sample sizes lead to large error bars. Neuroimage **180**, 68–77 (2018)
69. Zhang, G., Etemad, A: Deep recurrent semi-supervised EEG representation learning for emotion recognition. In: 2021 9th International Conference on Affective Computing and Intelligent Interaction (ACII), pp. 1–8. IEEE (2021)
70. Zhang, L., Lin, X.: Some considerations of classification for high dimension low-sample size data. Stat. Methods Med. Res. **22**(5), 537–50 (2013)
71. Zhao, Z.: A comparison review of transfer learning and self-supervised learning: definitions, applications, advantages and limitations. Expert Syst. Appl. **242**, 122807 (2024)
72. Zhou, Y.: Self-supervised pre-training tasks for an FMRI time-series transformer in autism detection. In: Bathula, D.R., et al. (eds.) MLCN 2024. LNCS, vol. 15266, pp. 145–154. Springer, Cham (2024). https://doi.org/10.1007/978-3-031-78761-4_14

Focus Detection Using EEG: Trends, Challenges, Advantages, Application Areas, Background, and Implementation

Teddy Marcus Zakaria[1,2](✉), Armein Z. R. Langi[2], Dimitri Mahayana[2], and Isa Anshori[3]

[1] Faculty of Smart Technology and Engineering, Universitas Kristen Maranatha, Bandung, Indonesia
teddy.marcus@it.maranatha.edu
[2] School of Electrical Engineering and Informatics, Institut Teknologi Bandung, Bandung, Indonesia
[3] Biomedical Engineering, Institut Teknologi Bandung, Bandung, Indonesia

Abstract. The detection of focus and unfocus is critical in education, healthcare, and human–computer interaction. Electroencephalography (EEG) offers a non-invasive and real-time approach to assessing brain activity related to attention, yet challenges persist due to individual variability, non-stationary signals, noise, and limited labeled datasets. This paper reviews current trends in EEG-based focus detection, with an emphasis on deep learning (e.g., CNN, LSTM), meta-learning (MAML), and self-supervised learning (SSL). Publication analysis shows a significant rise in interest, with deep learning studies increasing from 10 in 2015 to more than 3,000 in 2025, while SSL and meta-learning have rapidly emerged since 2020. Our contributions are threefold: (1) identification of major challenges in EEG-based attention detection, including data scarcity and adaptability across subjects; (2) comparative evaluation of learning strategies in terms of data requirements, adaptability, and computational complexity; and (3) discussion of implementation pathways and application areas spanning brain–computer interfaces, neurofeedback, education, mental health, and autonomous systems. This review highlights promising methodologies for improving accuracy, generalizability, and efficiency, underscoring the potential of adaptive AI-driven EEG systems to advance both research and real-world applications.

Keywords: Attention · Deep Learning · EEG · Meta Learning · Self Supervised Learning

Supplementary Information The online version contains supplementary material available at https://doi.org/10.1007/978-981-95-6304-3_20.

E. R. Kaburuan and S. Goundar (Eds.): HIS 2025, LNCS 16392, pp. 226–237, 2026.
https://doi.org/10.1007/978-981-95-6304-3_20

1 Introduction

1.1 Attention and Focus

Attention and focus are fundamental aspects of human cognition, directly influencing learning outcomes, productivity, and emotional stability. The ability to measure and detect focus levels accurately has broad applications in education, clinical psychology, and adaptive human–computer interfaces. Electroencephalography (EEG) provides a non-invasive, cost-effective, and portable method to monitor brain activity in real time, enabling quantitative analysis of attention states [1, 2]. EEG captures many brain wave types—delta, theta, alpha, beta, and gamma—reflecting unique patterns of cognitive and emotional activity.

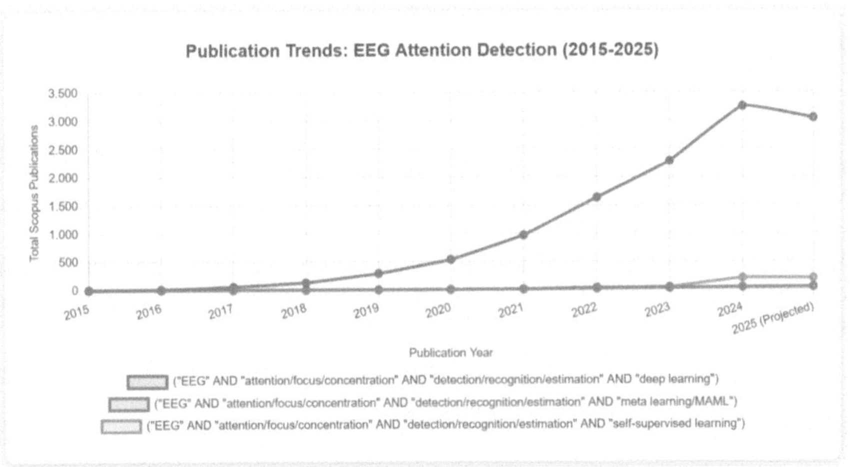

Fig. 1. Scopus Publication Trends: EEG Attention Detection (2015–2025). Note: Data for 2025 represents projected counts based on publications as of the query date. The search queries were executed on a scholarly database using keywords in the title, abstract, and keywords fields (TITLE-ABS-KEY). See Supplementary Material, Table 1, for the data.

Over the past decades, focus detection using EEG has evolved significantly. Early studies relied on handcrafted feature extraction methods and conventional classifiers such as Support Vector Machines and Linear Discriminant Analysis. With the rise of deep learning, convolutional and recurrent neural networks improved spatial-temporal feature modeling. More recently, meta-learning and self-supervised paradigms have introduced adaptive and data-efficient solutions, marking a new trend toward personalized, generalized, and minimally supervised attention detection systems (Fig. 1).

Despite substantial progress, EEG-based focus detection still faces several limitations, including inter-subject variability, low signal-to-noise ratio, and limited labeled datasets [3, 4]. This paper aims to present a structured review and methodological framework addressing these issues through a synthesis of technological advances, comparative analyses, and application case studies.

1.2 Research Questions and Contribution

Recent machine learning advances offer new solutions. CNNs and LSTMs can decode EEGs, but they need lots of labeled data. Meta-learning, especially Model-Agnostic Meta-Learning (MAML), lets models quickly adapt to new subjects with little calibration, addressing inter-subject variability. SSL uses massive unlabeled EEG datasets to develop meaningful representations without costly annotations. These methods represent a paradigm shift toward adaptive and data-efficient EEG-based attention detection. Based on these motivations, this study addresses the following research questions (RQs):

1. RQ1: What is the existing EEG-based focus detection methods and their effectiveness?
2. RQ2: How can self-supervised and meta-learning overcome challenges such limited labeled data and individual variability?
3. RQ3: Which applications are most promising for adaptive EEG-based focus detection systems?

This work makes three contributions:

- Our analysis focuses on EEG-based attention detection difficulties such as variabi-lity, signal non-stationarity, noise, and limited training data.
- We evaluate deep learning, meta-learning, and SSL, comparing flexibility, data requirements, and computing complexity.
- We discuss implementation methodologies and applications, including brain-computer interfaces, neurofeedback, education, clinical diagnostics, and autonomous systems.

Structure of the paper: Sect. 2 covers EEG basics and related studies, Sect. 3 discusses main methods, Sect. 4 compares, and Sect. 9 ends.

2 Background and Related Work

This section provides an overview of fundamental EEG and attention concepts, followed by an analysis of the evolution of detection methodologies. We trace the progression from early handcrafted feature extraction to contemporary AI-driven architectures, thereby situating our research within this advanced technological landscape.

2.1 EEG and Early Studies

EEG is a non-invasive, low-cost neuroimaging method that monitors brain electrical activity in real time using scalp electrodes. EEG signals are usually divided into five frequency bands: delta (0.5–4 Hz), theta (4–8 Hz), alpha (8–13 Hz), beta (13–30 Hz), and gamma. Alpha and beta rhythms are linked to cognition and attention. Beta power increases during persistent mental focus and active problem-solving, but alpha activity decreases during wakefulness [5]. The 10–20 and 10–10 electrode placement systems are used to measure cortical activity in frontal (Fz, Fp1–Fp2), parietal (Pz), and occipital (Oz) regions, which are involved in attention and executive function. Optimizing signal quality and separating attention-related brain processes requires electrode design.

Attention is the selective allocation of limited cognitive resources to relevant stimuli while filtering out distractors, which allows selective cognitive processing and influences perception, thinking, and action [6]. To manage sensory processing top-down, neuronal networks in the prefrontal cortex, parietal lobes, and thalamus operate. EEG studies have linked different oscillatory patterns to attentional states, such as elevated beta-band oscillations over frontal areas indicating active engagement and vigilance [5] and reduced alpha power indicating enhanced sensory processing and attentional focus [7, 8]. Theta-band activity is linked to working memory stress [9]. Alpha, beta, and theta oscillations are reliable attention biomarkers due to these neuro-physiological findings. Like biological systems, AI systems feature attention mechanisms, with first uses in machine translation allowing networks to focus on certain input segments, currently employed in vision and hearing models.

EEG uses in BCIs and brain function studies are longstanding. EEG has been shown to operate cursors and other devices by modulating brain activity since the early 1990s [10]. Estimating EEG band log-power is one way to extract information from recordings. BCI systems allow users to interact with their surroundings using cognitive signals or intents.

Early EEG-based BCI research showed brain signals could be processed into control commands [11]. To distinguish attentive and inattentive states, further investigations measured alpha and beta band spectral power variations. Klimesch established fundamental relationships between cognitive workload, arousal, and EEG spectral patterns [12].

These early systems verified EEG's potential as a quantitative measure of attention and provided routes for computational intelligence-based auto-classification, notwithstanding their limited accuracy.

2.2 Traditional Feature-Based Approaches

Before deep learning became popular, EEG analysis relied on feature extraction that was done by hand and traditional machine learning. A lot of different methods, like Fast Fourier Transform (FFT), Wavelet Transform (WT), and Common Spatial Pattern (CSP) were used to pull out patterns in time and space [13]. Support Vector Machines (SVM), Linear Discriminant Analysis (LDA), and k-Nearest Neighbors (kNN) were used to group these traits [14].

These methods were easy to understand and worked well with subject-specific data, but they were sensitive to noise and couldn't be used with a lot of people. They couldn't be used for real-time, generalized attention detection systems because they needed to be built by hand using small, labeled datasets and human feature engineering.

2.3 Evolution Toward AI-Driven Methods

Artificial intelligence has shaped EEG-based attention detection. Advanced CNN [15] and LSTM [16] architectures can automatically learn complicated spatiotemporal EEG representations. For non-stationary data, these algorithms outperform classic classifiers but require large-labeled datasets.

Meta-Learning can overcome data scarcity and inter-subject variability [17, 18]. Models can swiftly adapt to novel subjects with little calibration. SSL is popular for using unlabeled EEG data in pretext tasks and contrastive objects like contrastive predictive coding (CPC) [19]. These methods represent a paradigm change from static feature engineering to adaptive, data-driven EEG analysis for tailored neurotechnology.

EEG-based attention detection has evolved from handmade feature extraction to AI-driven frameworks. This study's methodological paradigm integrates EEG data processing with deep learning, self-supervised learning, and meta-learning.

3 Methodology

This section outlines the methodological components for EEG-based focus detection, including signal preprocessing, model architecture, and adaptive learning strategies.

3.1 EEG Signal Processing

Signal preprocessing typically involves band-pass filtering (4–30 Hz), artifact removal using ICA or WT, and normalization to mitigate inter-subject variation. Feature extraction may include spectral band power, entropy measures, and spatial filtering techniques such as CSP.

3.2 Deep Learning Approaches

CNN and LSTM networks handle spatial and temporal EEG data well. Spatial coherence and temporal dynamics improve performance in hybrid models and attention-based systems.

Convolutional neural networks (ConvNets) have revolutionized computer vision by learning directly from unprocessed input [10]. ConvNets for complete EEG analysis are gaining popularity [20]. The effective ConvNet architecture in computer vision has been updated for multi-channel EEG data analysis. Studies show that ConvNets, such as "Shallow ConvNet" and "Deep ConvNet," can read movement-related information from raw EEG data as accurately as Filter Bank Common Spatial Patterns (FBCSP) [21]. Additionally, ConvNets and LSTM RNN models have been used to handle sequential time series data from EEG. The temporal dependencies needed for attention detection are captured well by LSTMs. To use long-range information, the LSTM architecture incorporates the attention mechanism, which lets models focus on important signal areas [22].

3.3 Self-supervised Learning (SSL)

SSL is excellent for detecting patterns in unlabeled data to represent EEG signals [22, 23]. This can significantly reduce the need for expensive EEG annotations, a major EEG research restriction [23]. SSL features consistently outperform fully supervised deep neural networks with limited labeled input [22, 23]. SSL starts with temporal context prediction and contrastive predictive coding. CPC uses InfoNCE, a categorical cross-entropy loss, for end-to-end model training. SSL can identify sleep micro- and macrostructures and problems from unlabeled EEG [22, 23].

3.4 Meta-learning Methods

MAML adapts models to new subjects quickly with little training data. Meta-learning overcomes inter-subject variability in EEG-based research by considering each subject as a task. This paradigm improves participant generalization.

Meta-learning helps models learn "how to learn" and adapt quickly to new tasks with little input. Meta-learning's best algorithm is MAML. MAML improves a model's starting parameters to assure peak performance on a new job after parameter updates using one or more gradient steps using a limited dataset [3, 17, 24].

EEG data vary widely among individuals, making MAML particularly relevant [3, 25]. MAML treats each subject as a separate task, allowing it to quickly adapt to new persons without calibration data. MAML for sleep stage classification (MetaSleepLearner) improved performance in a few epochs with fine-tuning [3, 18, 22]. MAML is promising but suffers from base model sensitivity, training instability, and second-order gradient calculations that increase computing complexity. Using meta-learning for multi-stage loss optimization, proposed approaches aim to improve training stability and convergence [22, 26].

3.5 Mathematical Formulations and Pseudocodes

This section conceptually summarizes the mathematical formulations and pseudocodes of the major models employed in this study: CNN, LSTM, MAML, and SSL (see Supplementary Material, S1-S6, for the formulations and pseudocodes).

4 Comparative Analysis

Table 1 presents reported accuracy and performance trends for representative models across standard datasets to consolidate empirical information from EEG-based focus detection investigations. These figures are typical of current literature (2015–2025).

Table 1. Summary of Reported Results for EEG-Based Focus Detection

Method	Dataset	Reported Accuracy	Adaptability	Data Requirement	Ref
CNN	MEMA, EEG-Attention	85–92%	Low	High	[10, 15]
LSTM	EEG-Attention	78–88%	Medium	High	[16]
MAML	Multiple Subjects (Meta-Learning Benchmarks)	80–95%	Very High	Low	[17, 18]
SSL	Unlabeled EEG (Pretraining)	82–90%	High	Very Low	[19, 27]

Deep learning models (CNNs, LSTMs) perform well on subject-specific data, whereas meta-learning and SSL techniques are more adaptable and robust in cross-subject generalization. MAML-based frameworks personalize well with little calibration data, while SSL overcomes the lack of labeled EEG datasets. These results highlight the complementary benefits of adaptive and self-supervised paradigms for EEG-based focus detection. A comparative analysis of major learning paradigms—CNN, LSTM, MAML, and SSL—is summarized in Supplementary Material, Table 2.

5 Implementation Framework

The proposed implementation framework combines preprocessing, feature extraction, model training, and adaptive inference.

5.1 Data Flow Overview

The implementation pipeline follows a structured data flow: (1) EEG data acquisition (2) preprocessing and artifact removal (3) feature extraction (4) model training and validation (5) testing and adaptation.

This process ensures that raw EEG signals are transformed into meaningful representations suitable for AI models.

Data Acquisition and Preprocessing

Public EEG datasets with attention labels include MEMA [6], Mental Attention State EEG (Kaggle) [28], mEBAL [29], and EEG-Attention RSVP Experiment (OpenNeuro) [30]. Based on hardware, EEG waves are captured at 128–512 Hz. Pre-processing removes distractions from eye movements, muscle activity, and external interference. Pre-processing steps commonly include Band-pass filtering (4–30 Hz) to eliminate noise; ICA to remove artifacts; WT for sub-band decomposition; Signal normalization per participant to reduce inter-subject variability. These processes clean and normalize EEG data for downstream learning.

Feature Extraction

Band power and entropy measurements (Shannon, sample, permutation entropy) are handcrafted. To improve class separability, the Common Spatial Pattern (CSP) approach is extensively utilized. From raw EEG, CNNs, LSTMs, and Autoencoders may automatically extract spatio-temporal representations. Recent research uses Vision Transformers (ViTs) to learn EEG representations by capturing long-range dependencies.

Model Integration

The developed system integrates deep learning, meta-learning for optimal adaptability and Self-Supervised Learning. CNNs (e.g., EEGNet [17], CTCNN [17, 31], HS-CNN [32]) capture spatial structures and frequency information. LSTMs capture temporal dependencies across EEG epochs [33]. Hybrid CNN-LSTM architectures handle spatial and temporal patterns effectively. In small-sample EEG datasets, Batch Normalisation, Dropout, Exponential Linear Units (ELUs), and Layer Normalisation reduce overfitting and increase generalisation. SSL and MAML combination improve real-time EEG focus detection generalization and adaptability.

5.2 System Architecture

Figure 2 shows the EEG–AI integration framework's sequential signal capture to adaptive inference architecture.

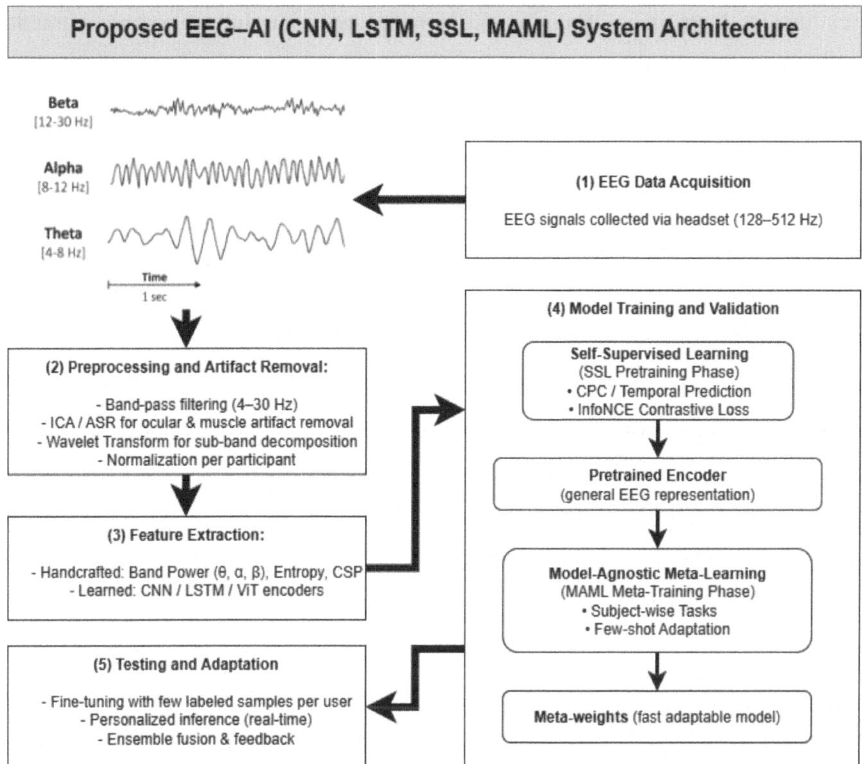

Fig. 2. EEG–AI system architecture showing sequential stages from EEG acquisition to adaptive inference. The pipeline begins with EEG preprocessing, proceeds through SSL-based feature representation, and ends with MAML-based subject adaptation, enabling real-time personalized focus detection.

6 Applications and Use Cases

This section analyzes and discusses focus and unfocus detection, emphasizing its advantages over conventional approaches and diverse implementation potential:

- Non-invasive, portable. Portable, non-invasive EEGs record brain activity. EEG equipment is becoming more portable and usable outside of clinical settings [23].
- High Temporal Resolution. EEG signals' great temporal resolution makes them suitable for research and diagnosis that requires quick brain activity detection [25].
- Real-time detection. Attention monitoring and brain-computer interfaces require real-time brain activity measurement, which EEG equipment can provide [11].

- Various applications. This technology could be used in healthcare, mental health, education, and interactive technology [34].
- Rapid Adaptation**.** Meta-learning methods like MAML enable models to adapt quickly to new subjects or tasks with minimal training data [17, 18, 25, 35].
- Automation: Deep learning methods extract discriminative features from physiological data without time-consuming and domain-dependent human feature extraction [25].
- Accuracy has improved due to advanced signal processing, deep learning, and meta-learning. Combining physiological signals accurately recognizes emotions [22].

7 Challenges and Limitations

EEG-based systems encounter inter-subject variability, signal noise, insufficient labeled data, computing needs, and model interpretability issues despite encouraging results. We need neuroscience, machine learning, and biomedical engineering collaboration to solve these problems.

8 Future Directions

Future research should aim to improve model interpretability, develop multimodal fusion frameworks (EEG with HRV and GSR) [1], and build standardized datasets for benchmarking. Advancements in wearable EEG hardware and cloud-based real-time processing can also support scalable deployment of adaptive focus detection systems.

9 Conclusion

This research reviewed EEG-based focus detection history, methods, problems, and implementation techniques. Deep learning, meta-learning, and self-supervised paradigms improve adaptability and data efficiency; therefore, it emphasized the move from traditional methodologies. EEG is a promising modality for understanding human attention, and data-driven modeling will improve focus detection systems for real-world applications.

Acknowledgments. The authors would like to thank the School of Electrical Engineering and Informatics, Bandung Institute of Technology (ITB), and Universitas Kristen Maranatha for their support and assistance in conducting this research.

Supplementary Materials. Additional materials related to this study are provided in separate supplementary documents, including detailed mathematical formulations, pseudocode of the CNN, LSTM, MAML, and SSL algorithms, extended comparison tables.

References

1. Zakaria, T.M., Langi, A.Z.R., Sophian Nazaruddin, M., Anshori, I.: Artificial intelligence (AI) in neurofeedback therapy using electroencephalography (EEG), heart rate variability (HRV), and galvanic skin response (GSR): a review. IEEE Access **13**, 133078–133112 (2025). https://doi.org/10.1109/ACCESS.2025.3582805
2. Souza, R.H.C., Naves, E.L.M.: Attention detection in virtual environments using EEG signals: a scoping review. Front Physiol. **12** (2021). https://doi.org/10.3389/fphys.2021.727840
3. Sharma, A., Miyapuram, K.: Evaluating fast adaptability of neural networks for brain-computer interface. In: 2024 International Joint Conference on Neural Networks (IJCNN), pp. 1–8. IEEE (2024). https://doi.org/10.1109/IJCNN60899.2024.10650562
4. Banluesombatkul, N., et al.: MetaSleepLearner: a pilot study on fast adaptation of bio-signals-based sleep stage classifier to new individual subject using meta-learning. IEEE J. Biomed. Health Inform. **25**, 1949–1963 (2021). https://doi.org/10.1109/JBHI.2020.3037693
5. Park, J., Kwon, H., Kang, S., Lee, Y.: The effect of binaural beat-based audiovisual stimulation on brain waves and concentration. In: 9th International Conference on Information and Communication Technology Convergence: ICT Convergence Powered by Smart Intelligence, ICTC 2018, pp. 420–423. Institute of Electrical and Electronics Engineers Inc. (2018). https://doi.org/10.1109/ICTC.2018.8539512
6. Lindsay, G.W.: Attention in psychology, neuroscience, and machine learning. Front Comput. Neurosci. **14** (2020). https://doi.org/10.3389/fncom.2020.00029
7. Sharma, A., Singh, M.: Assessing alpha activity in attention and relaxed state: an EEG analysis. In: Bisht, S., et al. (eds.) Proceedings on 2015 1st International Conference on Next Generation Computing Technologies, NGCT 2015, pp. 508–513. Institute of Electrical and Electronics Engineers Inc. (2016). https://doi.org/10.1109/NGCT.2015.7375171
8. Medvedeva, A., et al.: The development and testing of olfactory-based neurofeedback for the EEG alpha rhythm. Neurosci. Behav. Physiol. **54**, 177–186 (2024). https://doi.org/10.1007/s11055-024-01580-3
9. Aquino, V.G.U., Pacheco, J.Y.F., Córdoba, A.C., Huerta, K.C., Torres, B.T., Guzmán, A.S.: A comparative study of EEG signals from healthy subjects and medicated mental disorder patients while doing a selective attention task. In: Flores Cuautle, J.D.J.A., et al. (eds.) IFMBE Proceedings, pp. 463–470. Springer Science and Business Media Deutschland GmbH (2025). https://doi.org/10.1007/978-3-031-82123-3_44
10. Schirrmeister, R.T., et al.: Deep learning with convolutional neural networks for EEG decoding and visualization. Hum. Brain Mapp. **38**, 5391–5420 (2017). https://doi.org/10.1002/hbm.23730
11. Dutta, S., Banerjee, T., Roy, N.D., Chowdhury, B.: Development of a BCI-based application using EEG to assess attentional control. Adv. Intell. Syst. Comput. **1112**, 659–670 (2020). https://doi.org/10.1007/978-981-15-2188-1_52
12. Sauseng, P., Klimesch, W., Gerloff, C., Hummel, F.C.: Spontaneous locally restricted EEG alpha activity determines cortical excitability in the motor cortex. Neuropsychologia **47**, 284–288 (2009). https://doi.org/10.1016/j.neuropsychologia.2008.07.021
13. Seifeddine, B., Dib, N.: A single-channel EEG-based discrimination of major depressive disorder with wavelets features and machine learning. In: 6th International Conference on Networking and Advanced Systems, ICNAS 2023 (2023). https://doi.org/10.1109/ICNAS59892.2023.10330501
14. Tang, X., Wang, T., Du, Y., Dai, Y.: Motor imagery EEG recognition with KNN-based smooth auto-encoder. Artif. Intell. Med. **101**, 101747 (2019). https://doi.org/10.1016/j.artmed.2019.101747

15. Stock, S., et al.: Towards EEG-based objective ADHD diagnosis support using convolutional neural networks. In: CIBCB 2023 - 20th IEEE Conference on Computational Intelligence in Bioinformatics and Computational Biology (2023). https://doi.org/10.1109/CIBCB56990.2023.10264876
16. Chang, Y., Stevenson, C., Chen, I.-C., Lin, D.-S., Ko, L.-W.: Neurological state changes indicative of ADHD in children learned via EEG-based LSTM networks. J. Neural Eng. **19** (2022). https://doi.org/10.1088/1741-2552/ac4f07
17. Finn, C., Abbeel, P., Levine, S.: Model-agnostic meta-learning for fast adaptation of deep networks. In: Proceedings of the 34th International Conference on Machine Learning, Sydney, Australia (2017). https://doi.org/10.48550/arXiv.1703.03400
18. Javaid, M.H., Shah, I.A., Javaid, M.S., Bin Irshad, U., Halim, Z.: Model agnostic meta learning for EEG classification: multitask approach. In: 2023 IEEE IAS Global Conference on Emerging Technologies (GlobConET), pp. 1–4. IEEE (2023). https://doi.org/10.1109/GlobConET56651.2023.10150186
19. Yang, C., Xiao, C., Westover, M.B., Sun, J.: Self-supervised electroencephalogram representation learning for automatic sleep staging: model development and evaluation study. JMIR AI. **2**, 1–14 (2023). https://doi.org/10.2196/46769
20. Khan, S.A., Chaudary, E., Mumtaz, W.: EEG-ConvNet: convolutional networks for EEG-based subject-dependent emotion recognition. Comput. Electr. Eng. **116**, 1–13 (2024). https://doi.org/10.1016/j.compeleceng.2024.109178
21. Lin, C.-L., Chen, L.-T.: Improvement of brain–computer interface in motor imagery training through the designing of a dynamic experiment and FBCSP. Heliyon **9**, e13745 (2023). https://doi.org/10.1016/j.heliyon.2023.e13745
22. Lubianiker, N., Paret, C., Dayan, P., Hendler, T.: Neurofeedback through the lens of reinforcement learning (2022). https://doi.org/10.1016/j.tins.2022.03.008
23. Banville, H., Chehab, O., Hyvärinen, A., Engemann, D.-A., Gramfort, A.: Uncovering the structure of clinical EEG signals with self-supervised learning (2020). https://doi.org/10.48550/arXiv.2007.16104
24. Mahmud, S., Lim, K.H.: One-step model agnostic meta-learning using two-phase switching optimization strategy. Neural Comput. Appl. **34**, 13529–13537 (2022). https://doi.org/10.1007/s00521-022-07160-1
25. Duan, T., et al.: Meta learn on constrained transfer learning for low resource cross subject EEG classification. IEEE Access **8**, 224791–224802 (2020). https://doi.org/10.1109/ACCESS.2020.3045225
26. Yao, X., Zhu, J., Huo, G., Xu, N., Liu, X., Zhang, C.: Model-agnostic multi-stage loss optimization meta learning. Int. J. Mach. Learn. Cybern. **12**, 2349–2363 (2021). https://doi.org/10.1007/s13042-021-01316-6
27. Hu, K., Dai, R.-J., Chen, W.-T., Yin, H.-L., Lu, B.-L., Zheng, W.-L.: Contrastive self-supervised EEG representation learning for emotion classification. In: 2024 46th Annual International Conference of the IEEE Engineering in Medicine and Biology Society (EMBC), pp. 1–4. IEEE (2024). https://doi.org/10.1109/EMBC53108.2024.10781579
28. Acı, Ç.İ, Kaya, M., Mishchenko, Y.: Distinguishing mental attention states of humans via an EEG-based passive BCI using machine learning methods. Expert Syst. Appl. **134**, 153–166 (2019). https://doi.org/10.1016/j.eswa.2019.05.057
29. Daza, R., Morales, A., Fierrez, J., Tolosana, R.: mEBAL: a multimodal database for eye blink detection and attention level estimation (2020). https://doi.org/10.48550/arXiv.2006.05327
30. Robinson, A.K., Grootswagers, T., Shatek, S.M., Gerboni, J., Holcombe, A., Carlson, T.A.: Overlapping neural representations for the position of visible and imagined objects (2020). https://doi.org/10.48550/arXiv.2010.09932
31. He, H., Wu, D.: Transfer learning for brain-computer interfaces: a Euclidean space data alignment approach (2018). https://doi.org/10.48550/arXiv.1808.05464

32. Dai, G., Zhou, J., Huang, J., Wang, N.: HS-CNN: a CNN with hybrid convolution scale for EEG motor imagery classification. J. Neural Eng. **17**, 1–12 (2020). https://doi.org/10.1088/1741-2552/ab405f
33. Ngetich, V.K.: Familiarity detection from EEG signals using wavelet transform and LSTM (2021). https://doi.org/10.1007/978-981-33-4084-8_35
34. Belo, J., Clerc, M., Schön, D.: EEG-based auditory attention detection and its possible future applications for passive BCI (2021). https://doi.org/10.3389/fcomp.2021.661178
35. Hu, Z., Gan, Z., Li, W., Wen, J.Z., Zhou, D., Wang, X.: Two-stage model-agnostic meta-learning with noise mechanism for one-shot imitation. IEEE Access **8**, 182720–182730 (2020). https://doi.org/10.1109/ACCESS.2020.3029220

Machine Learning Approaches for Detection of Somatic Mutations and Copy Number Alterations: A Systematic Literature Review

Faisal Asadi(✉)

Computer Science Department, School of Computer Science, Bina Nusantara University, Jakarta 11480, Indonesia
Faisal.asadi@binus.ac.id

Abstract. The detection of somatic mutations and Copy number alterations (CNAs) in cancer cells is crucial for diagnosis and careful observation; however, existing traditional methods are both insufficient and inefficient. Examining the latest advances in Machine learning (ML) techniques, such as the Random forest algorithm, and ensemble models such as SomaticSeq, which turns out to have good mutation detection accuracy and efficiency. This method also proves capable of handling a variety of sample purity and sequencing strategies. Therefore, this method can offer good results and efficiency levels when compared to conventional approaches. Although there are still challenges, such as the need for a capable training dataset and high computational requirements, this ML model promises to make significant progress in cancer diagnosis, early detection, and personalized treatment. This review paper aims to review the ML methods that involve the detection of somatic mutations and (CNA). The results of the review showed that the ML method was promising in both implications, as proven by the minimum accuracy being above 70%.

Keywords: Artificial Intelligence · Cancer · Machine Learning · Mutation

1 Introduction

Cell mutations have constantly been increasing rapidly as humans grow and develop [1, 2]. Somatic mutations occur in non-reproductive cells, which will not be transmitted to their descendants. However, this mutation is the result of the human aging process that occurs over time. Therefore, studies on somatic mutations and how to overcome them continue to increase as the mutations vary in their nature. As the demands of medical treatment and research continue to expand, this requires excessive labor, resulting in low efficiency and frequently different diagnoses for clinicians with varying experiences. Take cancer, for example. Due to various factors, including tumor-normal cross-contamination, tumor heterogeneity, sequencing artifacts, and coverage biases, detecting a mutation in a cancer cell can be a time-consuming process. The primary disadvantage of traditional methods has been their reliance on statistical and algorithmic approaches,

E. R. Kaburuan and S. Goundar (Eds.): HIS 2025, LNCS 16392, pp. 238–250, 2026.
https://doi.org/10.1007/978-981-95-6304-3_21

which have been successful in detecting specific types of cancer. However, these methods are highly costly, subjective, and not scalable [3]. These methods often struggle to detect cancer due to variations in sample purity and sequencing strategies.

To address these limitations, recent advances in ML have been applied to the detection of somatic mutations. There are two approaches to handling this limitation. The first step involves using an unsupervised ML method to identify candidate driver genes from TCGA's mutation data, which includes both low and high-frequency occurrences from thousands of patients across over 30 cancer types [4, 5]. The second step involves a CNN-based approach for somatic mutation detection, marking a significant milestone. Unlike other deep learning-based methods focused on germline variants, the CNN-based approach can capture important mutation signals from the raw data and achieve high accuracy output for different sample purities and sequencing strategies. In this paper, we will conduct a literature review of papers that have implemented somatic mutation detection using an ML approach and their results.

2 Literature Review

Somatic mutations refer to genetic changes or variations that occur in tumor cells but not in normal cells of the body. These somatic mutations, such as single-nucleotide variants (SNVs), insertions or deletions (indels), or structural changes, are more complex in the tumor genome [3]. The explanation that seems to emphasize is that somatic mutations are literally genetic changes that occur in cancer cells and can influence the development of other diseases. Then, CNV primarily refers to changes in the copy number of specific regions of the genome, which are also associated with cancer [6]. The changes that occur in copy number refer to alterations in the copy number of a specific segment of the genome in tumor cells compared with normal cells. Such changes can take the form of amplifications, in which specific genome copies are increased, or deletions, in which specific genome copies are reduced in tumor cells. ML is used to detect and classify somatic mutations that occur, as well as to identify changes in the amount of genomic data from tumor specimens. ML methods were developed to distinguish genuine somatic variations from artifacts or false variations that may arise due to the complexity of the cancer genome or technical issues in genome analysis.

In cancer genome analysis, accurately and reliably identifying somatic variations is a significant challenge [7]. This is also due to the complexity of the cancer genome, technical variations in the sequencing process, and the presence of artifacts that may be introduced into the data. Currently, clinical laboratories still rely on manual screening methods to identify somatic variations based on sequencing data [4]. However, the problem is that this method is quite expensive, subjective, and difficult to implement on a large scale. To overcome these challenges, they proposed using ML to differentiate between true somatic variation cells and artifacts that may appear in sequencing data [4]. They also built a classification model using ML with three classification classes, namely true somatic variations, artifacts, and uncertain variations. The model development process will be carried out using a cohort of tumor sequencing data that has been collected. Each somatic variation will be manually inspected and labeled as either an actual variation or an artifact. A classification model will be trained using the training set, then adjusted to the validation set, and finally tested on the test set. The results of this study show that the optimized classification model has 100% specificity and 97% sensitivity on the test set [4]. This model is highly effective in identifying somatic variations with high accuracy, classifying false variations as artifacts, and assigning a third label, namely "uncertain," to variations that cannot be classified with certainty.

A thorough understanding of somatic mutations and copy number alterations is crucial for developing effective therapies for cancer treatment. ML methods can enhance somatic mutation detection by accurately identifying genetic anomalies, simplifying complex data analysis, and reducing the costs and time required for manual interpretation and validation of results. ML methods, such as "random forests," were found to be good at classifying within the "RFcaller" pipeline, helping to detect the presence of somatic mutations in typical tumor-paired samples. In addition, RFcaller, by utilizing somatic mutation sequencing data, can also track tumor tissue [8, 9]. The use of several different callers has also become common in many projects, aiming to achieve a more reliable set of mutations [8]. Methods such as NeoMutate utilize seven different ML algorithms to harness the power of calling across multiple variants, resulting in improved and optimal somatic variant detection rates [10]. However, this new method, which combines several callers, incurs additional costs because it requires substantial computing power and takes more time compared to conventional methods [8].

NeuSomatic is the latest innovation in somatic mutation detection, utilizing a CNN architecture to achieve high accuracy across multiple tumors and sequencing strategies. It effectively addresses the challenge of detecting somatic mutations and can also generate precise feature representations from raw genomic data [11]. Additionally, the use of Next-Generation Sequencing (NGS) technology facilitates rapid DNA/RNA sequencing to detect somatic mutations in the cancer genome. However, due to errors, the number of false positives often results in an overcount of true somatic mutations. To improve accuracy, the ensemble learning approach, SomanticSeq, combines several ML methods, also utilizing input from NGS data, aiming to produce better results compared to other individual detection algorithms [4]. One implementation of this importance is the use of somatic mutations and copy number variations (CNVs) in predicting the presence of breast cancer [6]. ML methods, especially the double kernel learning (MKL) method, to predict somatic mutations and CNVs with other molecular data such as gene expression, methylation, and protein expression. Their research aimed to improve the accuracy of predictions of breast cancer survival.

Before integration, we use the maximum relevance minimum redundancy (MRM) feature selection method. This method uses and selects features that have a reasonably high correlation with survival and have a low level of redundancy between the two in each type of data, including somatic mutations and CNV. Selecting the right features is crucial in this case because it can help identify the most relevant information and reduce the high dimensionality of the data. The results of this research, stemming from this implementation, show that the addition of somatic mutations and CNVs significantly improves the prediction performance in breast cancer survival. This also suggests that the information contained in somatic mutations and CNVs can have significant predictive value and contribute to improving prediction accuracy [6]. These features can also provide valuable additional insight into the prediction model.

Furthermore, other studies use somatic mutation data to predict the origin of cancer tissue. This research uses a random forest algorithm for feature selection and logistic regression for classification. The model obtained an average accuracy of 86.71% in predicting somatic mutation data from 13 other types of cancer. This means that the potential of ML methods in improving the detection and classification of somatic mutations, which proves to be very important in helping to diagnose cancer [1].

3 Methodology

In this methodology chapter, we will explain our systematic strategy that we used to create paper on somatic mutation detection and copy number changes using ML. We have outlined some of the literature search processes, selection criteria, and data extraction. Additionally, we present a flow diagram that illustrates the steps we took to create this paper.

3.1 Literature Search Strategies

Query Formulation. The keywords or phrases we applied to search for similar papers included somatic mutations, copy number alterations (CNA), ML, cancer genomics, and specific ML models (e.g., Random Forest, ensemble methods). We also frequently perform direct searches in scopus, such as "somatic mutation detection using machine learning", "copy number alterations in cancer genomics", "machine learning models for cancer diagnosis".

Search Engines and Databases. We searched the databases, including PubMed, IEEE Xplore, Google Scholar, and Scopus, which we knew had a large and comprehensive selection of papers. We also filtered search results based on publication date, namely, 2019 to the present, to ensure the inclusion of the latest research.

Research Criteria. The inclusion criteria for this review were peer-reviewed articles published between 2019 and 2025, written in English, that implemented ML algorithms for somatic mutation detection using human cancer data, and that reported quantitative performance metrics such as accuracy, sensitivity, and specificity. Furthermore, for the exclusion criteria included conference abstracts, letters, and editorials due to insufficient methodological detail; studies focused solely on germline mutations to maintain relevance to somatic mutation detection; articles without precise or reproducible methods; and studies using only synthetic data, as the review emphasized real-world human cancer applications.

3.2 Selection Process

Initial Screening. We review titles and abstracts to filter which papers are relevant and which are not. We also ensure relevance to established topics, namely somatic mutations and CNA, in cancer research.

Paper Screening. After screening, we evaluated the remaining relevant studies with their full texts to determine their suitability. This stage involves the methodology for extracting relevant data, the ML model used in the paper, its evaluation metrics, and the resulting outcomes.

Data Extraction. At this stage, we organize the extracted data into a structured format in an Excel file, making it easier for us to carry out comparisons and analysis between papers. We focus on analyzing comparisons in terms of models used, trends, strengths, and limitations of various ML approaches.

3.3 Flowchart of Research

We present the flow diagram below as an illustration of the entire systematic process for developing this paper, from the literature search to data extraction and the current writing stage (Fig. 1).

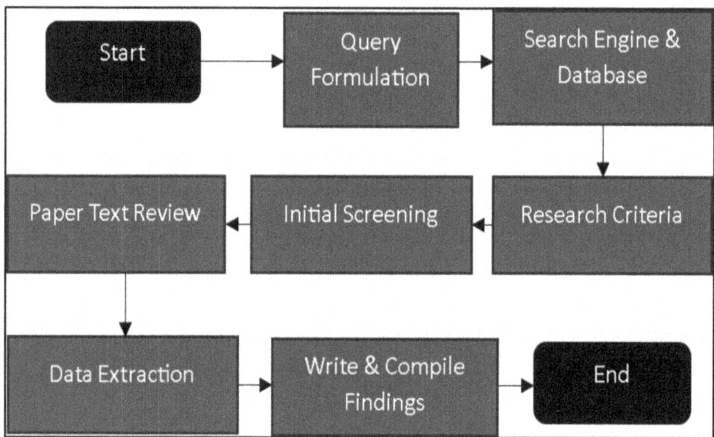

Fig. 1. Flowchart of Research.

4 Result

This chapter provides detailed information and analysis through a systematic literature review of previous studies on somatic mutation detection and copy number alterations using ML. We will attempt to compare the models used and analyze each one to provide an example of which model is most suitable for use under certain conditions.

In [3], which identified and validated somatic variants in pediatric cancer patients through Next Generation Sequencing (NGS [12]). This method stems from research conducted at the Children's Hospital of Philadelphia, with a focus on hematologic and solid tumors. More detailed research data were obtained from 291 patient samples using Agilent SureSelect QXT technology and sequenced on the Illumina MiSeq/HiSeq platform, using an average coverage of 1500x. To detect variants, it will be called using four different tools (Mutect, Scalpel, FreeBayes, and VarScan2), and variants detected by any of these tools will be retained. The criteria used for manual inspection were a high allele ratio, low mapping quality, and high strand bias, as observed and visually verified in three healthy control samples. The Random Forest model was also attempted to be used in the training, validation, and testing processes, utilizing existing libraries available in Scikit-learn Python, with features such as alternative allele coverage, strand bias, and variant allele fraction (Fig. 2).

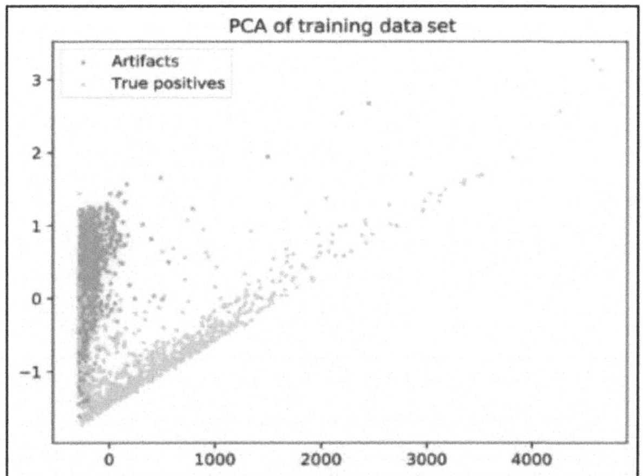

Fig. 2. Variants of training data represented the first two components from the principal component analysis. The plot indicates that the two classes are largely separable, despite a small degree of overlap [3].

The method used in [13] focuses on two main aspects: first, exploring the complex correlation between Copy Number Alterations (CNA) and gene expression in brain tumor samples from the TCGA pan-glioma cohort, also revealing significant differential expression patterns and identifying genes that unexpectedly increased. Second, using CNAPE as a multinomial logistic regression ML model with the Least Absolute Shrinkage and Selection Operator (LASSO), which aims to predict the status of CNA on gene expression data. This study also employed multilevel cross-validation to assess the performance and robustness of the model using data from the TCGA PancanAtlas dataset, which provides insight into the complex relationship between CNA and gene expression and offers a potential diagnostic tool in cancer genomics [9, 14] (Figs. 3 and 4).

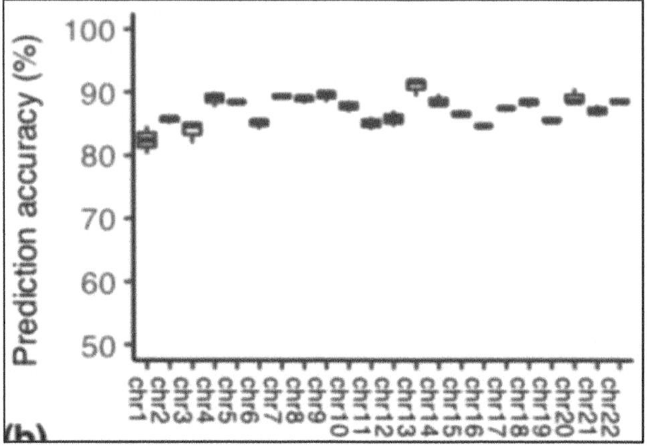

Fig. 3. Prediction accuracy of the chromosome-level models in the TCGA dataset [13].

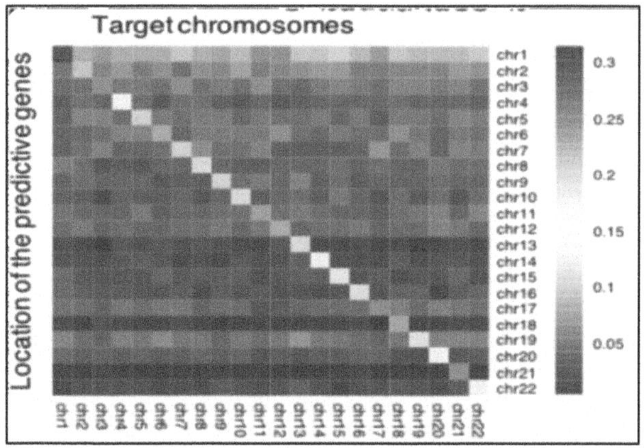

Fig. 4. Distribution of the feature genes for each chromosome-level model. Each column represents one prediction model, and for each model, the rows correspond to the locations of the feature genes. Each cell represents the proportion of feature genes on the corresponding chromosomes [13].

In another study, a multi-cohort approach was used to investigate the utility of circulating cell-free DNA (ccfDNA) for detecting early-stage Hepatocellular Carcinoma (HCC) in patients infected with Hepatitis B virus (HBV) [15, 16]. This consisted of a discovery cohort and two validation cohorts, which focused on early-stage HCC detection, with HBV-infected controls without cancer. Plasma DNA will be extracted for Illumina sequencing. Thereafter, Whole-Genome Sequencing (WGS) will be possible, with the estimation of tumor burden and detection of Somatic Copy Number Aberrations (SCNA). In the ML-based statistical modeling stage, a weighted random forest driving model was chosen, which was developed to analyze genome-wide SCNA in ccfDNA, by utilizing external data originating from The Cancer Genome Atlas (TCGA) and the International Cancer Genome Consortium (ICGC) [16]. Afterwards, the model performance will be evaluated using cross-validation and Receiver Operating Characteristic (ROC) curve analysis, with the raw sequencing data additionally deposited in a public repository.

The accuracy of each model varies between studies. Utilizing a dataset of 11,278 data points, a study using the Random Forest algorithm showed an accuracy of 96.6% [3]. Different studies using the same algorithm have produced accuracy rates of 88.2% [9, 7] and 73.4% [17]. A study using the NeoMutate framework, which incorporates seven different ML algorithms, achieved an average accuracy of 98.33% [10]. In contrast, a paper using a model named LICTOR achieved an accuracy of 83% [18]. Multiple Kernel Learning has also been utilized in another paper, achieving an accuracy of 98% [6]. NeuSomatic, a deep learning algorithm utilizing CNN, has also been employed, achieving an accuracy of up to 96.6% [11]. A study using CNAPE achieved an accuracy of over 90% [13]. Another study developed an SCNA-based, ML-driven model, which achieved an AUC of 0.893 [15]. SVMSomatic, a ML approach that employs SVM, is used in a study that achieved a precision of up to 97.1% [19]. Logistic Regression has also been utilized in a study, achieving an accuracy of 86.71% [1] (Table 1).

Table 1. Comparison of Each Paper's Evaluation Score.

Paper Number	Methods	Evaluation Score
Wu et al., [3]	Random Forest	Accuracy Score 96.6%
He et al., [6]	MKL	Accuracy Score 98%
He et al., [9]	Random Forest	Accuracy Score 88.2%
Anzar et al., [10]	NeuMutate	Accuracy Score 98.33%
Sahraeian et al., [11]	NeuSomatic	Accuracy Score 96.6%
Liu et al.,[1]	Logistic Regression	Accuracy Score 86.71%
Mu et al., [13]	CNAPE	Accuracy Score over 90%
Tao et al., [15]	SCNA-based	Accuracy Score 89,3%
Dragomir et al., [17]	Random Forest	Accuracy Score 73.4%
Garofalo et al., [18]	LICTOR	Accuracy Score 83%
Mao et al., [19]	SVMSomatic	Precision Score 97.1%

5 Discussion

In many of these studies, several discussion sections will focus on synthesizing the findings from our reference research, along with existing literature, and provide insights into the potential of this topic for the future.

5.1 Comparison of Existing Methods

Somatic Variant Detection. We have identified several methods that can detect and predict genetic changes in somatic cells, which is the primary goal. This mutation is the beginning of the spread of a malignant disease. It can occur naturally or be caused by external stimuli and factors. Due to the complexity of the underlying genomic data, conventional methods for somatic variation discovery often rely on statistical algorithms and heuristic approaches, which are less time-efficient and sometimes lead to errors. In this work, we demonstrate improvements in terms of accuracy and efficiency by comparing the performance of ML models with conventional approaches, to propose the use of advanced ML methods such as Convolutional Neural Networks (CNNs), which are shown to be more adept at dealing with variations in sample purity and sequencing schemes. This also leads to more accurate identification of mutations, especially in tumor samples that are heterogeneous and difficult to address with other traditional approaches.

Ensemble Methods. To improve overall performance, ensemble methods provide prediction results from multiple ML models. One implementation is the SomaticSeq model, which enhances the accuracy of somatic variant detection by integrating ML with various variant detection algorithms. Just like combining the advantages of multiple algorithms used, ensemble techniques such as SomaticSeq can mitigate the shortcomings of traditional single algorithms and provide better and more reliable detection results. In this work, we investigate whether the use of ensemble techniques can further enhance our ML models or whether traditional single models have their own advantages. Although ensemble approaches generally reduce variation and increase prediction accuracy, they also indirectly increase complexity and processing overhead [20].

5.2 Review of Novel Contribution

Innovative ML Techniques. This work contrasts with past thoughts on substantial transformation location and duplicate number modification (CNA) forecasting by employing a set of state-of-the-art ML algorithms. In contrast to routine procedures, which often rely on factual and computational strategies, our approach directly generates crude genomic information by utilizing advanced, deep learning structures, such as Convolutional Neural Networks (CNNs). The precision of change discovery across diverse test purities and sequencing strategies has made significant strides due to the remarkable capacity of CNNs to capture complex designs and features in large datasets. We also utilize numerous inclusion era methods that combine transcriptomic, epigenomic, and genomic information to create a multidimensional representation of the genetic landscape. The comprehensive strategy of our demonstration enables us to identify complex and subtle changes that conventional methods may overlook.

Integration of Somatic Mutations and CNAs. Our approach could be a significant development, as it combines the recognizable proof of CNAs with physical changes in a single, coherent system. Past considerations have regularly examined these genetic changes independently, which may have led to less thorough and nuanced outcomes. By coordinating the location of substantial transformations and predicting CNAs, our strategy provides a comprehensive understanding of the tumor's genetic composition [21, 22].

The development focuses on drugs and information regarding the total range of hereditary modifications that drive cancer progression, which depend on this integration. The bound-together framework, which enables the synchronous analysis of point mutations, additions, deletions, and quality copy number changes, provides a more comprehensive and accurate genomic profile [23, 24].

5.3 Clinical Implications

Application in Clinical Setting. The combination of ML models for detecting duplicate number changes and physical changes holds considerable potential for clinical applications. The accuracy and viability of hereditary investigation, which are fundamental for personalized cancer treatment, can be enhanced by these models. ML calculations can be utilized in clinical diagnostics to rapidly and accurately analyze genetic information from patients and identify mutations and variations that contribute to cancer progression. This may help oncologists treat patients better by selecting drugs based on the genetic characteristics of each patient's tumor [25]. Furthermore, these models can be applied in a variety of clinical settings, ranging from biopsy tests to profiling circulating tumor DNA, as they can accommodate different test purities and sequencing strategies [1, 26].

Early Detection and Monitoring. Furthermore, ML models offer valuable insights for cancer detection and early diagnosis. Early detection of cancer significantly increases the probability of successful treatment and survival. One example of how ML can be applied to early cancer detection is the investigation of circulating tumor DNA [15]. The models developed in this work can also be utilized to identify physical changes and numerical changes in blood tests, providing a non-invasive method for detecting cancer early. These models can also be utilized to track the progression of an infection and its response to treatment.

5.4 Limitations and Future Works

Challenges and Limitations. The quality and differences in preparing datasets are among the most significant deterrents to ML-based detection of substantial changes and duplicate number changes. Strong models suitable for various test types and sequencing strategies require training on high-quality, diverse datasets. In any case, due to protection concerns and the high cost of sequencing, collecting such datasets is often challenging. Furthermore, profound learning models can have substantial computational requirements for training and deployment, necessitating substantial investments in hardware and infrastructure. Another potential disadvantage is the risk of overfitting, where the model performs well on the training data but struggles to generalize to previously unseen information.

Future Directions. Future considerations may focus on a few key areas to address these challenges and limitations. To begin with, the more notable differences in populations and cancer types included in the training datasets would enhance the generalizability of the models. This development may be effectively supported by organizational collaboration and the establishment of centralized genetic databases. Investigating state-of-the-art

ML strategies and calculations, such as unified learning and transfer learning, helps overcome the limitations imposed by the size and diversity of the dataset. These strategies protect security and enable models to learn from decentralized information sources or utilize prior information from related tasks. Third, consolidating other types of genomic data, such as transcriptomic and epigenomic information, can enhance the capacity of models to identify and analyze substantial mutations and CNAs. Eventually, the execution of these modern ML models within the clinical setting may be encouraged by the improvement of effectively traversable programming devices and platforms, which would facilitate progress in cancer diagnosis and treatment [18].

6 Conclusions

From the many papers we observed, we found that detecting somatic mutations and CNA using ML has high potential at this time. Previous research by Wu et al. [3], which identified somatic variants using NGS, employed a variety of tools and manual methods, in another study investigating the quite complex relationship between Copy Number Alterations (CNA) and gene expression in brain tumor samples. Their methodologies include CNAPE and LASSO, which aim to predict CNA status based on gene expression data, as seen in another study investigating the usefulness of circulating cell-free DNA (ccfDNA). The random forest model analyzes Somatic Copy Number Aberrations (SCNA) in ccfDNA, utilizing TCGA and ICGC data. Overall, these studies hold promise for valuable applications and emphasize the importance of data, robust models, and the integration of ML in cancer research to enhance diagnostic accuracy and diseases understanding [15].

Data Availability.. The dataset is available on Zenodo at: https://doi.org/10.5281/zenodo.17265431.

References

1. Liu, X., et al.: Predicting cancer tissue-of-origin by a machine learning method using DNA somatic mutation data. Front. Genet. **11**, 1–11 (2020). https://doi.org/10.3389/fgene.2020.00674
2. Dou, Y., Gold, H.D., Luquette, L.J., Park, P.J.: Detecting somatic mutations in normal cells. Trends Genet. **34**, 545–557 (2018). https://doi.org/10.1016/j.tig.2018.04.003
3. Wu, C., et al.: Using machine learning to identify true somatic variants from next-generation sequencing. Clin. Chem. **66**, 239–246 (2020). https://doi.org/10.1373/clinchem.2019.308213
4. Fang, L.T.: SomaticSeq: an ensemble and machine learning method to detect somatic mutations. Methods Mol. Biol. **2120**, 47–70 (2020). https://doi.org/10.1007/978-1-0716-0327-7_4
5. Habibi, M., Taheri, G.: A new machine learning method for cancer mutation analysis. PLoS Comput. Biol. **18**, 1–30 (2022). https://doi.org/10.1371/journal.pcbi.1010332
6. He, Z., Zhang, J., Yuan, X., Zhang, Y.: Integrating somatic mutations for breast cancer survival prediction using machine learning methods. Front. Genet. **11**, 1–12 (2021). https://doi.org/10.3389/fgene.2020.632901

7. Sahraeian, S.M.E., et al.: Achieving robust somatic mutation detection with deep learning models derived from reference data sets of a cancer sample. Genome Biol. **23**, 12 (2022). https://doi.org/10.1186/s13059-021-02592-9
8. Díaz-Navarro, A., et al.: RFcaller: a machine learning approach combined with read-level features to detect somatic mutations. NAR Genomics Bioinforma. **5**, (2023). https://doi.org/10.1093/nargab/lqad056
9. He, B., et al.: A machine learning framework to trace tumor tissue-of-origin of 13 types of cancer based on DNA somatic mutation. Biochim. Biophys. Acta - Mol. Basis Dis. **1866**, 165916 (2020). https://doi.org/10.1016/j.bbadis.2020.165916
10. Anzar, I., Sverchkova, A., Stratford, R., Clancy, T.: NeoMutate: an ensemble machine learning framework for the prediction of somatic mutations in cancer. BMC Med. Genomics **12**, 63 (2019). https://doi.org/10.1186/s12920-019-0508-5
11. Sahraeian, S.M.E., Liu, R., Lau, B., Podesta, K., Mohiyuddin, M., Lam, H.Y.K.: Deep convolutional neural networks for accurate somatic mutation detection. Nat. Commun. **10**, 1041 (2019). https://doi.org/10.1038/s41467-019-09027-x
12. Lu, B.: Cancer phylogenetic inference using copy number alterations detected from DNA sequencing data. Cancer Pathog. Ther. **3**, 16–29 (2025). https://doi.org/10.1016/j.cpt.2024.04.003
13. Mu, Q., Wang, J.: CNAPE: a machine learning method for copy number alteration prediction from gene expression. IEEE/ACM Trans. Comput. Biol. Bioinforma. **18**, 306–311 (2021). https://doi.org/10.1109/TCBB.2019.2944827
14. Wang, Y., et al.: Detection of rare mutations, copy number alterations, and methylation in the same template DNA molecules. Proc. Natl. Acad. Sci. **120**, 1–9 (2023). https://doi.org/10.1073/pnas
15. Tao, K., et al.: Machine learning-based genome-wide interrogation of somatic copy number aberrations in circulating tumor DNA for early detection of hepatocellular carcinoma. EBioMedicine **56**, 102811 (2020). https://doi.org/10.1016/j.ebiom.2020.102811
16. Moser, T., Kühberger, S., Lazzeri, I., Vlachos, G., Heitzer, E.: Bridging biological cfDNA features and machine learning approaches. Trends Genet. **39**, 285–307 (2023). https://doi.org/10.1016/j.tig.2023.01.004
17. Dragomir, I., Akbar, A., Cassidy, J.W., Patel, N., Clifford, H.W., Contino, G.: Identifying cancer drivers using DRIVE: a feature-based machine learning model for a pan-cancer assessment of somatic missense mutations. Cancers (Basel). **13**, (2021). https://doi.org/10.3390/cancers13112779
18. Garofalo, M., et al.: Machine learning analyses of antibody somatic mutations predict immunoglobulin light chain toxicity. Nat. Commun. **12**, 3532 (2021). https://doi.org/10.1038/s41467-021-23880-9
19. Mao, Y.-F., Yuan, X.-G., Cun, Y.-P.: A novel machine learning approach (svmSomatic) to distinguish somatic and germline mutations using next-generation sequencing data (2021). https://doi.org/10.24272/j.issn.2095-8137.2021.014
20. Karim, M.R., Rahman, A., Jares, J.B., Decker, S., Beyan, O.: A snapshot neural ensemble method for cancer-type prediction based on copy number variations. Neural Comput. Appl. **32**, 15281–15299 (2020). https://doi.org/10.1007/s00521-019-04616-9
21. Sanjaya, P., et al.: Mutation-Attention (MuAt): deep representation learning of somatic mutations for tumour typing and subtyping. Genome Med. **15**, 1–18 (2023). https://doi.org/10.1186/s13073-023-01204-4
22. Anaya, J., Sidhom, J.W., Mahmood, F., Baras, A.S.: Multiple-instance learning of somatic mutations for the classification of tumour type and the prediction of microsatellite status. Nat. Biomed. Eng. **8**, 57–67 (2024). https://doi.org/10.1038/s41551-023-01120-3
23. Jose, A., Srivastava, A., Vinod, P.K.: DeepGraphMut: a graph-based deep learning method for cancer prognosis using somatic mutation profile. bioRxiv. 2024.12.03.626568 (2024)

24. Vilov, S., Heinig, M.: DeepSom: a CNN-based approach to somatic variant calling in WGS samples without a matched normal. Bioinformatics. **39**, (2023). https://doi.org/10.1093/bioinformatics/btac828
25. Shi, R., et al.: Integration of multiple machine learning approaches develops a gene mutation-based classifier for accurate immunotherapy outcomes. npj Precis. Oncol. **9**, (2025). https://doi.org/10.1038/s41698-025-00842-8
26. Koboldt, D.C., et al.: VarScan 2: somatic mutation and copy number alteration discovery in cancer by exome sequencing. Genome Res. **22**, 568–576 (2012). https://doi.org/10.1101/gr.129684.111

Air Quality Index During Coronavirus Disease 2019 Breakdown

Faisal Asadi[1,2](✉), Joko Pebrianto Trinugroho[2], and Arif Budiarto[1,2]

[1] Computer Science Department, School of Computer Science, Bina Nusantara University, Jakarta 11480, Indonesia
Faisal.asadi@binus.ac.id

[2] Bioinformatics and Data Science Research Center, Bina Nusantara University, Jakarta 11480, Indonesia

Abstract. Air Quality Index (AQI) has been a viral issue since the Coronavirus Disease 2019 (COVID-19) outbreak worldwide. Much research has been published on the topic of COVID-19 and its correlation with the air quality parameters such as Ozone (O3), Nitrogen Dioxide (NO2), Particulate Matter (PM) with microns size of 2.5, 10, and other parameters related to the measurement of the air quality. This paper research proposed and continued the issue of the correlation between the air quality parameters with the pandemic of COVID-19 and compared it to the improvement of the traffic location in Jakarta. We used several air quality parameters to measure the AQI in Jakarta during COVID-19. The air quality parameters are NO2, SO2, CO, O3, and PM10. The results showed a significant improvement in the air quality parameters when compared pre and during COVID-19. Some locations of research that are Kebon Jeruk and Kelapa Gading, have the better air quality since the pandemic COVID-19 meanwhile, other research locations that are Lubang Buaya, Jagakarsa, and Thamrin, did not have a significant impact on the COVID-19.

Keywords: Artificial Quality Index (AQI) · AQI Parameters · COVID-19

1 Introduction

Much research on Air Quality Index (AQI) was happening during the outbreak of COVID-19 [1, 2]. Several countries gain research deeply in the AQI impact the correlation with the air pollutant, such as AQI research from India, Bangladesh, China, Germany, Taiwan, and the USA [1–7]. The main point of most research highlights the correlation between the impact of the lockdown of the COVID-19 pandemic and AQI exposure science [1]. The other main point researched deeply was the meteorological factors correlating the air-pollutant during the better AQI to the COVID-19 pandemic [8–10]. Same as in Indonesia, the research on AQI during the pandemic of COVID-19 also being a viral topic because the researcher found significant value in their research. The significant factors such as the parameters of the AQI such as Nitrogen Dioxide (NO2), Nitrogen Monoxide (NO), Sulfur Dioxide (SO2), Carbon Monoxide (CO), Ozone (O3),

E. R. Kaburuan and S. Goundar (Eds.): HIS 2025, LNCS 16392, pp. 251–259, 2026.
https://doi.org/10.1007/978-981-95-6304-3_22

Metana (CH4), and PM 2.5 and 10 are shown to be better index. At the same time, the outbreak of COVID-19 [2] because Large-Scale Social Restriction (LSSR) phase that impacted decreased the pollutant [6, 11, 12].

Several pieces of research from Indonesia related to the impact of the outbreak of COVID-19 on the AQI have been researched from several cities in Indonesia Yogyakarta, Surabaya, Palembang, and the last is Jakarta as the capital city [11–17]. Nevertheless, the top city that researched the AQI index related to the outbreak of COVID-19 is Jakarta [17, 18]. The research from Handayani T discovers that there are dependent variables between AQI the meteorological factors such as temperature, humidity, wind speed, PM10, O3, and CO3 [17]. Related to this research, similar research was proposed by E. R. Sihayuardhi et al., given the analysis of the effect of COVID-19 on the AQI parameters, which are SO2, CO, and NO2. The result showed that the AQI increased during the outbreak of COVID-19 [19]. Furthermore, based on the explanation of the research in COVID-19 and AQI, we stated that this research aims to analyze the parameters of the AQI, which are sulfur dioxide (SO2), carbon monoxide (CO), nitrogen dioxide (NO2), ozone (O3), and PM10, during the outbreak of COVID-19 in Jakarta.

2 Previous Work

Time series visualization of PM 2.5 in Jakarta denotes an air quality improvement. From January to April 2020, the improvement happened only in the first two weeks in March, indicating the early lockdown days [15]. The concentration is still categorized as unhealthy, according to the AQI [17]. As the fact that Jakarta's air quality had improved was assured by the Bureau of Meteorological, Climate, and Geophysics (BMKG), Rahutomo and Pardamean continued the study focused on developing a pipeline to generate [11].

The same research that was gained deeply in the AQI improvement during COVID-19 has been discussed by M. Rendana et al. The data that analysis was collected since the period of LSSR was eased. The research observed that during the LSSR, the AQI parameter was increased by 59.4%, 21.2%, 16.2%, and 1.0% for NO2, PM2.5, O3, and CO [12, 20]. The research from S. Suhardono et al. also discussed the same issue related to the AQI correlation with the LSSR. The statistical analysis showed that CO was reduced to 19.7%, 14.9%, and 21% [18]. Besides, the different result research from A. Jakob et al. showed the empirical evidence pre and during COVID-19 and compared the parameters of PM2.5 and PM10 is misleading, and there is no significant effect from pre and during COVID-19 in correlation to the AQI improvement in Jakarta [15].

3 Methodology

3.1 Data Collection

There are two types of datasets used in this research. The first dataset is a series of particle concentration measurements recorded by The Provincial Government of Jakarta. The dataset was generated from air quality observation from five districts representing each municipality in Jakarta. Each observation area collected particle concentration measurements: PM10, O3, CO, SO2, and NO2. From January 2020 to June 2020, the observation collected over 900 timestamped and categorized air quality records. In addition, the second dataset is traffic information extracted from semi-structured Twitter data. These tweets data were sourced from one official Twitter account of Jakarta's local police department @TMCPoldaMetro. The tweets from this account, especially those containing traffic reports, are considered semi-structured data because of the implementation of a specific format for this kind of content. To collect the text of these historical tweets, an open-source Python library called GetOldTweets was used.

To give a comparison view of different periods during the pandemic, all collected data were dated from January 2020 to June 2020, divided into three divisions that are division 1 from January-February 2020 was considered as a pre-pandemic period, division 2 from March-April 2020 was considered as the early pandemic period, and division 3 form May- June 2020 was the peak of the pandemic among these six months.

Related to twitter data for air quality research, some research also proposed and conducted in several analysis. The first research was proposed by Gurajala et al., that gain deeper research in using tweet analysis to understand public reaction to air quality. The research discover that health concerns dominated public response when air quality degraded [21]. Besides, the other research using the same data has proposed by Kumbalaparambi et al., [22], with analyzing the urban air quality from twitter data using self-attention network and multilayer classification network. The result showed that the accuracy of the classification network was achieved around 80–99%. The last research that involved the Twitter data was proposed by Kwilas et al. The research assessing the feasibility of Twitter to monitor outdoor air pollutant in Lodon. The research suggests that social media may provide additional resources for detecting and monitoring policing in rural areas [23].

3.2 Data Processing

Different data pre-processing procedures were applied to both datasets. Simple missing values and anomaly data removal were performed to clean the air quality data. Unfortunately, all data during March indicates the measurement error. Therefore, these anomaly data were filtered out. On the other hand, a more complex data pre-processing was conducted to extract the tweets data. Firstly, the duplicate data were removed from the dataset as they can inflate the traffic score for specific locations. The table below shows the research location for the data collected (Table 1).

Table 1. Location of Research Data

No	Location	Region
Location 1	Kebon Jeruk	West Jakarta
Location 2	Kelapa Gading	North Jakarta
Location 3	Lubang Buaya	East Jakarta
Location 4	Jagakarsa	South Jakarta
Location 5	Thamrin	Central Jakarta

3.3 Data Processing

Different data pre-processing procedures were applied to both datasets. Simple missing values and anomaly data removal were performed to clean the air quality data. Unfortunately, all data during March indicates the measurement error. Therefore, these anomaly data were filtered out. On the other hand, a more complex data pre-processing was conducted to extract the tweets data. Firstly, the duplicate data were removed from the dataset as they can inflate the traffic score for specific locations. The table below shows the research location for the data collected.

3.4 Statistical Analysis

The statistical analysis was done using Python statistical packages scipy.stats and scikit_posthocs.

4 Results and Discussion

4.1 Traffic and Air Quality in Each Location

As a general overview, two series of chi-square tests were performed to obtain the correlation between traffic status and COVID-19 periods and air quality status and COVID-19 periods. Table II and Table III show these two sets of correlations. Table I clearly shows significant differences in traffic status in each location. During the Pre of COVID-19 period, high traffic occurred on almost all the reported days. On the other hand, a significant improvement in traffic conditions happened during the COVID-19 pandemic [1, 24, 25]. This result indicates the effect of the lockdown policy during the pandemic, drastically reducing the use of cars and motorcycles in these locations [1, 26, 27]. However, surprisingly, the air quality measurements in some locations indicate insignificant disparities between the two phases. Table III indicates air quality improvements during the COVID-19 pandemic, given less hectic traffic conditions in Kebon Jeruk and Jagakarsa. Around 80% of reported dates in these two locations denote unhealthy air quality. The table below is the statistical result of traffic comparison pre-COVID-19 and during COVID-19 in each location.

4.2 Air Quality Parameters Pre and During COVID-19 in Each Location

Referring to Table IV, we tested the data using a statistical student test (t-test) to evaluate the significance of the AQI parameters improvement in each of the research locations. We evaluate the P-value for testing the significance of the AQI parameters. Table IV shows the significant result by p-value in each location. We found in location 1 and location 2 that all the AQI parameters significantly improved during the COVID-19 pandemic. Besides, in location 3, the significance of the AQI parameters was only O3. In location 4, the significance was NO2, CO, and O3, and last, in location 5, the AQI parameters that significance was NO2, SO2, CO, and O3. In the sum of Table IV, from the five research locations observed, we concluded that only location 3 (Lubang Buaya) did not significantly improve air quality during the pre and COVID-19 periods in Jakarta.

In contrast, the other locations 1, 2, 4, and 5 (Kebon Jeruk, Kelapa Gading, Jagakarsa, Thamrin) significantly improved the air quality when compared pre and during COVID-19.

In other words, the air quality in the fourth location increased during COVID-19 and the policy of LSSR in Jakarta [11, 12, 28]. Moreover, based on Table V, we can compare AQI parameters in each location based on the traffic situation. Based on the p-value, we conclude that AQI parameters have significance with the traffic in location 1(Kebon Jeruk). The AQI parameters are NO2, SO2, CO, and O3. In location 2 (Kelapa Gading), the significant AQI parameters were NO2, SO2, CO, O3, and PM10. In location 3 (Lubang Buaya), the improved AQI parameters were SO2, CO, O3, and PM10. Moreover, in Location 4 (Jagakarsa), the AQI parameters that improved were CO and O3, and the last was in Location 5 (Thamrin). The AQI improvement (Tables 2, 3 and Figs. 1 and 2).

Table 2. Traffic Comparison Pre and During COVID-19 Periods in Each Location

Location	Season	Low Traffic	High Traffic	P-Value
Kebon Jeruk	PreCovid	1	25	6.13E-09*
	Covid	38	16	
Kelapa Gading	PreCovid	1	9	2.66E-08*
	Covid	41	1	
Lubang Buaya	PreCovid	3	22	6.84E-06*
	Covid	17	5	
Jagakarsa	PreCovid	0	11	8.66E-05*
	Covid	14	5	
Thamrin	PreCovid	0	17	3.12E-09*
	Covid	30	6	

*Statistically significant at p-value < 0.05

Table 3. Air Quality Comparison Pre and During COVID-19 Periods in Each Location

Location	Season	Low Traffic	High Traffic	P-Value
Kebon Jeruk	PreCovid	5	21	1.42E-01
	Covid	4	50	
Kelapa Gading	PreCovid	6	4	2.47E-04*
	Covid	2	40	
Lubang Buaya	PreCovid	7	18	1.04E-02*
	Covid	0	22	
Jagakarsa	PreCovid	2	9	1.00E + 00
	Covid	4	15	

(*continued*)

Table 3. (*continued*)

Location	Season	Low Traffic	High Traffic	P-Value
Thamrin	PreCovid	13	4	2.17E-02*
	Covid	13	21	

*Statistically significant at p-value < 0.05

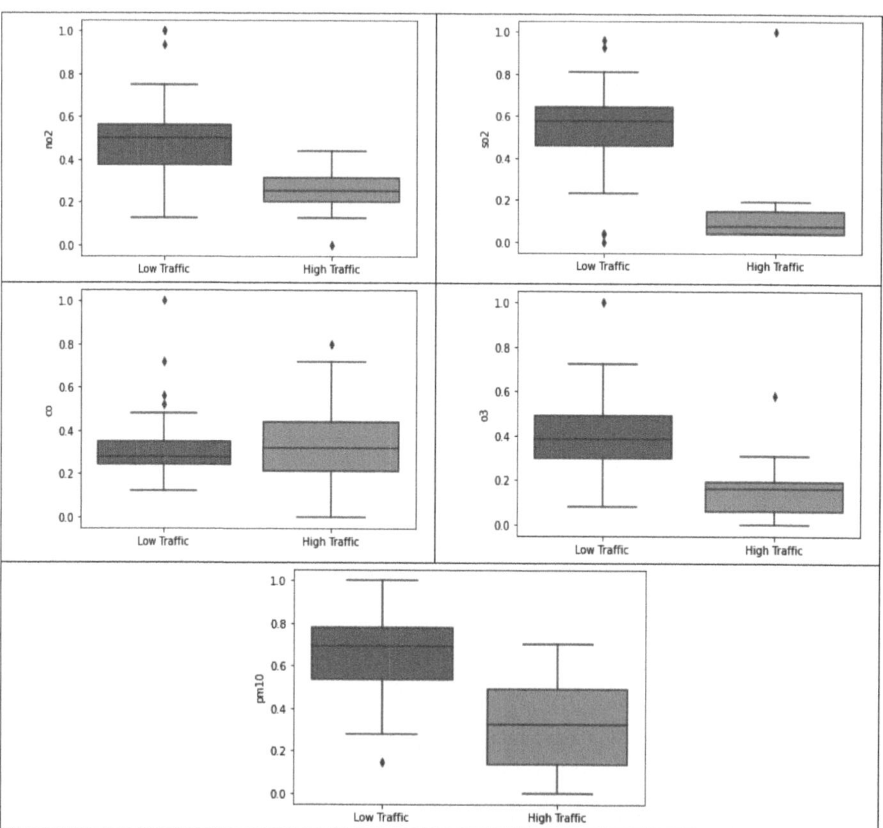

Fig. 1. Box plot the traffic correlation with the AQI parameter in Loc 2 (Kelapa Gading).

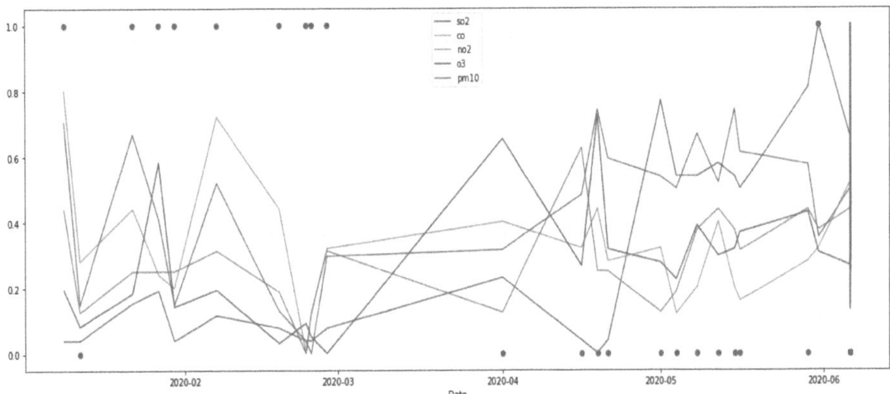

Fig. 2. The main plot of the traffic correlation with the AQI parameter in Loc 2 (Kelapa Gading).

5 Conclusion

Based on the result and statistical analysis from the comparison of the AQI parameters pre and during the pandemic COVID-19, and the comparison of the AQI parameters' improvement to traffic in five locations around Jakarta, we concluded that there is a significant improvement in the air quality pre and during of the pandemic of the COVID-19 in five of the research locations in Jakarta. We found that the minimum air quality improvement happened in location 3 (Lubang Buaya), with the significance of the p-value only containing one parameter, Ozone (O3). In addition, we found that the minimum improvement of the air quality during COVID-19 happened related to the traffic location in Jakarta in locations 4 and 5 (Jagakarsa and Thamrin). In these locations, we found only two AQI parameters that improved the locations compared to other locations. The parameters that improved were Nitrogen Dioxide (SO2), Carbon Monoxide (CO), and Ozone (O3).

Author Contributor

Conceptualization, F.A.; methodology, F.A.; data acquisition, F.A.; data curation, F.A; data analysis F.A. J.P.T., A.B; investigation, F.A.; writing-original draft preparation, F.A., J.P.T.; supervision, F.A.; project administration, F.A.; All authors reviewed the manuscript.

Data Availability.. The dataset is available in Zenodo with access at: https://doi.org/https://doi.org/10.5281/zenodo.17276303.

References

1. Burns, C.J., et al.: Research on COVID-19 and air pollution: a path towards advancing exposure science. Environ. Res. **212**, 113240 (2022). https://doi.org/10.1016/j.envres.2022.113240

2. Ravindra, K., Singh, T., Vardhan, S., Shrivastava, A.: Since January 2020 Elsevier has created a COVID-19 resource centre with free information in English and Mandarin on the novel coronavirus COVID- 19. The COVID-19 resource centre is hosted on Elsevier Connect , the company ' s public news and information. J. Infect. Public Health. **15**, 187–198 (2020)
3. Jiang, Z., et al.: Modeling the impact of COVID-19 on air quality in southern California: Implications for future control policies. Atmos. Chem. Phys. **21**, 8693–8708 (2021). https://doi.org/10.5194/acp-21-8693-2021
4. Cui, H., Ma, R., Gao, F.: Relationship between meteorological factors and diffusion of atmospheric pollutants. Chem. Eng. Trans. **71**, 1417–4122 (2018). https://doi.org/10.3303/CET1871237
5. Kayes, I., Shahriar, S.A., Hasan, K., Akhter, M., Kabir, M.M., Salam, M.A.: The relationships between meteorological parameters and air pollutants in an urban environment. Glob. J. Environ. Sci. Manag. **5**, 265–278 (2019). https://doi.org/10.22034/gjesm.2019.03.01
6. Gope, S., Dawn, S., Das, S.S.: Effect of COVID-19 pandemic on air quality: a study based on Air Quality Index. Environ. Sci. Pollut. Res. **28**, 35564–35583 (2021). https://doi.org/10.1007/s11356-021-14462-9
7. Caraka, R.E., et al.: Did noise pollution really improve during covid-19? Evidence from Taiwan. Sustain **13**, 1–12 (2021). https://doi.org/10.3390/su13115946
8. Şahin, M.: The association between air quality parameters and COVID-19 in Turkey. Pharm. Biomed. Res. **6**, 49–58 (2020). https://doi.org/10.18502/pbr.v6i(s1).4402
9. Khalis, M., et al.: Relationship between meteorological and air quality parameters and COVID-19 in Casablanca Region, Morocco. Int. J. Environ. Res. Public Health. **19**, (2022). https://doi.org/10.3390/ijerph19094989
10. Rad, A.K., et al.: Machine learning for determining interactions between air pollutants and environmental parameters in three cities of Iran. Sustain **14**, (2022). https://doi.org/10.3390/su14138027
11. Pardamean, B., Rahutomo, R., Cenggoro, T.W., Budiarto, A., Perbangsa, A.S.: The impact of large-scale social restriction phases on the air quality index in Jakarta. Atmosphere (Basel). **12**, 1–14 (2021). https://doi.org/10.3390/atmos12070922
12. Rendana, M., Idris, W.M.R., Rahim, S.A.: Changes in air quality during and after large-scale social restriction periods in Jakarta city, Indonesia. Acta Geophys. **70**, 2161–2169 (2022). https://doi.org/10.1007/s11600-022-00873-w
13. Pramana, S., et al.: Air pollution changes of Jakarta, Banten, and West Java, Indonesia during the first month of COVID-19 pandemic Setia PRAMANA 1, Dede Yoga PARAMARTHA 2, Yustiar ADHINUGROHO 3, Mieke NURMALASARI 4. J. Bus. Econ. Environ. Stud. **10**, 15–19 (2020). https://doi.org/10.13106/jbees.2020.vol10.no4.15
14. Santoso, M., et al.: Multiple air quality monitoring evidence of the impacts of large-scale social restrictions during the covid-19 pandemic in Jakarta, Indonesia. Aerosol Air Qual. Res. **21**, (2021). https://doi.org/10.4209/aaqr.200645
15. Jakob, A., Hasibuan, S., Fiantis, D.: Empirical evidence shows that air quality changes during COVID-19 pandemic lockdown in Jakarta, Indonesia are due to seasonal variation, not restricted movements. Environ. Res. **208**, (2022). https://doi.org/10.1016/j.envres.2021.112391
16. Rahutomo, R., Pardamean, B.: Data engineering pipeline to analyse Jakarta's air quality during covid-19-caused lockdown periods. IOP Conf. Ser. Earth Environ. Sci. **794**, 012112 (2021). https://doi.org/10.1088/1755-1315/794/1/012112
17. Handhayani, T.: An integrated analysis of air pollution and meteorological conditions in Jakarta. Sci. Rep. **13**, 5798 (2023). https://doi.org/10.1038/s41598-023-32817-9
18. Suhardono, S., et al.: Changes in the distribution of air pollutants (Carbon Monoxide) during the Control of the COVID-19 Pandemic in Jakarta, Surabaya, and Yogyakarta, Indonesia. J. Ecol. Eng. **24**, 151–162 (2023). https://doi.org/10.12911/22998993/159508

19. Sihayuardhi, E.R., Brontowiyono, W., Maziya, F.B., Hakim, L.: The effect of the COVID-19 pandemic on ambient air quality in Yogyakarta urban area parameters SO2, CO and, NO2with inverse distance weighting (IDW). IOP Conf. Ser. Earth Environ. Sci. **933**, (2021). https://doi.org/10.1088/1755-1315/933/1/012013
20. Caraka, R.E., Chen, R.C., Yasin, H., Suhartono, Lee, Y., Pardamean, B.: Hybrid vector autoregression feedforward neural network with genetic algorithm model for forecasting space-time pollution data. Indones. J. Sci. Technol. **6**, 243–268 (2021). https://doi.org/10.17509/ijost.v6i1.32732
21. Gurajala, S., Dhaniyala, S., Matthews, J.N.: Understanding public response to air quality using tweet analysis. Soc. Media Soc. **5**, 1–14 (2019). https://doi.org/10.1177/2056305119867656
22. Kumbalaparambi, T.S., Menon, R., Radhakrishnan, V.P., Nair, V.P.: Assessment of urban air quality from Twitter communication using self-attention network and a multilayer classification model. Environ. Sci. Pollut. Res. **30**, 10414–10425 (2023). https://doi.org/10.1007/s11356-022-22836-w
23. Kwilas, A.R., Donahue, R.N., Tsang, K.Y., Hodge, J.W.: 乳鼠心肌提取 HHS public access. Cancer Cell **2**, 1–17 (2015). https://doi.org/10.1016/j.ypmed.2019.02.005.Feasibility
24. Du, W., Wang, G.: Indoor air pollution was nonnegligible during covid-19 lockdown. Aerosol Air Qual. Res. **20**, 1851–1855 (2020). https://doi.org/10.4209/aaqr.2020.06.0281
25. Rahutomo, R., Purwandari, K., Hidayat, A.A., Pardamean, B.: South jakarta's air quality using PM 2.5 data at the beginning of COVID-19 Restriction. In: Proceedings of 2021 International Conference on Information Management and Technology, ICIMTech 2021. pp. 517–521 (2021). https://doi.org/10.1109/ICIMTech53080.2021.9535044
26. Shihab, A.S.: Investigating the relationship between air pollutants and meteorology: a canonical correlation analysis. Polish J. Environ. Stud. **31**, 5841–5849 (2022). https://doi.org/10.15244/pjoes/151908
27. Caraka, R.E., et al.: Impact of COVID-19 large scale restriction on environment and economy in Indonesia. Glob. J. Environ. Sci. Manag. **6**, 65–84 (2020). https://doi.org/10.22034/GJESM.2019.06.SI.07
28. Rahutomo, R., Purwandari, K., Sigalingging, J.W.C., Pardamean, B.: Improvement of Jakarta's air quality during large scale social restriction. IOP Conf. Ser. Earth Environ. Sci. **729**, 012132 (2021). https://doi.org/10.1088/1755-1315/729/1/012132

In the Digital Age, Branding for Sustainable Healthcare

Wahyu Sardjono[1(✉)], Deltu Ariesa[2], Maryani[3], Trias Septyoari Putranto[4], Azani Cempaka Sari[5], Ilham Radito[6], and Hasyiya Karimah Adli[7]

[1] Information Systems Management Department, BINUS Graduate Program – Master of Information Systems Management, Bina Nusantara University, Jl. K. H. Syahdan No. 9, Kemanggisan, Palmerah, Jakarta 11480, Indonesia
wahyu.s@binus.ac.id

[2] Master of Management in the Faculty of Economics and Business, Airlangga University, Surabaya, Indonesia
deltu.ariesa-2024@feb.unair.ac.id

[3] Information Systems Department, School of Information Systems, Bina Nusantara University, Jakarta 11480, Indonesia
yanie@binus.edu

[4] Hotel Management. Department Faculty of Digital Communication, Hotel & Tourism, Bina Nusantara University, Jakarta 11480, Indonesia
tputranto@binus.edu

[5] Computer Science Department, School of Computer Science, Bina Nusantara University, Jakarta 11480, Indonesia
acsari@binus.edu

[6] School of Computer Science, Faculty of Engineering, The University of Sydney, Sydney, Australia
irad0511@uni.sydney.edu

[7] Faculty of Data Science and Computing, Universiti Malaysia Kelantan City Campus, Pengkalan Chepa, Kelantan, Malaysia
hasyiya@umk.edu.my

Abstract. Healthcare branding is increasingly central to reputation, trust, and service quality. This PRISMA-guided systematic review synthesizes 34 peer-reviewed studies (2019–2025) identified from Scopus and related sources. Findings show dominance of quantitative designs using SEM/PLS-SEM, rising digital and AI-driven branding, and hospital-focused contexts, with growing attention to telemedicine and medical tourism, especially in developing countries. Bibliometric mapping (VOSviewer) and thematic analyses consolidate key theories, Brand Equity, Service Quality, Brand Trust, and Smart/Digital Branding. We outline gaps in qualitative evidence, cross-cultural comparisons, and explainable AI, and practical implications for strategies aligned with SDGs 3, 10, and 17.

Keywords: Healthcare Brand · Digital Brand · Sustainable Development Goals

E. R. Kaburuan and S. Goundar (Eds.): HIS 2025, LNCS 16392, pp. 260–271, 2026.
https://doi.org/10.1007/978-981-95-6304-3_23

1 Introduction

1.1 Background

The healthcare industry has undergone a paradigm shift, with branding emerging as a crucial strategic tool for competitiveness. Healthcare branding encompasses hospital brand image, clinic identity, medical professionals' personal branding, and patient perception, enhancing institutional reputation and supporting universal health coverage (UHC) in line with SDG 3: Good Health and Well-being. Recent research highlights branding's role in medical tourism, hospital brand equity, and digital marketing, emphasizing trust, service quality, and patient satisfaction while aligning with SDG 9: Industry, Innovation, and Infrastructure. A systematic literature review (SLR) synthesizes studies from developed and developing markets, analyzing methodologies such as SEM, PLS-SEM, content analysis, and PRISMA, with tools like SPSS, AMOS, and SmartPLS driving research advancements. Healthcare branding also supports SDG 10: Reduced inequalities by ensuring equitable access to quality services and SDG 17: Partnerships for the Goals through collaborations among hospitals, pharmaceutical companies, and digital health platforms. By examining research methodologies and trends, this study provides insights for academics, healthcare practitioners, and policymakers to develop effective branding strategies that enhance service delivery, patient satisfaction, and institutional credibility, with further sections detailing the research methodology, key findings, and future directions in healthcare branding and sustainability.

1.2 Research Question

This review addresses three questions:

RQ1: Which theories, constructs, methods, and analytic tools dominate healthcare branding research (2019–2025)?
RQ2: How do digital/AI-driven branding strategies affect patient trust, reputation, and perceived service quality?
RQ3: How do country- and setting-level contexts (developing vs. developed; hospitals vs. other healthcareservices) shape branding strategies and outcomes linked to SDG 3, 10, 17?

2 Literature Review

2.1 Healthcare Branding Concepts and Importance

Healthcare branding plays a critical role in influencing patient decisions, shaping institutional reputation, and differentiating healthcare services in an increasingly competitive market [1, 2]. Beyond hospitals, healthcare branding encompasses clinics, medical professionals, pharmaceutical companies, and digital health services. Recent research highlights that brand image, service quality, and patient trust are key factors influencing healthcare service quality and patient loyalty [3].

Several studies emphasize the importance of digital transformation in branding, particularly with the growing reliance on online branding strategies, AI-driven branding, and digital engagement [4] and trust-building mechanisms [5].

2.2 Theoretical Foundations in Healthcare Branding

Several branding theories have been widely applied in healthcare research, including:

- Service Quality Theory: Establishes a link between branding strategies, perceived service excellence, and patient satisfaction.
- Brand Trust Theory: Explains how patients develop loyalty and trust toward healthcare institutions based on their branding strategies.
- Brand Equity Theory: Highlights how branding influences perceived value, patient loyalty, and hospital reputation.
- Smart Branding Theory: Investigates the impact of AI, digital branding, and online platforms in shaping modern healthcare branding.
- Brand Positioning Theory: Analyzes how hospitals and clinics position themselves in highly competitive healthcare markets.

Recent healthcare branding research highlights a shift toward technology-driven strategies. Key trends include the growing influence of digital branding through social media, AI and big data for brand positioning, and the role of branding in medical tourism, especially in developing countries. Additionally, patient testimonials, word-of-mouth marketing, and online reviews are crucial in shaping trust and brand perception.

3 Research Method

3.1 Research Design

This study adopts a Systematic Literature Review (SLR) methodology to synthesize existing research on healthcare branding across different markets. The SLR follows the Preferred Reporting Items for Systematic Reviews and Meta-Analyses (PRISMA) framework, ensuring a rigorous and transparent selection process. The objective is to consolidate theoretical perspectives, methodological approaches, and key findings in healthcare branding research, thereby identifying research gaps and future directions.

Given the increasing role of digital branding and AI-driven healthcare marketing, this review also explores recent technological advancements and their impact on branding strategies in the healthcare sector. Following PRISMA, we identified 103 records in Scopus; after removing 2 duplicates, 20 automation-flagged ineligible items, 12 off-tier records, and 3 without abstracts, 66 records were screened with 10 excluded, 56 full texts were sought with 22 not retrieved, leaving 34 articles assessed for eligibility none excluded, resulting in 34 studies included in the final review (see Appendix 1, PRISMA Flow).

3.2 Data Source

This study follows a rigorous selection process based on the PRISMA framework, ensuring a systematic and transparent approach. Articles are sourced from Scopus, Web of Science, ScienceDirect, and Google Scholar, focusing on healthcare branding topics using keywords like "hospital branding,", "clinic branding", "healthcare branding", and "AI-driven healthcare branding." The study includes peer-reviewed journal articles, case studies, and systematic reviews published between 2019 and March 2025, emphasizing digital branding strategies, AI applications, and healthcare service marketing. Only English-language publications are considered for consistency. The scope covers hospitals, clinics, telemedicine platforms, and other healthcare facilities, ensuring a comprehensive analysis of branding strategies in the healthcare sector.

3.3 Research Instrument

A structured coding framework was developed to systematically extract and categorize key data from the selected studies, ensuring a comprehensive and consistent review process. The extracted data included publication details (author(s), year, and journal name), research methodology (quantitative, qualitative, or mixed-methods), and data collection techniques such as surveys, interviews, case studies, content analysis, and systematic reviews. Analytical tools were examined, with statistical methods like Structural Equation Modeling (SEM), Partial Least Squares SEM (PLS-SEM), and descriptive statistics, while qualitative approaches included content analysis, sentiment analysis, and thematic analysis. Bibliometric techniques, including keyword co-occurrence and citation mapping using VOSviewer, were used to analyze research trends. The study also identified key theoretical frameworks such as Service Quality Theory, Brand Trust Theory, Smart Branding Theory, Brand Equity Theory, and Brand Positioning Theory, providing insights into branding's impact on healthcare institutions, patient perceptions, and service quality. The findings synthesized branding effectiveness in healthcare, highlighting research gaps in digital branding, AI integration, and cross-cultural perspectives, emphasizing the need for future studies to enhance patient engagement, institutional reputation, and market competitiveness.

3.4 Data Analysis

This study combines quantitative and qualitative analysis to evaluate healthcare branding research. Using bibliometric analysis with VOSviewer (see Fig. 1 Appendix 4), it identifies key authors, institutions, and emerging trends. Content analysis categorizes branding strategies, including brand positioning, service quality, patient trust, and digital marketing, with a focus on medical tourism and telemedicine. A comparative case study examines branding practices in hospital chains, AI-driven healthcare platforms, and telemedicine services, highlighting best practices and areas for improvement. Data is analyzed through qualitative content analysis and descriptive statistics to assess recurring themes, theoretical contributions, and methodological trends.

3.5 Research Methodologies in Healthcare Branding

The methodologies employed in healthcare branding research exhibit considerable diversity, reflecting the multidisciplinary nature of the field. A predominant approach among existing studies is quantitative research, particularly survey-based investigations utilizing Structural Equation Modeling (SEM) and Partial Least Squares SEM (PLS-SEM) as key analytical techniques. These statistical methods enable researchers to assess complex relationships between branding constructs, patient perceptions, and institutional reputation, offering robust insights into healthcare branding dynamics.

Beyond traditional statistical modeling, recent advancements have incorporated artificial intelligence-based sentiment analysis, particularly in the context of telemedicine branding, to evaluate patient perceptions of healthcare brands in digital platforms. The integration of AI-based methodologies underscores the increasing reliance on data-driven branding analytics within the healthcare sector.

In addition to quantitative approaches, qualitative methodologies have played a crucial role in exploring branding narratives and patient experiences. Case studies and content analysis have been widely used to provide an in-depth understanding of branding strategies, enabling researchers to capture contextual nuances and patient-driven insights. Furthermore, systematic literature reviews employing the Preferred Reporting Items for Systematic Reviews and Meta-Analyses (PRISMA) methodology have facilitated the synthesis of existing knowledge, allowing for the identification of theoretical and empirical gaps within the healthcare branding domain.

To support these methodological approaches, various software applications have been utilized for data analysis. SPSS, AMOS, and SmartPLS have been extensively employed for statistical modeling, hypothesis testing, and structural equation modeling, providing researchers with advanced tools for validating branding-related hypotheses. Additionally, VOSviewer has been widely applied for bibliometric analysis, enabling the examination of research trends, keyword co-occurrences, and citation networks within healthcare branding literature. The integration of these analytical tools underscores the methodological rigor applied in contemporary healthcare branding research, facilitating a systematic and empirical exploration of branding strategies and their implications for healthcare institutions.

4 Results

4.1 Number of Publication

The annual output shows a U-shaped trajectory with a sharp surge in 2024 (see Fig. 2, Appendix 4). Publications decline from 2019 (9 articles) and 2020 (8 articles) to a trough in 2021–2022 (4 each), rebound in 2023 (9 articles), and then peak in 2024 (16; 75–80% above 2023), indicating intensified scholarly attention to the topic. The low count in early 2025 reflects partial-year data and should not be interpreted as a reversal. Overall, the pattern suggests post-2022 recovery and consolidation, culminating in a 2024 acceleration likely driven by maturing methods and expanding digital/AI themes in the field.

This review identifies the number of studies is still relatively low compared to research on other marketing topics, especially in healthcare management. Through research, researchers can identify the most effective brand design or implementation strategy so that it can generate optimal revenue in the healthcare industry.

4.2 Types of Reserach

Based on data analysis from the research (see Fig. 3, Appendix 4) on healthcare brands, it can be seen that the research trend uses more quantitative methods compared to qualitative or mixed methods. Of the 34 studies listed, 27 studies used a quantitative approach, while only 5 studies used a qualitative approach, and 1 study used mixed methods. This shows that research on healthcare brands tends to be predominantly carried out using a quantitative approach.

Quantitative research has the advantage of measuring variables objectively and producing data that can be analyzed statistically. In the context of healthcare brands, a quantitative approach allows researchers to measure the impact of various factors such as brand image, service quality, patient loyalty and patient satisfaction numerically. This approach allows researchers to test hypotheses and produce generalizable findings.

In the healthcare industry, verifiable and measurable data is critical for making strategic decisions. Quantitative research provides data that hospital management or healthcare providers can use to improve their branding strategies. For example, research by [6] in China used quantitative methods to measure the impact of service quality, brand image and perceived value on patient loyalty in private dental clinics. The data generated from this research can be used to develop more effective marketing strategies.

Quantitative research often uses methods such as Structural Equation Modeling (SEM) or regression to test relationships between variables. This is particularly relevant in healthcare brand research, where researchers often want to understand how factors such as service quality, trust and brand image influence each other. For example, research by [7] in Iran used SEM to examine the role of service quality, trust, and loyalty in building hospital brand equity.

With technological developments, quantitative data such as patient surveys, social media usage data, and health transaction data have become more easily accessible. This makes it easier for researchers to conduct extensive quantitative research. For example, research by [8] in Indonesia used survey data to measure the impact of social media marketing on beauty clinic brand equity.

Quantitative research allows researchers to produce findings that can be generalized to a larger population. This is especially important in the context of healthcare brands, where branding strategies often need to be implemented broadly. The findings from this research can be used by other hospitals to improve the quality of their services.

4.3 Research Subjects

It can be seen from Fig. 4 (Appendix 4), Research subjects that focus on hospitals dominate with a total of 24 publications. Other healthcare facilities besides clinics are pharmaceutical, herbal healthcare, healthcare organizations, medical tourism, and traditional medicine. This result may be related to increasingly fierce competition between hospitals, which involves greater resources compared to other healthcare services. Hospitals are the main healthcare centers that handle complex medical cases, requiring significant investments in technology, human resources, and branding strategies. Additionally, the role of hospitals in medical tourism has further intensified the need for strong brand positioning to attract international patients. The complexity of internal and external factors, such as patient satisfaction, trust, and regulatory challenges, also makes hospitals a rich subject for research. Therefore, the dominance of hospitals as research subjects reflects their critical role in the healthcare ecosystem and the need for continuous innovation in branding strategies.

Hospitals are primary healthcare centers that handle complex medical cases and require large resources. This makes hospitals a rich research subject in terms of variables, such as service quality, patient trust, loyalty, and brand image. For example, a study in Iran examined the role of service quality, trust, and loyalty in building hospital brand equity. This complexity makes hospitals an interesting research subject.

Hospitals also play a significant role in the medical tourism industry, where patients from different countries choose a particular hospital based on its reputation and brand image. A study by [9] in Turkey explored how hospital brand image influences medical tourists' decisions. This suggests that hospitals are not only competing locally but also globally, increasing the urgency of building a strong brand.

Hospitals are often pioneers in adopting the latest technologies and innovations, such as the use of artificial intelligence (AI) and digital platforms to enhance the patient experience. A study in Spain explored how hospitals are using digital tools and AI to build their brands. The large investment in these technologies makes hospitals a relevant and interesting subject for research.

4.4 Healthcare Brand Theories Selected

Brand theory is one of the topics in marketing management. However, there is a difference in implementing brand strategy in healthcare compared to other industries. Based on the analysis, digital and online branding theory is currently having a high trend. This is driven by the rapid development of digital technology, especially the use of social media and mobile applications, which have transformed how hospitals and healthcare providers interact with patients. For instance, research in Spain explores how hospitals use digital tools and artificial intelligence (AI) to build their brands. Meanwhile, other research also involves brand positioning theory, brand trust and loyalty theory, and service branding theory, although they are not as prominent as digital and online branding. The increasing use of social media in branding, the need for personalization and interactivity, the importance of online reputation, and the integration of technology in healthcare services are key factors driving the trend of digital and online branding in healthcare. Therefore, while some publications focus on a single topic, others highlight multiple aspects of branding, reflecting the complexity and diversity of healthcare branding strategies.

Brand theory is one of the important topics in marketing management (see Fig. 5, Appendix 4). However, there are differences in the implementation of branding strategies in the healthcare sector compared to other industries. Based on data analysis from the research table on healthcare brands, it can be seen that digital and online branding theories are currently experiencing a high trend. This can be seen from the many studies that raise topics related to the use of social media, mobile applications, and digital technology in building brands in the healthcare sector. Meanwhile, several other theories such as brand positioning theory, brand trust and loyalty theory, and service branding theory are also quite widely used in research, although not as popular as digital and online branding theories.

The rapid development of digital technology, especially in the use of social media and mobile applications, has changed the way hospitals and healthcare providers interact with patients. Research by Medina in Spain explored how hospitals use digital tools and artificial intelligence (AI) to build their brands. This shows that digital technology is an effective tool for increasing patient engagement and loyalty.

Social media has become a very effective platform for building brand image and interacting with patients. Research by Hung, et al. in Taiwan shows how integrating social media into branding strategies can increase patient engagement [10]. Social media allows hospitals to quickly disseminate information, build communities, and respond to patient feedback in real-time.

Patients today expect a more personalized and interactive experience when interacting with healthcare providers. Research by Parrish and Nevins in the United States explores how personalized branding can increase patient engagement [11]. Digital technology allows hospitals to offer more personalized and responsive services, thereby increasing patient satisfaction and loyalty.

Technologies such as telemedicine, health apps, and other digital platforms have become an integral part of modern healthcare. A study by AlSaleh in Kuwait explored how technology-based services can enhance a hospital's brand equity [12]. This technology integration not only improves service quality but also strengthens the hospital's brand image as an innovative service provider.

4.5 Types of Country

Based on data analysis from the research on healthcare brands (see Fig. 6, Appendix 4), it can be seen that research trends are carried out more in developing countries compared to developed countries. The majority of research was conducted in countries such as India, Malaysia, Indonesia, Vietnam and Turkey, while there were relatively fewer studies in developed countries such as the United States, England and other European countries. This phenomenon is interesting to study in more depth, considering that developed countries are usually considered centers of innovation and research in various fields, including health. However, data shows that interest in healthcare brands is actually higher in developing countries.

The adoption of health technology (healthtech) in developing countries is increasing, especially with the widespread use of smartphones and the internet. This opens up new opportunities for health brands to reach consumers through digital platforms. Research on healthcare brands often focuses on how these brands can leverage technology to increase consumer engagement and loyalty. For example, research in Indonesia and Brazil shows how social media and digital tools are used to build brand equity in healthcare [13].

Regulatory of developing countries often have dynamic business environments, which influence how health brands operate. The research was conducted to understand how brands can adapt to changing regulations, market competition and evolving consumer expectations. For example, research in India and Thailand shows how healthcare brands seek to maintain patient loyalty through service quality and brand image [14].

Awareness and education about health is increasing, especially among the younger generation. This encourages health brands to be more active in building image and trust through in-depth research into consumer behavior and preferences. For example, research in China and Indonesia shows how health brands seek to build emotional connections with patients through effective branding strategies [15].

Experienced significant healthcare market growth in recent years. This is driven by increased awareness of the importance of health, population growth, and increased access to health services. Along with this, health brands are competing to understand the needs of consumers in these countries, thus encouraging a lot of research related to branding and marketing strategies in the health sector. For example, research in India and Indonesia suggests a focus on how health brands can position themselves in competitive markets [16].

Developing countries often face complex health challenges, such as infectious diseases, lack of access to basic health services, and a double burden of disease (communicable and non-communicable diseases). This condition creates a need for innovative and affordable health solutions. Research on healthcare brands helps companies and governments to develop effective communication and marketing strategies to face these challenges. For example, research in Iran and Turkey shows how healthcare brands seek to build patient loyalty through service quality and brand image.

4.6 Data Collection Instruments

In Fig. 7, Appendix 4. Surveys are the most widely used data collection instrument in healthcare branding research, with 20 studies employing this method. They are preferred for their efficiency in gathering data from large respondent groups and their flexibility in aligning questions with research objectives. Surveys enable researchers to quantitatively measure key variables such as brand perception, patient loyalty, and service quality. While they remain the most effective and popular tool due to their ability to generate statistically analyzable data, future research could benefit from combining quantitative and qualitative methods for a more comprehensive understanding of healthcare branding dynamics.

4.7 Data Analysis Methods

Structural Equation Modeling (SEM) is the most widely used data analysis method in healthcare branding research, with 18 studies employing it as the primary approach. SEM is preferred for its ability to test complex relationships between branding variables, such as brand perception, patient loyalty, service quality, and the influence of social media on brand equity. It allows researchers to analyze causal relationships between latent and manifest variables while incorporating mediation and moderation effects. Although other methods like descriptive analysis, multiple regression, and content analysis are used, they are less common. SEM remains the dominant analytical tool due to its effectiveness in testing complex theoretical models, but future research could benefit from integrating qualitative methods for a more comprehensive understanding of healthcare branding dynamics (see Fig. 8, Appendix 4).

5 Discussion

This study identifies key trends in global healthcare branding, emphasizing the dominance of quantitative methods, hospital-focused research, and the rise of digital branding. Analysis of 34 studies shows healthcare branding is growing, especially in developing countries, with surveys and SEM as preferred methods. While these provide insights into brand image and patient loyalty, the lack of qualitative approaches limits understanding of patient experiences. Research mainly focuses on hospitals, overlooking other sectors like clinics and pharmaceuticals. Digital branding, driven by social media and AI, is reshaping healthcare marketing, particularly in medical tourism, but aspects like trust and positioning need further study. Most studies are in developing countries, highlighting rapid market growth, while research in developed nations remains limited. Integrating qualitative methods could provide a deeper understanding of healthcare branding dynamics.

Beyond the survey/SEM core, qualitative evidence highlights (i) patient trust narratives built through transparent communication and consistent service cues, (ii) experience cues (staff empathy, waiting-time clarity, safety signals) that convert functional satisfaction into reputation and loyalty, (iii) peran digital touchpoints (UGC, reviews, social platforms) sebagai arena ko-kreasi makna merek; temuan ini menegaskan bahwa strategi branding berbasis AI/digital efektif bila dipasangkan dengan meaning-making kualitatif yang peka konteks [18].

In developing countries, rapid platform adoption, limited health literacy, and evolving data/AI governance encourage cost-efficient blends of owned and earned media and SDG-17 partnerships to expand reach and build trust; in developed contexts, the emphasis shifts to data governance, transparency/XAI, and the integration of outcome-based metrics (trust, quality) across channels. These differences require context-sensitive branding playbooks to ensure more equitable impacts on SDGs 3 and 10 [4, 9, 17].

Limitations. This article was constrained by the journal's template and formatting limits (page/word count and citation style), so some sources consulted during the review could not be listed in the References. For transparency, the complete bibliography is provided in the Appendix/Supplementary materials.

6 Conclusion

This study explores healthcare branding trends, highlighting the dominance of quantitative methods, hospital-focused research, and digital branding. Surveys and SEM are preferred for measurable data, but the lack of qualitative methods limits insight into patient experiences. While hospitals dominate research, clinics and pharmaceutical companies are underexplored. Digital branding, especially in medical tourism, is growing, though brand trust needs more attention. Most studies focus on developing countries, reflecting market growth, while research in developed nations remains limited. Expanding methodologies and innovation are crucial for a deeper understanding of healthcare branding.

This review identifies a survey- and SEM-centric field with accelerating digital/AI-driven branding, underscores qualitative mechanisms of trust and reputation, and proposes context-sensitive strategies to advance SDG 3, 10, and 17 while strengthening institutional credibility.

Acknowledgments. We would like to express our deepest gratitude to Bina Nusantara University for the opportunity to receive the BINUS International Research Grant - Applied 2025 and for the invaluable facilities in fostering collaboration and stimulating in-depth discussions during this research work.

Open Data. https://doi.org/10.5281/zenodo.17392748.

Author Contributor. *Wahyu Sardjono*, abstract and introduction. *Deltu Ariesa*, literatur review, *Maryani*, methodology. *Trias Septyoari Putranto*, result. *Azani Cempaka Sari*, discusion. Ilham Radito, managing data via Zenodo, and Hasyiya Karimah Adli, conclusion.

References

1. Cham, T.H., Cheng, B.L., Low, M.P., Cheok, J.B.C.: Brand image as the competitive edge for hospitals in medical tourism. Eur. Bus. Rev. **33**(1), 31–59 (2021)
2. Adlakha, K., Sharma, S.: Brand positioning using multidimensional scaling technique: an application to herbal healthcare brands in Indian market. Vision **24**(3), 345–355 (2019)
3. Górska-Warsewicz, H.: Consumer or patient determinants of hospital brand equity—a systematic literature review. Int. J. Environ. Res. Public Health **19**(15), 9026 (2022)
4. Medina Aguerrebere, P., Medina, E., González Pacanowski, T.: Building smart brands through online and artificial intelligence tools: a quantitative analysis about the best hospitals in Spain. Online J. Commun. Media Technol. **14**(1), Art. no. e202407 (2024)
5. Kumar, P., Mittal, S., Kumar, S.: Building healthcare brand: Role of service, image, and trust. Asia Pac. J. Health Manag. **19**(1), (2024)
6. Lin, W., Yin, W.: Impacts of service quality, brand image, and perceived value on outpatient's loyalty to China's private dental clinics with service satisfaction as a mediator. PLoS ONE **17**(6), e0269233 (2022)
7. Kalhor, R., Khosravizadeh, O., Kiaei, M.Z., Shahsavari, S., Badrlo, M.: Role of service quality, trust, and loyalty in building patient-based brand equity: Modeling for public hospitals. Int. J. Healthc. Manag. **14**(4), 1389–1396 (2020)
8. Warbung, C.J.E., Wowor, M.C., Walean, R.H., Mandagi, D.W.: The impact of social media marketing on beauty clinic brand equity. Int. J. Prof. Bus. Rev. **8**(4), e01389 (2023)
9. Demir, Y., Dağ, E., Aydın Kılınç, Z., Karakuş, P., Özpinar, S: Hospital brand image and determinants in medical tourism: the case of Samsun. Geoj. Tour. Geosites **53**(2), 413–420 (2024)
10. Hung, C.L., et al.: Enhancing healthcare services and brand engagement through social media marketing: integration of Kotler's 5A framework with IDEA process. Inf. Process. Manag. **60**(4), 103379 (2023)
11. Parrish, F., Nevins, S.: Mass personalisation: a strategy for building brand equity in the healthcare sector. J. Brand Strategy **12**(1), 6–24 (2023)
12. AlSaleh, D.A.: The role of technology-based services in establishing brand equity within the private hospital sector in Kuwait. J. Transnatl. Manag. **24**(1), 21–39 (2019)

13. de Assis, W.M., Vilela, B.: The impact of social media marketing influence on value co-creation, brand equity, and customer engagement. Strateg. Dir. **40**(8), 8–10 (2024)
14. Wathanakom, N., Juicharoen, N., Saranrom, A.: The cause-and-effect model of service quality of private hospital on brand loyalty, mediated by customer satisfaction. Pak. J. Life Soc. Sci. **22**(1), 5248–5261 (2024)
15. Aji, H.M., Muslichah, I.: Is halal universal? The impact of self-expressive value on halal brand personality, brand tribalism, and loyalty: case of Islamic hospitals. J. Islam. Mark. **14**(4), 1146–1165 (2023)
16. Mandagi, D.W., Rampen, D.C., Soewignyo, T.I., Walean, R.H.: Empirical nexus of hospital brand gestalt, patient satisfaction and revisit intention. Int. J. Pharm. Healthc. Mark. **18**(2), 215–236 (2024)
17. Woods, B., Fox, A., Sculpher, M., Claxton, K.: Estimating the shares of the value of branded pharmaceuticals accruing to manufacturers and to patients served by health systems. Health Econ. (2021). https://doi.org/10.1002/hec.4393
18. Kennedy, D.M.: Managing the mayo clinic brand: a case study in staff-developed service performance standards. J. Brand Manag. (2019). https://doi.org/10.1057/s41262-018-00148-0

Managing Health Insurance in Indonesia: Developments, Obstacles, and Industry 4.0's Impact on Claim Processing

Wahyu Sardjono[1](✉), Dwi Putra Kasoema[2], Maryani[3], Trias Septyoari Putranto[4], Azani Cempaka Sari[5], Ilham Radito[6], and Hasyiya Karimah Adli[7]

[1] Information Systems Management Department, BINUS Graduate Program – Master of Information Systems Management, Bina Nusantara University, Jl. K. H. Syahdan No. 9, Kemanggisan, Palmerah, Jakarta 11480, Indonesia
wahyu.s@binus.ac.id

[2] Master of Management in the Faculty of Economics and Business, Airlangga University, Surabaya, Indonesia
dwiputrakasoema@mail.ugm.ac.id

[3] Information Systems Department, School of Information Systems, Bina Nusantara University, Jakarta 11480, Indonesia
yanie@binus.edu

[4] Hotel Management. Department Faculty of Digital Communication, Hotel and Tourism, Bina Nusantara University, Jakarta 11480, Indonesia
tputranto@binus.edu

[5] Computer Science Department, School of Computer Science, Bina Nusantara University, Jakarta 11480, Indonesia
acsari@binus.edu

[6] School of Computer Science, Faculty of Engineering, The University of Sydney, Sydney, Australia
irad0511@uni.sydney.edu

[7] Faculty of Data Science and Computing, Universiti Malaysia Kelantan City Campus, Pengkalan Chepa, Kelantan, Malaysia
hasyiya@umk.edu.my

Abstract. In the current landscape of economic uncertainty and escalating healthcare costs, health insurance plays a pivotal role as a vital financial tool. The projected surge in healthcare expenditures in Indonesia, as outlined by the Mercer Marsh Benefits Trend Health 2023 report, underscores the urgency for robust health insurance solutions to mitigate the financial risks associated with unpredictable health events. This paper explores the evolving dynamics of health insurance in Indonesia against the backdrop of rising healthcare costs and the growing awareness among the populace regarding the significance of financial protection. We also delve into the burgeoning field of Industry 4.0 and its implications for health insurance claim processing, emphasizing the role of Optical Character Recognition (OCR) technology in automating and streamlining claim administration processes. The study underscores the criticality of optimizing service quality within health insurance companies and delineates the claim decision process, elucidating the pivotal role of technological advancements such as OCR in enhancing

E. R. Kaburuan and S. Goundar (Eds.): HIS 2025, LNCS 16392, 272–285, 2026.
https://doi.org/10.1007/978-981-95-6304-3_24

efficiency and accuracy. Furthermore, we offer insights into the challenges and considerations associated with OCR implementation and present a comparative analysis of claim decision processes with and without OCR. Overall, the research underscores the importance of leveraging technology and expert human oversight to navigate the complexities of health insurance in Indonesia and ensure swift, equitable, and cost-effective claim resolutions.

Keywords: OCR (Optical Character Recognition) · health insurance · claim administration · industry 4.0

1 Introduction

In the era of economic uncertainty and rising healthcare costs, health insurance has become a crucial financial instrument. According to Mercer Marsh Benefits Trend Health 2023, the projected increase in healthcare costs in Indonesia for the year 2023 is expected to reach 13.6%, surpassing Asia's projection of 11.5% and exceeding Indonesia's financial inflation rate of 5.5% in 2022 [1]. This increase is influenced by several factors, including medical cost inflation, advancements in healthcare technology, and treatment delays during the pandemic. This situation has heightened awareness among the public regarding the need for financial protection against unpredictable health risks. The potential for private health insurance products in Indonesia is significant and continues to grow, despite government programs such as BPJS Kesehatan with limited coverage. Many Indonesians seek additional protection through private health insurance to access better services and broader coverage. Awareness of the importance of health protection is increasing, as indicated by the results of the 2023 Populix survey titled "Indonesia's Perceptions and Attitude Towards Health & Life Insurance Products. "The survey indicates that 73% of Indonesians consider having insurance to be very important, especially for health security with notes that the COVID-19 pandemic has heightened awareness of health risks, with 3 out of 10 Indonesians starting to have insurance in the past 1–2 years [2] (Fig. 1).

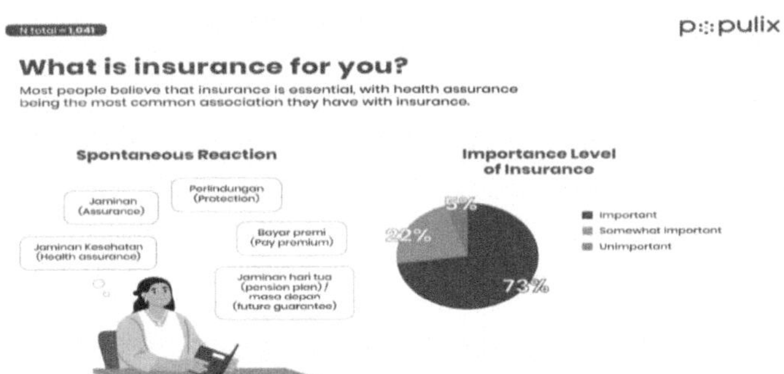

Fig. 1. The result of the Populix survey on the importance level of insurance (https://info.populix.co/product/consumer-trend-report/download?report=2023-01-indonesias-perceptions-and-attitude-towards-health-life-insurance-products)

According to the Asosiasi Asuransi Jiwa Indonesia (AAJI) reported that health insurance claims reached Rp 15.24 trillion in the third quarter of 2023, which grew by 32.9 percent annually compared to the same period last year, amounting to Rp 11.47 trillion [3].

Table 1. Total Health Insurance Claims Paid in 2022 - 2023

Quarter	Total Health Insurance Claims Paid (IDR trillion)		Change (%)
	2022	2023	
Q1 [4]	3.32	4.6	+38.6%
Q2 [5]	6.94	9.39	+35.3%
Q3 [6]	11.47	15.24	+32.9%
Q4 [7]	16.41	N/A	N/A
Average			+35.6%

Meanwhile, the world is currently undergoing a significant change, known as the Fourth Industrial Revolution (Industry 4.0). Industry 4.0 represents a change in the mechanisms of producing goods and services, characterized by the use of the Internet of Things (IoT), big data, automation, robotics, cloud computing, and artificial intelligence (AI) [8]. With the increasing number of healthcare claims, there is a need for a revolution in processing and validating health insurance claims from manual processes of paper checking to automation using Optical Character Recognition (OCR). OCR is process of classification of optical patterns contained in a digital image corresponding to alphanumeric or other characters [9]. OCR helps digitize printed texts to enable data extraction, process insurance claims, and build better solutions. In other words, OCR enables users to obtain information and further modify it. It is a reliable method that allows various industries to derive maximum value from data.

2 Literature Review

The origins of OCR trace back to 1809 with the development of reading devices for blind individuals and telegraph reading, followed by Emanuel Goldberg's invention in 1914 of a machine capable of converting printed characters into standard telegraph code, claimed as the inception of OCR technology, later named the "statistical machine" in 1927, alongside Edmund Fourier's creation of the Optophone, a portable scanning device producing sound corresponding to printed characters, leading to widespread utilization of OCR by libraries in the 1990s to digitize historical newspapers, with the digitization of historical books and primary reference sources flourishing in the 21st century due to rapid advancements in hardware, software, and the internet [10]. However, managing the substantial volume of such documents necessitates significant time and space resources for storage and organization. While transitioning to paperless document management is ideal, the process of scanning documents into images presents its own set of challenges. This method often requires manual intervention and is inherently laborious and time-consuming. Moreover, the digitization of document content often results in image files containing hidden text. Unlike text documents, text within images cannot be easily processed by conventional word processing software. Herein lies the importance of Optical Character Recognition (OCR) technology [11].

The diagram below illustrates the types of OCR systems, which typically guide how OCR will be applied during conversion via online or offline modes and predict the positions of characters on the page. Recognizing handwritten characters can sometimes pose a challenge due to the varying writing styles of users and the different pen movements used for certain characters. The accuracy of handwritten character recognition is typically lower due to the variations in shapes and types of handwriting. Additionally, differences in characters across languages, such as Mandarin, Japanese, and other Kanji writings, also significantly impact recognition accuracy. Online written documents are less complex as they can capture temporal or time-based information. In contrast, offline recognition systems operate on static data, where the input is an electronic image, making the recognition process more difficult. Offline character recognition systems first generate documents, digitize them, and store them in a computer before processing. On the other hand, for online character recognition systems, characters are processed directly during their creation. External factors such as writing speed affect offline systems. Both offline and online systems can be applied to optical as well as handwritten character recognition [12] (Fig. 2).

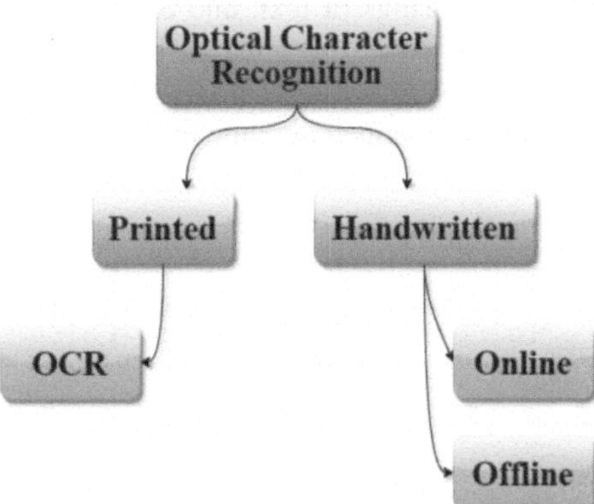

Fig. 2. Types of OCR (https://www.jetir.org/papers/JETIR2104193.pdf)

Optical Character Recognition (OCR) functions through a series of systematic steps, each contributing to the accurate conversion of images containing text into machine-readable data. Here's a breakdown of the key stages in the OCR process [13]:

1. Image Acquisition.

   OCR begins with the acquisition of images, typically done through scanning devices. These devices convert documents into binary data. The scanned image is then analyzed by OCR software, where bright areas are identified as background and dark areas as text.

2. Pre-processing.

   Pre-processing involves various operations performed on the scanned or input image to enhance its quality and suitability for segmentation. This includes removing noise, improving character clarity, and enhancing image rendering.

3. Segmentation.

   Following pre-processing, the image is segmented into distinct components. This typically involves dividing the image into lines, words, and individual characters. Segmentation is crucial for isolating characters and preparing them for feature extraction and recognition.

4. Feature Extraction.

   Feature extraction plays a critical role in identifying and distinguishing characters within the segmented image. Two primary methods are employed: pattern matching and feature extraction. Pattern matching compares character images to stored glyphs, while feature extraction breaks down characters into distinctive features such as lines, circles, and intersections.

5. Training and Recognition.

   OCR systems employ various techniques for pattern recognition, including template matching, statistical methods, syntactic analysis, and artificial neural networks. Training the system involves teaching it to recognize patterns and mitigate issues related to incomplete vocabulary.

6. Post-processing.

   The final stage involves activities such as grouping, error detection, and correction. Symbols are associated with strings of text, and errors are identified and rectified where possible. Following analysis, extracted text data is converted into editable files. Certain OCR systems can generate annotated PDF files containing both pre- and post-processed versions of scanned documents.

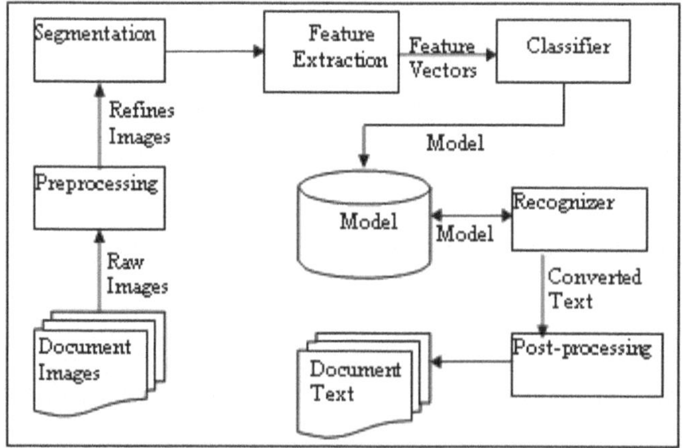

Fig. 3. Modules of OCR. (https://www.irjet.net/archives/V6/i6/IRJET-V6I6736.pdf)

There are several compelling reasons for selecting OCR systems over alternative scanning methods [14] (Fig. 3):

1. Searchable Immutable Files.
   PDF files and textual electronic images often lack searchability and editability, rendering the information within them inaccessible. OCR technology facilitates the conversion of static text into machine-readable data, allowing for efficient searching.
2. Ease of Edits.
   OCR transforms unalterable files into editable text documents, enabling seamless editing. This adaptability is crucial for accommodating changes in business operations.
3. Error Prevention.
   OCR not only facilitates editing and searching within documents but also helps identify and rectify incorrect or misprinted information. By detecting and resolving human errors, OCR technology enhances accuracy and reliability.
4. Time and Cost Savings.
   OCR significantly reduces the time and resources required for manual data entry. By automating the scanning process, businesses can save both time and money, thereby improving efficiency.
5. Space Efficiency.
   Digitizing paper documents through OCR eliminates the need for physical storage space, freeing up valuable office space. This transition to digital documents promotes organization and efficiency in the workspace.

Despite its numerous benefits, OCR technology presents several challenges that can affect its accuracy and performance [15]:

1. Scene Complexity.
   Images captured by cameras often contain complex backgrounds or objects, making text recognition challenging. Non-textual elements in the scene can interfere with OCR preprocessing and character recognition.

2. Uneven Lighting Conditions.
   Variations in lighting and shadows in outdoor environments can degrade image quality, impacting OCR accuracy. Uneven lighting complicates character detection and segmentation, favoring scanned documents over camera-captured images.
3. Skewness (Rotation).
   Images captured by handheld devices may exhibit rotation or skewing, affecting OCR performance. Techniques such as Fourier transformation and Hough transform can be employed to address this issue.
4. Blurring and Degradation.
   Blurring and degradation in images, caused by factors such as distance, movement, and focusing issues, pose challenges for OCR. Sharpness is essential for accurate character segmentation and recognition.
5. Font and Style Variations.
   Overlapping characters in connected scripts or italicized fonts can impede OCR segmentation and recognition. Multilingual environments with diverse character sets further complicate the process.
6. Multilingual Environments.
   Languages with extensive character sets, such as Chinese or Arabic, present challenges for OCR segmentation and recognition. Connected scripts and similar characters require specialized handling to ensure accurate recognition.
7. Damage Documents. Old or damaged documents may contain noise or missing characters, hindering OCR accuracy. Noise removal techniques must be applied carefully to preserve essential content.

3 Research Method

The methodology for this paper employs a qualitative analysis approach, utilizing literature review as the foundation for analysis. This involves gathering data and information by examining research journals, reference books, literature, and credible sources, both in print and digital form, relevant to the topic of discussion. The study was conducted by conducting a comprehensive search of literature and online sources related to the discussed problem, in this case, OCR (Optical Character Recognition), for subsequent analysis. The primary objective of this literature search is to acquire pertinent information and ascertain the extent of interconnectedness among the gathered information, whether they complement or contradict each other. The methodology consists of the following steps:

1. Collecting existing literature and sources of information from various sources such as books, the internet, previously published papers, personal experiences, and other materials related to the topic of discussion.

2. Thoroughly review and read the collected sources to understand their content and relevance to the research topic.
3. Assessing the information obtained to determine its relevance to the topics that will be discussed in the paper.
4. Summarize the key points and findings from each relevant literature source to extract essential insights.
5. Compiling and organizing the important points obtained from the literature review into a structured format suitable for inclusion in the paper.

By following these steps, the paper ensures a comprehensive review of existing literature and sources of information relevant to the research topic, thereby laying a solid foundation for the subsequent analysis and discussion.

4 Results and Discussion

Claim administration is a critical function within insurance and financial services companies. It involves fulfilling the commitments made by insurers to policy owners. When individuals purchase insurance, they rely on the insurer's promise to provide a specified amount in the event of certain conditions. For policyholders, receiving a claim payment signifies the fulfillment of the promise made at the time of purchasing the policy. Therefore, insurers have a responsibility to promptly and fairly settle all legitimate claims, as required by laws in most jurisdictions. Claim administration processes aim to facilitate swift settlements while maintaining appropriate controls to ensure the legitimacy of claims [16]. There are two methods of reimbursing money to customers as insured parties in the claims process: reimbursement and cashless. Broadly speaking, the fundamental difference between these methods lies in the cashless method, where the customer does not have to spend any money during the treatment or care process, except in cases of claim excess where costs incurred are beyond the agreed benefit coverage in the policy. Through the cashless method, the customer as the insured party coordinates with the hospital partner of the insurer using a card provided by the insurance company as the insurer. In settling the claim excess, the insured party can do so using personal funds or coordinate benefits with another insurance company if the insured party has more than one health insurance. On the other hand, if there is no claim excess, then the customer can go home directly. In the process of reimbursing money, the insured party first uses their own funds to carry out outpatient or inpatient treatment processes. Then in the claim submission for reimbursement of costs from the treatment and medical care process [17].

Insurers typically establish four key objectives for each claim analyst involved in examining and deciding on claims [18]:

1. Sensitivity.
   Claim analysts must demonstrate sensitivity to each claimant's situation, recognizing their potential loss. This involves training in product information, claim handling procedures, and customer service etiquette to ensure polite and empathetic interactions.
2. Equitable decision making.
   Analysts gather necessary information to make fair decisions consistent with policy provisions. While some claims can be handled quickly, complex cases may require extensive investigation to ensure accurate outcomes.
3. Timely processing.
   Insurers aim to handle claims promptly, mindful of statutory requirements for timely settlements. However, processes are in place to prevent hasty decisions that may lead to paying unfounded claims.
4. Cost-effectiveness.
   Efficient claim administration relies on well-trained staff and ongoing education to stay abreast of industry changes. Insurers implement guidelines and utilize technology to streamline processes, reduce errors, and facilitate rapid and accurate claims disbursement.

The effectiveness of claim administration hinges on the skills and attitudes of claim staff, as well as the management of claim processes within the insurer. The claim decision process within an insurance company involves several sensitive and critical activities. Regardless of the type or amount of claim, claim analysts follow a standardized process aimed at ensuring accurate and fair outcomes. The key activities in claim administration include [19]:

1. Verifying Policy Status.
   Claim analysts verify whether the insurance policy was active at the time of the incurred loss. This typically involves checking electronic records to confirm premium payments and policy status.
2. Verifying the Insured.
   Analysts confirm that the individuals suffering the loss are covered under the policy. While this is usually straightforward, occasional clarifications may be necessary.
3. Verifying the Loss.

Analysts ascertain whether the claimed loss indeed occurred. While submitted information often suffices, additional verification may be needed in certain cases, such as contacting healthcare providers for confirmation.

4. Verifying Policy Coverage of the Loss.

   Claim analysts ensure that the claimed loss is covered under the policy's provisions. This may involve detailed policy review to determine coverage eligibility.

5. Verifying Recipients of Benefits.

   Analysts determine the rightful recipients of policy benefits, which can sometimes be complex. Situations involving multiple beneficiaries or changes in beneficiary status require thorough investigation.

6. Calculating Benefit Amount.

   Analysts calculate the amount of benefits due, adhering closely to policy provisions. While straightforward in most cases, certain claims may require assessing multiple factors to determine benefit amounts accurately.

B. Infromasi Perawatan

1.	**Tanggal masuk**	: 20-May-2021	5.	**Lama Perawatan**	: 9 Hari	
2.	**Nama Rumah Sakit**	: Royal Taruma, RS	6.	**Kamar Perawatan**	: **Kelas** : 1	**Rp** : 750.000
3.	**Dokter yang Merawat**	:	7.	**Jumlah Tempat Tidur**	: 2	
4.	**No. Rekam Medis**	:	8.	**Estimasi Biaya Rawat Inap**	:	

C. Nilai Jaminan

Manfaat Polis	Biaya Diajukan	Biaya Dijamin	Biaya Tidak Dijamin
Biaya Unit Perawatan Intensif(ICU)	6.750.000,00	6.750.000,00	0,00
Biaya Kunjungan Dokter Umum	110.000,00	110.000,00	0,00
Biaya Kunjungan dr. Spesialis	2.565.000,00	2.565.000,00	0,00
Biaya Aneka Perawatan	26.557.053,00	26.455.165,00	101.888,00
TOTAL	35.982.053,00	35.880.165,00	101.888,00

Tidak dijamin : tensivask

*Bila pasien menempati kamar perawatan di atas manfaat yang dimiliki maka pasien wajib membayar selisih yang timbul dan biaya yang tidak dijamin setelah menjalani perawatan Rumah Sakit

Fig. 4. Example of an insurance benefit calculation decision letter

Optimizing service quality within health insurance companies is paramount due to the direct reliance of nearly all customers on interactions with providers and the company itself. Research reveals six key factors influencing participant satisfaction, encompassing organizational aspects, insurance types, benefit packages, sociodemographic elements, health services, and personal consumer factors. Globally, service quality, participant expectations, and utilization of health services emerge as the most significant influences [20] (Figs. 4 and 5).

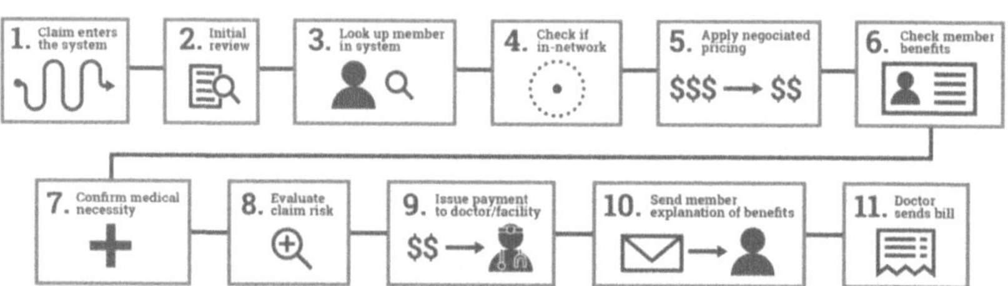

Fig. 5. The Journey of a Claim. (https://www.6degreeshealth.com/healthcare-claims-processing-steps-sdh/)

The author attempts to create a simple calculation comparing the claim decision process with and without OCR. Using the Health Insurance Claims Paid in Q3 2023 in Table 1 and estimating the OCR cost at USD 500,000 with a monthly maintenance of USD 40,000, the calculation according to Table 2 is obtained.

From Table 2, it can be seen that the total claim per month with the use of OCR is cheaper compared to without OCR, which may be a consideration for insurance companies. Research conducted by Pasalli (2022) to determine the resolution of national health insurance claims shows that among the supporting factors in claim resolution is the accuracy of claim settlement while inhibiting factors include staff lacking qualifications in processing claims [21]. This can be mitigated by the combination of OCR usage, which processes low to medium-difficulty claim cases, while high-difficulty claim cases are assigned to trained claim analysts. Nonetheless, intricate claims necessitate the expertise of trained claim analysts to ensure meticulous assessment and accurate decision-making.

Table 2. Cost Comparison With and Without OCR

	Expense Without OCR/bulan (IDR)	Expense With OCR/bulan (IDR)	Description
Total Health Insurance Claims Paid in Q3 2023 (a)	15.240.000.000.000	15.240.000.000.000	
Estimated Claim Paid/hospitalization (b)	30.000.000	30.000.000	
Total Claims/month (c)	56.444	56.444	((a)/(b))/9
Man Power Needed (Claim Analyst)/month (d)	7.056	1.411	((c)/8), assuming 1 claim requires 60 min (1 working day = 8 h) of work by claim analyst, OCR can handle 80% of the total cases
Claim Analyst Salary/month	52.916.666.667	10.583.333.333	Claim Analyst Salary/month = IDR 7,500,000
OCR Price	0	7.500.000.000	Estimated OCR Price = USD 500,000. 1 USD = IDR 15,000
OCR Maintenance/month	0	600.000.000	OCR Maintenance/month = USD 40,000. 1 USD = IDR 15,000
Total Cost/month	52.916.666.667	18.683.333.333	

5 Conclusion

The landscape of health insurance is evolving rapidly, driven by economic uncertainties, rising healthcare costs, and technological advancements. The projected increase in healthcare costs in Indonesia underscores the importance of optimizing service quality within health insurance companies to meet the needs and expectations of customers. As evidenced by the Mercer Marsh Benefits Trend Health 2023 report, healthcare costs are expected to rise significantly, prompting individuals to seek additional financial protection through private health insurance. Moreover, the Fourth Industrial Revolution (Industry 4.0) presents opportunities for innovation in claim processing through technologies like Optical Character Recognition (OCR). Research indicates that the combination of OCR technology and trained claim analysts can enhance claim resolution efficiency, mitigating inhibiting factors such as staff qualifications.. By leveraging technology and human expertise effectively, insurers can navigate the complexities of the claim decision process and deliver on their commitment to policyholders.

Acknowledgments. We would like to express our deepest gratitude to Bina Nusantara University for the opportunity to receive the BINUS International Research Grant - Applied 2025 and for the invaluable facilities in fostering collaboration and stimulating in-depth discussions during this research work.

Open Data. https://doi.org/10.5281/zenodo.17374810.

Author Contributor. *Wahyu Sardjono*, abstract and introduction. *Dwi Putra Kasoema*, literatur review, *Maryani*, methodology. *Trias Septyoari Putranto*, result. *Azani Cempaka Sari*, discusion. Ilham Radito, managing data via Zenodo, and Hasyiya Karimah Adli, conclusion.

References

1. Mercer Marsh Benefits, "MMB Health Trends 2023," October 2022
2. Populix, "Indonesia's Perceptions and Attitude Towards Health & Life Insurance Products," January 2023
3. Respati, A.R.: Klaim Asuransi Kesehatan Melonjak, Masyarakat Diminta Berasuransi," kompas.com, 29 Nov 2023
4. Asosiasi Asuransi Jiwa Indonesia, "Siaran Konfrensi Pers Kinerja Industri Asuransi Jiwa Indonesia Kuartal 1 2023," aaji.or.id, May 29, 2023
5. Asosiasi Asuransi Jiwa Indonesia, "Press Release Laporan Kinerja Industri Asuransi Jiwa Semester I 2023," aaji.or.id, Sep. 10, 2023
6. Asosiasi Asuransi Jiwa Indonesia, "Siaran Pers – Kinerja IAJ Periode Januari - September 2023," aaji.or.id, 14 December 2023
7. Asosiasi Asuransi Jiwa Indonesia, "Press Release Laporan Kinerja Industri Asuransi Jiwa Full Year 2022," aaji.or.id, 08 March 2023
8. Slack, N., Brandon-Jones, A., Burgess, N.: Operations Management 10th edition., 10th ed. S.L.: Pearson Education Limited, pp. 259–260 (2022)
9. Chaudhuri, A., Mandaviya, K., Badelia, P., Ghosh, S.K.: Optical Character Recognition Systems for Different Languages with Soft Computing. Springer, p. 9, (2016)
10. Firdaus, A., Kurnia, M.S., Shafera, T., Firdaus, W.I.: Implementasi optical character recognition (OCR) Pada Masa Pandemi Covid-19. Jupiter **13**(2), 188–194 (2021)
11. Wahono, S.: Sistem Keamanan Parkir Berbasis RFID dan Plat Nomor Kendaraan Menggunakan Metode Leptonica, Tugas Akhir, Universitas Dinamika (2020)
12. Thanki, J.D., Davda, P.D., Swaminarayan, P.: A review on OCR technology. Int. J. Emerg. Technol. Innov. Res. (www.jetir.org) **8**(4), 716–720 (2021)
13. Awel, M.A., Abidi, A.I.: Review on optical character recognition. Int. Res. J. Eng. Technol. (IRJET) **06**(06), 3666–3669 (2019)
14. Raj, A., Sharma, S., Singh, J., Singh, A.: Revolutionizing data entry: an in-depth study of optical character recognition technology and its future potential. Int. J. Res. Appl. Sci. Eng. Technol. **11**(2), 645–653 (2023)
15. Avyodri, R., Lukas, S., Tjahyadi, H.: Optical character recognition (OCR) for text recognition and its post-processing method: a literature review. In: 2022 1st International Conference on Technology Innovation and Its Applications (ICTIIA), Tangerang, Indonesia, pp. 1–6 (2022)

16. Ku, A., Misra, P.S.N., Ghadai, S.K.: Claim settlement: the moment of truth in health insurance. Int. J. Recent Technol. Eng. **8**(2), 581–585 (2019)
17. Goretti, M., Aditya, K.: Kajian Perlindungan Konsumen di Sektor Jasa Keuangan: Asuransi Kesehatan. Otoritas Jasa Keuangan (OJK), pp. 61–64 (2019)
18. Brown, J.L., Herrod, J.W., Maxwell, M.R.: Claim Administration, 3rd ed. United States of America: International Claim Association (2001)
19. Kongstvedt, P.R.: Health insurance and managed care : what they are and how they work, 5th ed. Burlington, Ma: Jones & Bartlett Learning, pp. 185–188 (2020)
20. Abigael, S.C.: Faktor-Faktor Yang Memengaruhi Kepuasan Peserta Asuransi Kesehatan Di Berbagai Negara: Literature Review, Skripsi, Fakultas Kesehatan Masyarakat Universitas Indonesia (2022)
21. Pasalli, R.R.: Penyelesaian Klaim Asuransi Kesehatan Nasional Di Berbagai Negara: Literature Review, Skripsi, Fakultas Kesehatan Masyarakat Universitas Indonesia (2022)

Dissemination of Sustainable Development Goals for the Third Indicator (Good Health and Well-Being) Through the Knowledge Management Systems

Wahyu Sardjono[1(✉)], Hasyiya Karimah Adli[2], Maryani[3], Trias Septyoari Putranto[4], Azani Cempaka Sari[5], and Ilham Radito[6]

[1] Information Systems Management Department, BINUS Graduate Program – Master of Information Systems Management, Bina Nusantara University, Jl. K. H. Syahdan No. 9, Kemanggisan, Palmerah, Jakarta 11480, Indonesia
wahyu.s@binus.ac.id

[2] Faculty of Data Science and Computing, Universiti Malaysia Kelantan City Campus, Pengkalan Chepa, Kelantan, Malaysia
hasyiya@umk.edu.my

[3] Information Systems Department, School of Information Systems, Bina Nusantara University, Jakarta 11480, Indonesia
yanie@binus.edu

[4] Hotel Management. Department Faculty of Digital Communication, Hotel and Tourism, Bina Nusantara University, Jakarta 11480, Indonesia
tputranto@binus.edu

[5] Computer Science Department, School of Computer Science, Bina Nusantara University, Jakarta 11480, Indonesia
acsari@binus.edu

[6] School of Computer Science, Faculty of Engineering, The University of Sydney, Sydney, Australia
irad0511@uni.sydney.edu

Abstract. The government's policy on sustainable development is that there are sustainable development goals that aim to improve the welfare of the world community and preserve nature through 17 main factors with 169 agreements as targets. The third program of sustainable development goals is better health and well-being. This goal talks about better health and well-being for all people, guaranteeing access to basic health services, and protecting all people for well-being. This program needs to be disseminated to the whole community through various means including online by utilizing information technology. This research was conducted to evaluate the knowledge management system which contains a substance on SDG: 3, data analysis was carried out using factor analysis and regression analysis was also used to build mathematical models. The results of this study show that new factors have been formed, namely: socialization culture, socialization innovation, socialization technology, and socialization governance that need to be considered for the success of SDG 1 performance measurement: socialization without poverty through the use of knowledge management systems in the future.

E. R. Kaburuan and S. Goundar (Eds.): HIS 2025, LNCS 16392, pp. 286–296, 2026.
https://doi.org/10.1007/978-981-95-6304-3_25

Keywords: sustainable development goal · third indicator · evaluation model

1 Introduction

The condition of maternal mortality in Indonesia is compared to countries around ASEAN.

The risk of death during childbirth mostly occurs in women who marry at a young age, but it can also be caused by other problems, such as financial conditions so economic factors can also be a cause.

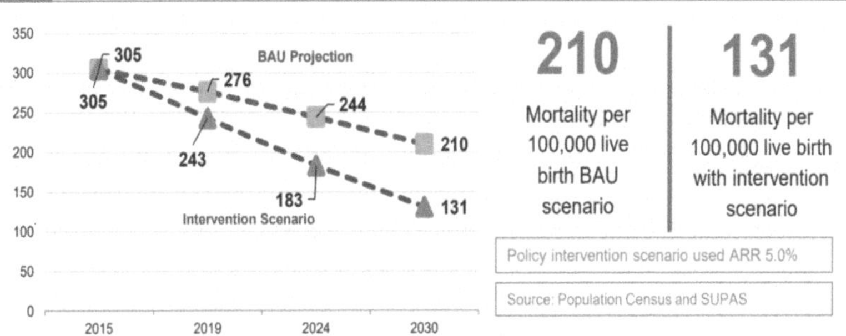

Fig. 1. Maternal mortality per 100,000 live births

In Indonesia, the role of midwives who help deliver a mother is very important to prevent maternal death [1]. However, in reality, there is still a gap between the availability of skilled birth attendants in various regions. For the conditions in the Java-Bali region, it is around 52%, while in other areas it is only 42%. For this reason, the role of skilled birth attendants really needs to be significantly increased so that the reduction in maternal mortality in 2030 can be fulfilled. Lack of access to quality health services can also increase maternal mortality. Access to quality health services is not only hampered by the absence of health service providers but also related to geographic barriers, especially for people living in rural areas [2]. Ultimately, competent midwives and functioning maternal referral systems have an important role to play in preventing maternal deaths.

1.1 (a) Infant Mortality Per 1,000 Live Births

For conditions in Indonesia, the infant mortality rate is still the highest among ASEAN countries, although a significant reduction has been achieved, the infant mortality rate in Indonesia is 4.6 times higher than the condition in Malaysia, and 1.8 times higher than in Thailand. It even turns out to be 1.3 times higher than the Philippines. For this reason, Indonesia's target of reducing infant mortality to 12 deaths per 1,000 live births in 2030 will be a challenge, because the causes of infant mortality are now becoming increasingly complicated because they are related to maternal health during pregnancy and in the first month of care after delivery. Most of the infant deaths occur in the

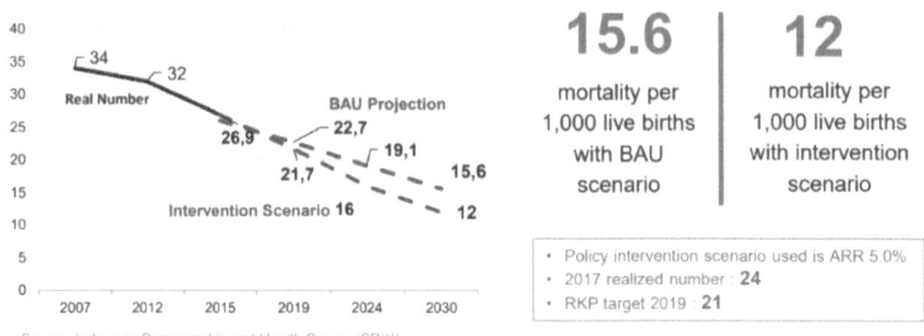

Fig. 2. Infant Mortality per 1,000 live births

neonatal period [3]. For this reason, the quality of care during labor and after delivery and postpartum care in the first month is very important. Immunization efforts in infants also play a major role in reducing infant mortality and improving infant health. An example of the conditions above is a health and welfare problem in the global community, including Indonesia, which must be known by the public, so it needs to be disseminated so that there is a concern for this problem. Through a knowledge management system that contains substance from the third indicator of the Sustainable Development Goal (SDGs), namely better health and well-being, dissemination can be carried out more effectively and efficiently. This research was conducted to create a model for evaluating the success of dissemination of the third indicator SDGs program to increase better dissemination in line with future population growth [4] (Fig. 2).

2 Literature Review

Knowledge Management Development

All knowledge management is a collection of strategic frameworks or systems designed to help both organizations and individuals analyze, record, create, use and reuse knowledge to achieve competitive advantage (Fig. 3).

Knowledge Management System (KMS)

Knowledge Management System (KMS) is a technological and systematic infrastructure that supports the collection, organization, and distribution of knowledge within an organization. KMS facilitates the creation, access and use of existing knowledge to increase organizational efficiency and effectiveness [6].

According to Fernandez Knowledge Management System (KMS), the process has a cycle that can be described as follows (Fig. 4):

The explanation of the knowledge management cycle is:

1. Creates means creating knowledge through new ways of doing things.
2. Captures is identifying and capturing new knowledge.
3. Refine is placing knowledge in a certain place so that it can be used/repaired.
4. Stores is placing knowledge into storage.
5. Manage is the existence of review activities for accuracy and relevance.
6. Disseminate means making existing knowledge available at any time to anyone who needs it.

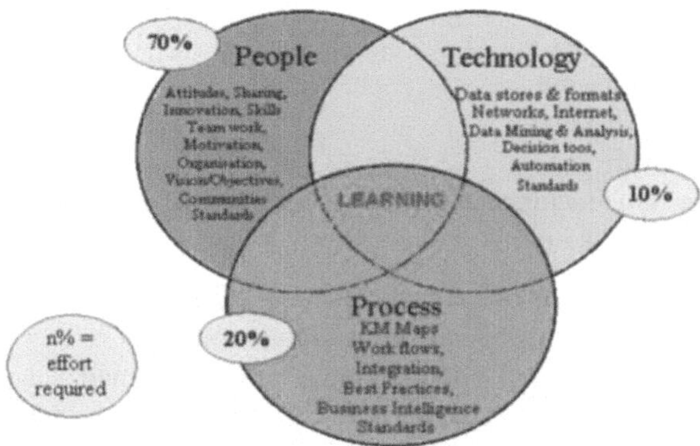

Fig. 3. Knowledge Management Relationship [5]

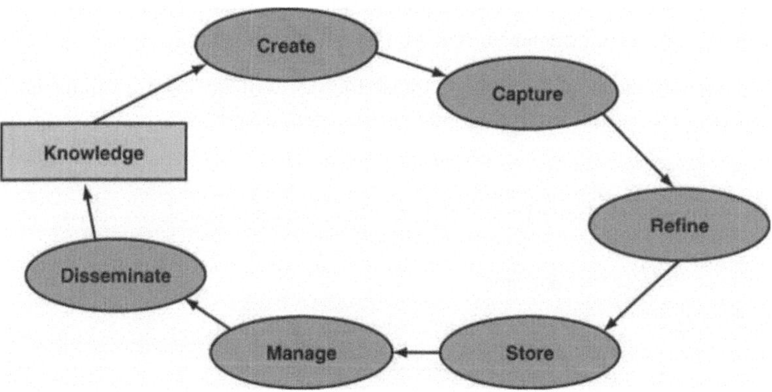

Fig. 4. Knowledge Management System [6]

Knowledge Management Solution and Foundation

Knowledge management depends on two aspects, namely knowledge management solution and knowledge management foundation as shown in Fig. 1. Knowledge management solution is a way to facilitate knowledge-sharing activities, which is divided into 2 (two) parts, namely the knowledge management process and the knowledge management system. Meanwhile, the knowledge management foundation is a broad organizational aspect that supports knowledge management in the short and long term. The knowledge management foundation consists of technology and knowledge management mechanisms as well as knowledge management infrastructure [7].

Based on the concept of the Knowledge Management Systems Cycle [8], it can be explained several stages for further analysis in the development of research instruments:

1. The first stage. Based on the theory above, it is known that there are a number of main factors that support the knowledge management systems cycle development which is the basis for e-learning development, including:

1. Create knowledge factor
2. Capture knowledge factor
3. Refine knowledge factor
4. Store knowledge factor
5. Manage knowledge factor
6. Disseminate factor

Having obtained the factors that affect student interest in learning to be looking for the next most influential factor.

2. The second stage. Analysis that is based on the factors mentioned in the first stage to obtain the indicators that will be the basis of questionnaires.
3. The third stage. The next step is distributing questionnaires and data processing, then analyzing the data with factor analysis to refine the existing indicators as well as to obtain new factors that most affect student interest and learning outcomes using E-Learning.
4. The fourth stage. The output of the data analysis process can be used as input to the next process, namely prepared to be the result of research that produces conclusions that can be useful for education, research and further research object.

The results of the construction of these factors will be used as material for the evaluation of SDG's dissemination which was developed as a research instrument. Table 1.

Table 1. Research instrument development

Factor	Indicator	Ref.e
Create Knowledge	Addition of new knowledge (CK1)	[10]
	Experiences and skill (CK2)	[11]
	Determine new ways of doing thing (CK3)	[12]
Capture Knowledge	Knowledge Repositories to capture knowledge (CP1)	[13]
	Represented in a reasonable way (CP2)	[14]
	Must be identified as valuable (CP3)	[15]
Refine Knowledge	Actionable (RK1)	[16]
	New knowledge is to be place in contex (RK2)	[17]
	Refine a long with explicit knowledge (RK3)	[18]
Store Knowledge	Codification store in knowledge database (SK1)	[19]
	Understandable knowledge store (SK2)	[20]
	Store knowledge quality (SK3)	[21]
Manage Knowledge	Knowledge must be keep manage (MK1)	[22]
	Reviewed to verify that is relevant and accurate (MK2)	[23]
	Knowledge should be keep up to date (MK3)	[24]
Disseminate Knowledge	Communication or distribution of knowledge (DK1)	[25]

(continued)

Table 1. (*continued*)

Factor	Indicator	Ref.e
	Sharing and collaboration acquired knowledge (DK2)	[26]
	Useful format (DK3)	[27]
	Relevant contens to user (DK4)	[28]

3 Research Method

3.1 Population and Sample

The population of respondents in this study were students in Jakarta and the sample used in this study were students of University who were taken randomly from various study programs. By looking at a large population and researchers cannot study everything in the population, because of limited funds, energy, and time, researchers use samples taken from that population [29]. So the number of samples that will be used will depend on the level of desired accuracy or error. The university has 23.486 students' active period from 2017/to 2018. Based on the formula with a standard error of at least 5% the sample that will be used in this study is approximately 348 students. The questionnaire was distributed to 348 students who returned the questionnaires, while as many as 332 students.

3.2 Methods of Data Analysis

This research used a questionnaire as a data collection instrument. Questionnaires were distributed to college students University. The questions in the questionnaire were designed according to the needs of the information required for testing factor analysis in this study. The scaling technique used in this study is itemized rating scales using a Likert scale (1–5). According to [30], the Likert scale is used to measure attitudes, opinions, and perceptions of a person or group of people about social phenomena.

The questionnaire consisted of two parts, the first part is to collect respondent data. Respondent data required are as follows: Gender, Age, Know the topic of e-learning, Faculty, Generation, and Current learning media assessment.

And the second part is the part that is formed by factor analysis points statement built by a number of factors, which factors in question are all factors that have been discussed previously.

4 Results and Discussion

4.1 Respondents Profile

We received 348 questionnaires from our respondents, of which 332 were returned. This indicates that the data collected was comprehensive and met the research's requirements. The data that can be further processed is the number. A summary of the study participants is provided below. No respondent in this research was determined to be younger than or equal to 18 years old, according to dimensions calculated by dividing the respondent's age by the age range. 234 respondents were between the ages of 18 and 21, 79 respondents were between the ages of 22 and 25, and 19 respondents were beyond 25. According to the results, most responders were between the ages of 18 and 21 Table 2.

Table 2. Respondents Profile

Total samples	**332**	*Region*	
		Jakarta	73 (22%)
Gender		Bandung	56 (17%)
Male	170 (51%)	Semarang	28 (8%)
Female	162 (49%)	Surabaya	46 (14%)
		Bali	48 (15%)
Age Year)		Lombok	38 (11%)
< 18 Year	0 (0%)	Makasar	43 (13%)
18 - 21	234 (70%)		
21-25	79 (24%)	*Generation*	
> 25	19 (6%)	< 2016	7
		2016	34

1. The first new factor is **knowledge sharing (X_1)**, namely the ability of an organization with its community to create a knowledge-sharing situation. This new factor represents several grouped indicators, namely the indicators:
   a. Distribution of knowledge or communication (DK1)
   b. Content that is pertinent to the user (DK4)
   c. Knowledge has to be updated (MK3)
   d. Acquired knowledge sharing and collaboration (DK2)
2. The second new factor is **managing knowledge (X_2)**, namely the importance of the organization and its community in managing the knowledge they have, both organizationally and individually. This factor represents the level of importance of the organization to:

a. Represented in a reasonable way (CP2)
b. Knowledge codification stored in the knowledge database (SK1)
c. Useful format (DK3)
d. Knowledge must be kept managed (MK1)

3. The third new factor is **understanding knowledge (X_3)**, namely the process of determining the knowledge to be disseminated and increasing understanding for the community. This factor represents the level of importance of the organization to:
   a. Refine a long with explicit knowledge (RK3)

a. New knowledge is to be placed in context (RK2)
b. Actionable (RK1)
c. Store knowledge quality (SK3)

4. The fourth new factor is **utilization knowledge (X_4)**, namely the process of using existing knowledge and developing new knowledge innovations. This factor represents the level of importance of the organization to:
   a. Addition of new knowledge (CK1)
   b. Experiences and skill (CK2)
   c. Must be identified as valuable (CP3)

After a regression model is created using the newly generated factors, the results of the analysis of student interest and learning outcomes related to the implementation of e-learning can be seen. This model can then be used to predict future interest and identify strategies for boosting it. Regression analysis methods can be used to process data by assessing student interest and learning outcomes as dependent variables and factor scores as independent variables. This process yields a regression equation that can be used as a formula to describe the effect of using e-learning media on participant interest and learning outcomes.

$$Y(x) = \mathbf{7.199} + \mathbf{0.186}X_1 + \mathbf{0.001}X_2 + \mathbf{0.115}X_3 + \mathbf{0.153}X_4$$

This formula is interpreted in a model that can be seen in Fig. 5.

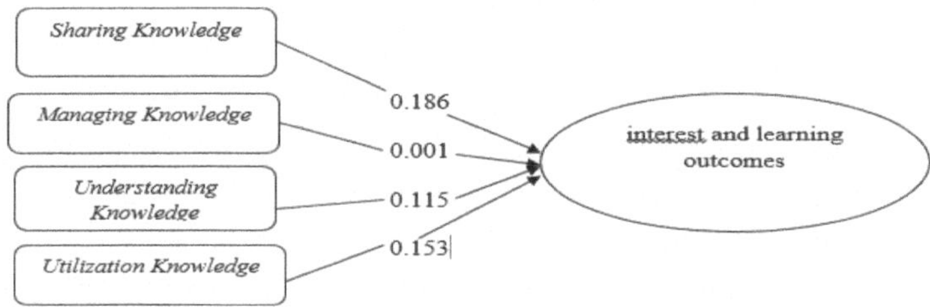

Fig. 5. Relation between dependent variable and independent variable

The components X2 and X3 have a high importance, namely 99% and 37%, according to the findings of the statistical test. The two aforementioned variables, which have an impact on student learning outcomes and interests, cannot be included in the model since the significance level was more than the standard error, which is 0.5% in general. Thus, the following are the student learning outcomes and the model of interest:

$$Y(x) = \mathbf{7.199} + \mathbf{0.186}\,X1 + \mathbf{0.153}\,X4$$

From formula interpreted a model as shown below (Fig. 6):

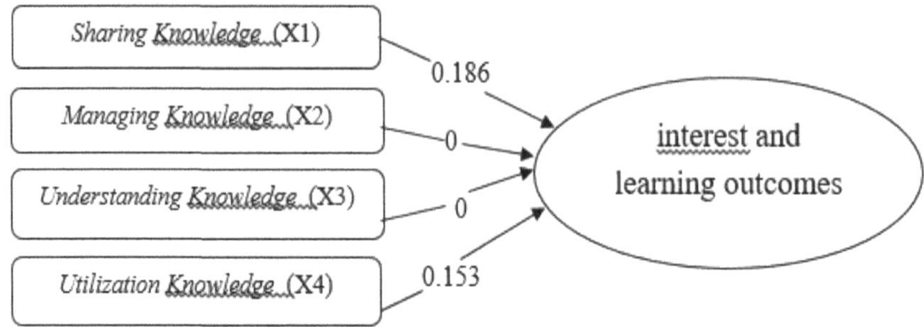

Fig. 6. Factors Affecting Interests and Student Learning Outcomes Solution

5 Conclusion

It takes a skilled delivery attendant to save the lives of mothers. Still, there remains a regional disparity in the availability of expert birth attendance. While coverage was just 42% in other regions, it was 52% in the Java-Bali region. To reduce maternal mortality by 2030, a large increase in the coverage of skilled birth attendance is necessary. Maternal mortality is also increased by limited access to high-quality healthcare. The lack of healthcare professionals and geographic barriers, especially for those residing in distant places, both hinder access to high-quality healthcare. Furthermore, important to note are the important roles that capable midwives and an efficient system of maternal referrals play in reducing the rate of maternal death. The importance of socializing the issue of sustainable development requires its way of conveying it to the community. A strong understanding of knowledge management is needed for successful dissemination that must reach the community completely and correctly.

Acknowledgments. We would like to express our deepest gratitude to Bina Nusantara University for the opportunity to receive the BINUS International Research Grant - Applied 2025 and for the invaluable facilities in fostering collaboration and stimulating in-depth discussions during this research work.

Data Available.

https://zenodo.org/records/17294592.

Authors Contribution. *Wahyu Sardjono,*

For all research processes and results to produce articles published in national and international reputable journals and coordinate research activities with research members including lecturers.

Hasyiya Karimah Adli,

Provide theoretical direction that is the basis of research, develop research instrument designs, and determine research methods and ensure the output of research results.

Maryani,

Build theories that are the basis of research, Develop research instrument designs, and determine research methods and conduct surveys on research objects.

Trias Septyoari Putranto,

Provide basic research direction in Developing research instrument designs, and determining research methods and ensuring the output of research results.

Azani Cempaka Sari.

Data collection, documentation, publication preparation, process execution, and monitoring.

Ilham Radito,

Provide basic research direction in Developing research instrument designs, and determining research methods and ensuring the output of research results.

References

1. Mosharraf, M., Taghiyareh, F.: Qualitative development of eLearning environments through a learner relationship management methodology. Knowl. Manag. E-Learn. **5**(1), 56–65 (2013)
2. Ching, Y.H., Hsu, Y.C.: "Collaborative learning using VoiceThread in an online graduate course. Knowl. Manag. E-Learn. **5**(3), 298–314 (2013)
3. Olaniran, B.A.: Discerning culture in e-learning and in the global workplaces. Knowl. Manag. E-Learn. **1**(3) (2009)
4. Larsen, T.J., Olaisen, J.: Innovating strategically in information and knowledge management: applications of organizational behavior theory. Management **33**(5), 764–774 (2013)
5. Cloonan, M.R., Cloonan, D.J., Fingeret, A.L.: Learners with experience in surgical scrub benefit from additional education with an interactive e-learning module. J. Am. College Surgeons **20**(4), 196
6. McGibbon, C., Ophoff, J., Van Belle, J.-P.: Our building is smarter than your building: the use of competitive rivalry to reduce energy consumption and linked carbon footprint. Knowl. Manag. E-Learn. **6**(4), 464–471 (2014)
7. Liang, D., Jia, J., Wu, X., Miao, J., Wang, A.: Analysis of learners' behaviors and learning outcomes in a massive open online course. Knowl. Manag. E-Learn. **6**(3), 281–298 (2014)
8. Sardjono, W., Firdaus, F.: Readiness model of knowledge management systems implementation at the higher education. ICIC Express Lett. **14**(pp), 477–487 (2020)
9. Sardjono, W., Laksmono, B.S., Yuniastuti, E.: The social welfare factors of public transportation. ICIC Express Lett. **14**(4), 361–368 (2020)
10. Flowers, S., Meyer, M.: How can entrepreneurs benefit from user knowledge to create innovation in the digital services sector? J. Bus. Res. **119**, 122–130 (2020)
11. Bert, F., Pompili, E., Siliquini, R.: Empowering seizure management skill: knowledge, attitudes, and experiences of school staff trained in administering rescue drugs in northern Italy. Epilepsy Beh. **114**(Part A) (2020) Article 107362
12. Schwan, K.J., Fallon, B., Milne, B.: The one thing that actually helps: art creation as a self-care and health-promoting practice amongst youth experiencing homelessness. Child Youth Serv. Rev. **93**, 355–364 (2018)
13. Konys, A.: Knowlegde repository of ontology learning tools from text. Procedia Comput. Sci. **159**, 1614–1628 (2019)
14. Lorio, A.D., Rossi, D.: Capturing and managing knowledge using social software and semantic web technologies. Inf. Sci. **432**, 1–21 (2017)
15. Farshidi, S., Jansen, S., van der Werf, J.M.: Capturing software architecture knowledge for pattern-driven design. J. Syst. Software **169** (2020). Article 110714
16. Arnott, J.C., Mach, K.J., Wong-Parodi, G.: Editorial overview: the science of actionable knowledge. Curr. Opin. Environ. Sustain. **42**, a1–a5 (2019)
17. Bardi, M.: How can I make something interesting for me relevant for the wider community? – An ethnographic exploration of Romanian researcher's adjustment to research communication standards. J. Engl. Acad. Purposes **49** (2020). Article 100943
18. Ge, R., Garcia, R.: Refining semantics for multi-stage programming. J. Comput. Langu. **51**, 222–240 (2020)

19. García-Muiña, F.E., Pelechano-Barahona, E., Navas-López, J.E.: Knowledge Codification and technological innovation success: empirical evidence from Spanish biotech companies. Technol. Forecast. Soc. ChangeJanuary **76**(1), 141–153 (2020)
20. Alhomoud, F.K., Alsadiq, Y., Alhomoud, F.: Pharmacy student's knowledge and practices concerning the storing and disposal of household medication in Saudi Arabia. Curr. Pharm. Teach. Learn. **13**(1), 5–13 (2020)
21. Rajan, N.S., Gouripeddi, R., Facelli, J.C.: Computer Meth. Programs Biomed. **177**, 193–201 (2019)
22. Riedel, R., Jacobs, G., Sprehe, J.: Managing knowledge and parameter dependencies with MBSE in textile product development processes. Procedia CIRP **91**, 170–175 (2020)
23. Hussain, M., Afzal, M., Lee, S.: Acquiring guideline-enabled data-driven clinical knowledge model using formally verified refined knowledge acquisition method. Comput. Meth. Programs Biomed. **197** (2020). Article 105701
24. Bag, S., Gupta, S., Sivarajah, U.: An integrated artificial intelligence framework for knowledge creation and B2B marketing rational decision making for improving firm performance. Ind. Mark. Manage. **92**, 178–189 (2019)
25. Georgescu, M., Popescul, D.: The impact of new information and communication technologies on the creation and dissemination of knowledge inheritance. Procedia. Soc. Behav. Sci. **188**, 122–129 (2015)
26. Chatterjee, S., Chaudhuri, R., Piccolo, R.: Enterprise social network for knowledge sharing in MNCs: examining the role of knowledge contributors and knowledge seekers for cross-country collaboration. J. Int. Manag. **27**(1) Article 100827 (2021)
27. Fuller,C.D., van Dijk, L.V., Thomas, C.R.: Meeting the challenge of scientific dissemination in the era of COVID-19: Toward a Modular Approach to Knowledge-Sharing for Radiation Oncology. Int. J. Radiat. Oncol. Biol. Phys. **108**(2), 496–505 (2020)
28. Tejeda-Lorente, Á., Porcel, C., Herrera-Viedma, E.: A quality based recommender system to dissemination information in a university digital library. Inf. Sci. **261**, 52–69 (2014)
29. Sardjono, W., Erna, S., Gia Perdana, W.: The application of the factor analysis method to determine the performance of IT implementation in companies based on the IT balanced scorecard measurement method. J. Phys. Conf. Ser. **1538** (2020)
30. Sardjono, W., Selviyanti, E., Perdana, W.G., Maryani: Modeling of development of performance evaluation on health information systems implementation. J. Phys. Conf. Ser. **1465**(012025) (2020)

What Users Want: Insights from Indonesian Mobile Health Applications Reviews

Devi Karolita[1(✉)], Indra Fiqi Ripani[1], Ariesta Lestari[1], Felicia Sylviana[1], and Angeline Novia Toemon[2]

[1] Informatics Engineering Department, Palangka Raya University, Palangka Raya, Indonesia
{devikarolita,ariesta,feliciasylviana}@it.upr.ac.id, indrafr9@mhs.eng.upr.ac.id

[2] Immunology Histology Department, Palangka Raya University, Palangka Raya, Indonesia
angeline_toemon@med.upr.ac.id

Abstract. Mobile health applications are increasingly used in Indonesia, yet little is known about how users evaluate and experience these tools. This study aims to identify user needs, challenges, and expectations from popular Indonesian mHealth applications by analysing publicly available app reviews. We applied a mixed-methods approach, combining automated preprocessing with qualitative thematic coding. The dataset included 100,000+ user reviews from leading mHealth apps, with analysis supported by inter-rater reliability checks and AI-assisted keyword identification. The findings reveal recurring issues of usability, reliability, and trust, alongside user expectations for affordable services, responsive customer support, and integration with the national healthcare system. Based on these insights, we propose prioritised design and policy recommendations, considering implementation complexity, success metrics, and cultural context. This study contributes to the design of inclusive, trustworthy mHealth platforms in low- and middle-income countries, and informs both academic research and practitioner development.

Keywords: mobile health · user reviews · human-centred design · recommendations

1 Introduction

The development of digital technology in Indonesia has experienced rapid growth, particularly over the past decade. The Digital 2025 report by We Are Social and Meltwater notes that internet users in Indonesia are projected to reach 212 million in 2025, a significant increase from 185.3 million users in the previous year [6,7]. This growth has influenced various sectors, including healthcare, which has undergone accelerated digital transformation as a result of the

E. R. Kaburuan and S. Goundar (Eds.): HIS 2025, LNCS 16392, pp. 297–310, 2026.
https://doi.org/10.1007/978-981-95-6304-3_26

COVID-19 pandemic. The pandemic, in particular, prompted Indonesians to utilise digital health services as an alternative to conventional healthcare [21,23].

In Indonesia, mobile health (mHealth) applications (apps) were first introduced in 2010 [24], but their usage increased markedly in the post-pandemic period. These platforms are now widely used for medical consultations, accessing health information, and managing chronic conditions. Reported benefits include improved affordability, greater accessibility to healthcare professionals, and enhanced opportunities for self-monitoring [21,24]. The four most widely used mHealth apps in Indonesia are Halodoc, Alodokter, SATUSEHAT Mobile, and mobile JKN, each consistently ranking among the top free mHealht apps on the Google Play Store. On this platform, users can provide ratings and write reviews about their experiences using the apps.

As mHealth apps become increasingly adopted, user reviews on platforms such as the Google Play Store offer a valuable source of experiential insight. These reviews reflect user satisfaction, highlight usability issues, and express expectations, ranging from praise for well-designed features to criticism of technical or service-related shortcomings. Apps with a high volume of positive reviews often benefit from increased trust among prospective users, whereas negative reviews may deter potential adoption [14].

Given this context, we analyse publicly available user reviews from the Google Play Store to gain a deeper understanding of user experiences with mHealth apps in Indonesia. These insights can inform efforts to improve user satisfaction, identify usability barriers, and guide future enhancements in the design and delivery of digital health services. Through the analysis of user reviews, we aim to address the following two research questions:

RQ1. What topics are frequently discussed in user reviews of mHealth apps in Indonesia? This question seeks to identify recurring themes, concerns, and experiences shared by users, thereby uncovering their priorities and perceptions of mHealth services.

RQ2. What are the reported benefits and challenges of using mHealth apps in Indonesia, based on user reviews? This question explores perceived strengths and limitations from the users' perspective, providing insights into design and implementation gaps within the Indonesian mHealth context.

This study makes three key contributions. First, we extend prior work by identifying 12 technical aspects relevant to the Indonesian context and uncovering three additional non-technical aspects that reflect local user needs. Second, we propose empirically grounded recommendations to improve the design and refinement of mHealth apps in Indonesia. Third, we provide a comprehensive replication package[1] that includes the raw dataset, aspect-specific keyword lists, and analysis code, enabling transparency and reproducibility.

Overall, this study advances user-centred design and evidence-based mHealth development, particularly in low- and middle-income settings. The findings and recommendations presented here offer actionable insights for developers,

[1] https://doi.org/10.5281/zenodo.17009246.

policymakers, and researchers seeking to enhance the usability, accessibility, and trustworthiness of digital health services in Indonesia and similar contexts.

The remainder of this paper is structured as follows. Section 2 reviews prior studies on mHealth adoption and user experience in low- and middle-income contexts. Section 3 outlines the dataset, preprocessing steps, analytical approach, and key findings from both quantitative and qualitative analyses. Section 4 interprets these findings and derives design and policy recommendations, while Sect. 5 presents the limitations of the study. Finally, Sect. 6 summarises the main contributions and outlines directions for future research.

2 Related Work

The adoption of mHealth apps in low- and middle-income countries (LMICs) has expanded rapidly, driven by increasing mobile penetration and demand for accessible healthcare solutions [5]. These technologies offer promising avenues for overcoming traditional healthcare barriers, including geographic distance, cost, and healthcare workforce limitations. However, successful implementation depends not only on technological infrastructure but also on users' trust [13], literacy [8], and contextual needs [26].

User experience (UX) and satisfaction are central to the sustained use and effectiveness of mHealth services. Prior studies have shown that design factors such as ease of use, responsiveness, and perceived usefulness significantly influence user retention and engagement [16]. Particularly in LMICs, usability issues such as poor performance, low compatibility with local devices, or inadequate customer support can lead to rapid app abandonment. Despite the increasing body of work on mHealth usability, many studies rely on surveys or interviews with small samples and often neglect large-scale, naturally occurring feedback available on public platforms.

App store reviews have become a valuable resource for understanding user behaviour and expectations in real-world contexts. Recent research in software engineering and health informatics has shown the potential of mining user-generated reviews to identify feature requests, detect usability issues, and guide app evolution [11,20]. Specifically, Haggag et al. [11] classified 13 main issues mHealth apps, which are: Privacy, Stability, Requests, Advertising, Uninstallation, Payments, Compatibility, Resources, Connectivity, Account and Logging, Notification, Updates, and Internationalisation. However, the study focuses mostly on technical aspects or quality evaluation in high-income countries. In Indonesia, there is a need for empirical studies that leverage large-scale user reviews to derive actionable design insights. This is particularly important given the country's diversity and low-income settings, where limited resources present unique challenges that require tailored approaches.

3 Method

This study employed a mixed-methods approach to analyse user reviews of three popular mHealth apps in Indonesia: Halodoc, Alodokter, SATUSEHAT Mobile, and mobile JKN. The research design combined quantitative and qualitative techniques to identify key themes, usage patterns, and user concerns across different dimensions of app use. The method consisted of five main steps: data collection and filtering, text pre-processing, aspect-based labeling, and data analysis. Figure 1 illustrates the overall research design.

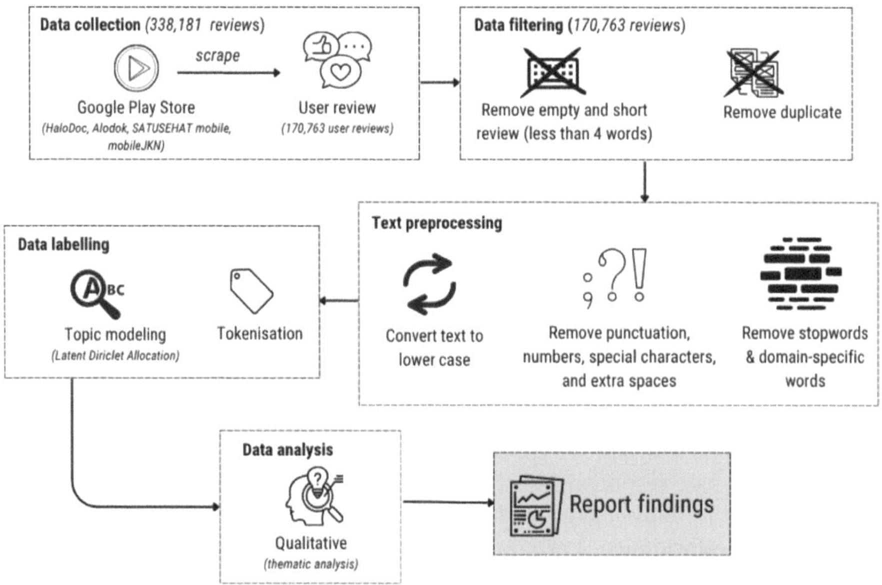

Fig. 1. Research design.

3.1 Data Collection, Filtering, and Preprocessing

User reviews were collected from the Google Play Store for four major Indonesian mHealth applications—Halodoc, Alodokter, SATUSEHAT Mobile, and Mobile JKN—totalling 338,181 entries. The review period spanned January 2021–June 2025 for Halodoc and Alodokter, April 2023–June 2025 for SATUSEHAT Mobile, and January 2021–August 2025 for Mobile JKN. After removing duplicates and reviews containing four words or fewer, 170,763 unique reviews remained (Mobile JKN: 118,135; Alodokter: 19,478; Halodoc: 18,272; SATUSEHAT Mobile: 14,878). The dataset covers roughly 70% of all available reviews for Indonesia's leading mHealth apps, representing a broad and diverse user base. Each review included metadata such as rating score, submission date, and app version, which supported subsequent analyses.

The text was then preprocessed by converting all reviews to lowercase, removing punctuation, numbers, special characters, and excessive white space. Non-standard words were normalised using a manually curated mapping, and stopwords along with domain-specific common terms (e.g., "aplikasi") were removed to reduce noise. This produced a clean and standardised corpus optimised for keyword analysis, word cloud generation, and content interpretation.

3.2 Aspect-Based Labelling and Topic Modelling

Subsequently, the reviews were filtered using keywords relevant to each aspect. These keywords were identified through three approaches: referencing prior research [11], leveraging generative AI (GPT-4), and applying manual reasoning based on the likely occurrence of terms within each aspect. The reviews were then labelled into 12 aspects introduced by Haggag et al. [10]: Privacy, Stability, Requests, Advertising, Uninstallation, Payments, Compatibility, Resources, Connectivity, Account and Logging, Notification, and Updates. We excluded the aspect *Internationalisation*, as the mHealth apps analysed are specifically designed for Indonesia.

Following the labelling, we applied tokenisation and conducted topic modelling using Latent Dirichlet Allocation (LDA) [3]. Each aspect was linked to a curated set of keywords representing common UX issues. For instance, terms such as *"bayar"*, *"biaya"*, or *"gopay"* were mapped to the Payments aspect, while *"login"*, *"akun"*, or *"verifikasi"* were associated with Account and Logging. We refer to these as the technical aspects of mHealth apps. The aspects and their associated keywords are summarised in Table 1.

Aside from the 12 predefined aspects, 76,683 user reviews did not fall into these categories. The aim was to explore whether additional aspects could emerge beyond the predefined ones. We applied topic modelling to these reviews and identified four additional aspects: Perceived Usefulness and User Satisfaction, Teleconsultation and Service Quality, Technical and Access Issues, and Healthcare Administration and Insurance Management. After manual inspection, we merged the *Technical and Access Issues* aspect into *Account and Logging*, leaving three newly identified aspects. These aspects reflect non-technical UX dimensions with mHealth apps in Indonesia. In total, 15 aspects were derived from the user reviews. Table 2 presents the newly identified aspects with their associated keywords.

The most frequently mentioned aspect in the user reviews was *Account and Logging* (63,295), followed by *Perceived Usefulness and User Satisfaction* (27,416) and *Stability* (24,258). Other commonly discussed aspects included *Requests* (21,904), *Updates* (14,008), *Teleconsultation and Service Quality* (13,373), *Payments* (13,277), and *Healthcare Administration and Insurance Management* (11,856). In contrast, the least frequently mentioned aspects were *Connectivity* (3,782), *Uninstallation* (2,689), *Notification* (1,959), *Privacy* (1,452), *Compatibility* (578), *Resources* (264), and *Advertising* (112).

3.3 Thematic Analysis

In addition to the quantitative analysis, a thematic analysis [4] of user reviews was conducted to explore the benefits and challenges of mHealth app usage in Indonesia. To reduce bias, codes were iteratively reviewed by the research team,

Table 1. Technical aspects of mHealth apps

Aspect	**Keywords**	**User review sample**
Privacy	privacy, leaked, my data, personal data, data security, confidential	*My number keeps getting calls from loan apps, even though I've never used any of them. Incapable of protecting people's privacy on social media networks. Don't use the Peduli Lindungi registration validation rules.*
Stability	loading, bug, crash, eror, error, slow	*The app keeps getting stuck loading whenever I try to select a feature. Come on, app developers—please improve the app's performance so that Indonesian citizens can use it comfortably and enjoy the services.*
Requests	please, add/increase, suggestion/recommendation, fix, if possible, suppose, kindly	*Unable to download the vaccination certificate file and update profile data, among many other issues. Please fix this immediately. The file is needed to complete my job application documents. I gave five stars not because I'm satisfied, but so that my review stays relevant and people know that there's no point in installing this broken app.*
Advertising	advertisement, ads	*A pop-up ad appears that cannot be closed.*
Uninstallation	uninstall, delete application	*Makes my phone glitch. Can't go back, and when I try to purchase multiple medicines, the app crashes right away. Can't return to the main menu. I have to restart the phone first, and even then I have to wait a long time for Halodoc to load. So I had to uninstall it... it's really frustrating.*
Payments	pay, purchase, top up, refund, free, price, cost, premium, gopay, dana	*Already paid to chat with a doctor, but it failed and the balance disappeared. This is a scam app. There's no help option. What kind of fraudulent app is this?.*
Compatibility	compatible, do not support, android	*Not compatible with [redacted].*
Resources	battery, memory, cache	*Notifications keep appearing, constantly asking to turn on GPS. Very annoying and drains the battery.*
Connectivity	signal, connection, network, internet, wifi, 4G, 5G, connect	*I appreciate that the app exists, but it takes hours just to log in by entering a PIN. Does it need a 5G signal or what just to log in? So many people have complained already—it's down to a 3-star rating—how come there's still no improvement?*
Account and Logging	login, signin, signup, verification, account, otp	*It's so hard to log in, when verifying via email the code never gets sent. Then when I try using my phone number, it says the account isn't available.*
Notification	notif, notification	*I booked a consultation well in advance, only for it to be suddenly cancelled unilaterally without any follow-up confirmation or notification? It's not about the money. It's about respecting the patient's time and sense of urgency. Really disappointed. If you can't take patients, then don't make consultation slots available.*
Updates	notif, notification	*Please fix this because after the update the app can't be opened and has become slow.*

Table 2. Non-technical aspects of mHealth apps

Aspect	Keywords	User review sample
Perceived Usefulness and User Satisfaction	helpful, easy, beneficial, simple, useful, health service, accessible, gratitude, convenient, supportive	💬*Extremely helpful for health consultations.*
Teleconsultation and Service Quality	doctor, consultation, response, chat, prescription, medicine, clear explanation, friendly, fast service, patient care, satisfaction	💬*I feel helped because the health issues I experienced could be addressed.*
Healthcare Administration and Insurance Management	healthcare facility, BPJS, insurance, administration, participant data, membership, card, registration, transfer, verification, online service, bureaucratic process	💬*Even though my business went bankrupt after COVID, I could still transfer healthcare facilities easily.*

though no formal inter-rater reliability statistic was calculated. The categorised dataset, grouped into 15 aspects, primarily reflected functional and technical issues, while analysis of the uncategorised dataset revealed broader insights into usability, interface design, and overall user interaction with mHealth applications.

From the categorised dataset, we analysed user reviews across 15 identified aspects of mHealth apps in Indonesia. The analysis reveals recurring themes of compliments and criticisms that reflect users' lived experiences, expectations, and frustrations when engaging with these platforms.

Account, access, and compatibility. Users appreciated smooth account creation, prompt verification, and updates that improved device support. However, recurring issues with failed logins, verification loops, incompatibility with certain Android versions or lower-spec devices, and frequent update disruptions often left users locked out of their accounts.

Performance, stability, and resources. Positive experiences included fast loading, efficient memory and battery use, and reliable operation. In contrast, endless loading, frequent crashes, excessive resource consumption, and bugs introduced by updates were among the most frequent complaints, often leading to app abandonment or uninstallation.

Notifications, payments, privacy, and requests. Well-timed reminders, smooth payments, and secure handling of personal data fostered user trust, while affordable fees encouraged continued use. Yet gaps in critical notifications, failed transactions, refund difficulties, data privacy fears, and unresolved user requests reduced confidence in the platforms and their developers.

Teleconsultation, service quality, and healthcare administration. Users valued courteous doctors, clear explanations, timely prescriptions, and the digitalisation of administrative tasks such as insurance checks and online registrations. However, slow or superficial consultations, appointment cancellations, and difficulties with card downloads or data synchronisation undermined these perceived benefits.

Perceived usefulness and overall value. Across apps, users praised convenience, practical value, and the integration of multiple features into one platform, describing them as "one-stop solutions." Still, satisfaction declined when workflows were cumbersome, navigation unclear, or inclusivity limited, especially for older users, those abroad, or those with lower-end devices.

To complement the categorised analysis, we conducted a thematic analysis towards the uncategorised data of user reviews to understand how users experience mHealth apps in Indonesia, particularly in terms of practical value, quality of interaction, and integration with existing health systems. The analysis highlights both the reported benefits that drive continued use and the challenges that limit adoption or satisfaction, illustrated with representative user review excerpts.

☺ *Convenient access to healthcare.* A recurring benefit was the ease of accessing health services without the need for hospital visits or long queues. Users valued the ability to consult with doctors and order medicines directly from home, describing the apps as 🗩*"very helpful and making things easier in emergency conditions."* Such convenience was especially appreciated during urgent or high-risk situations.

☺ *Time-saving and efficient service.* Efficiency was another strong positive theme. Many users highlighted fast responses from doctors and quick delivery of prescriptions or medicines. One review praised that 🗩*"delivery is very fast [and the order] processed immediately,"* underscoring that digital platforms can outperform traditional health facilities in terms of speed.

☺ *Helpful and professional medical advice.* Users frequently commended the quality of teleconsultations. Doctors were often described as friendly, patient, and detailed in their explanations. For example, one review noted that online consultations 🗩*"were very helpful... to keep my spirits up to recover."* Such interactions built trust in the apps as credible healthcare services.

☺ *Broad range of services and features.* The integration of consultations, electronic prescriptions, medicine delivery, and vaccination records was widely regarded as valuable. Users appreciated having a 🗩*"one-stop solution"* for health needs, especially when features such as vaccination certificates or rare medicines functioned as intended.

☹ *Account setup and profile management issues.* Many users struggled with registration, profile updates, and verification. Some encountered bugs that made critical fields (e.g., gender or date of birth) unresponsive, while others faced repeated login requests after updates. Such onboarding difficulties undermined accessibility.

☹ *User interface glitches and navigation problems.* Non-responsive buttons, blank screens, and confusing navigation flows were common complaints. One user described the interface as 🗨*"unclear and too complicated,"* reflecting a broader frustration with poor UI reliability and design.

☹ *Performance and stability issues.* Slow loading, frequent crashes, and errors were among the most cited problems. Some reviews reported that features like vaccine certificate downloads failed repeatedly, while others complained that constant updates introduced new bugs instead of fixes.

☹ *Complex workflows and cumbersome processes.* Rather than simplifying tasks, several app processes were described as 🗨*"troublesome"*. Users noted lengthy steps for accessing free check-ups, difficulties cancelling medicine orders, and burdensome offline verification requirements. These workflow issues reduced the apps' perceived usefulness.

☹ *Support and communication gaps.* Users often reported ineffective or unresponsive help channels. Failed transactions and generic, template-like responses left users feeling abandoned. For instance, one user criticised that after losing money to a failed payment, 🗨*"there's no help option, what kind of app is this?"* Such gaps eroded trust in the platforms.

☹ *Accessibility and inclusivity limitations.* Finally, inclusivity challenges emerged. Reviews highlighted the inability to register with international phone numbers, restrictions based on age criteria for health programmes, and difficulties for less tech-savvy or older users. Device optimisation issues also excluded users with low-end smartphones.

4 Recommendations for mHealth Apps Improvements

The findings from both the categorised and uncategorised analyses point to two overarching areas where mHealth apps in Indonesia can be improved: **technical** enhancements that ensure reliability and usability, and **non-technical** measures that build trust, inclusivity, and long-term engagement.

From a **technical perspective**, several priorities emerge. First, account and authentication systems must be strengthened to reduce frustrations with failed verification and login loops. This can be achieved by incorporating *redundant verification mechanisms* such as SMS, email, or biometric checks, alongside clear and accessible account recovery workflows [15]. Importantly, user data should be preserved through updates so that accounts remain intact without forcing re-registration.

Second, app performance and stability need to be optimised [19]. Users consistently reported problems with crashes, freezes, and excessive battery drain, particularly on lower-spec devices that are common in rural Indonesia. Developers should adopt lightweight architectures, efficient resource management, and comprehensive performance testing across a diverse device range to ensure smooth and reliable use. Similarly, compatibility and connectivity must be enhanced by maintaining backward compatibility with older devices and operating systems, while also offering *offline or low-bandwidth modes* so that critical features remain accessible in low-connectivity environments [9].

Another technical challenge lies in the update process. Updates should undergo rigorous quality assurance through phased rollouts, regression testing, and rollback options [27]. Clear update notes would help users anticipate changes and build trust in the app's reliability. Related to this, user interfaces must be simplified and made more accessible in order to minimise users' cognitive load [18]. By reducing workflow complexity, adopting designs similar to familiar messaging platforms, and providing *multimodal content* (e.g., icons, short videos, and audio captions in local languages) apps can better accommodate users with diverse literacy levels and experiences.

Financial transactions represent another key area. Payments must be transparent and reliable [12], with multiple options available, instant confirmations, and automated refunds in cases of failure. Clarity around fees and pricing is essential to reinforce user confidence. Equally, privacy must be safeguarded by design [2]. This requires collecting only essential data, providing *clear and transparent privacy policies*, and giving users control over their information, including options for deletion or export. Notification systems also demand refinement: critical alerts should always be delivered reliably [28], while promotional notifications must be limited and subject to user control, ensuring that health-related reminders take priority.

In addition to these technical improvements, **non-technical measures** are equally vital for sustainable adoption. One recurring theme was the lack of effective customer support. Stronger communication and support systems are needed [17], with responsive in-app chat, helplines, and user-friendly FAQs. Automated template responses should be avoided in favour of personalised assistance, while proactive communication about cancellations, outages, or system changes would further reduce frustration [22].

Beyond service delivery, trust and transparency must be actively fostered [25]. Collaborations with trusted institutions (e.g., the Ministry of Health, BPJS, or accredited hospitals) can provide validation and credibility, reassuring users that the apps are safe and official which will affect users' adoption decision towards the apps [13]. At the same time, inclusivity and accessibility should be prioritised to ensure broader adoption [1]. This includes supporting older adults, individuals with limited digital literacy, and marginalised groups through *simplified registration, larger fonts, local languages, and minimal technical requirements.* These can be made possible by employing adaptive user interface (UI) so the each user can customise the UI based on their needs [26].

Overall, the high-priority recommendations address core usability, reliability, and inclusivity issues that most directly affect UX, while the medium-priority actions focus on sustaining long-term trust and institutional credibility. Together, they provide a roadmap for developers, policymakers, and healthcare providers seeking to design culturally responsive and technically robust mHealth solutions for Indonesia (see Table 3).

Table 3. Prioritised design recommendations for Indonesian mHealth Apps

Recommendation	Priority	Complexity	Success Metrics	Cultural Considerations
Simplify and localise user interfaces (familiar layouts, multimodal content)	High	Moderate – UI/UX redesign, translation	Higher usability, faster task completion	Support users with low literacy and diverse languages
Strengthen authentication systems (redundant verification, recovery workflow)	High	Moderate – system redesign	Fewer login failures, higher successful registrations	Reflect common verification methods (OTP, WhatsApp codes)
Optimise performance and stability (lightweight design, device testing)	High	High – re-engineering required	Fewer crashes, higher app ratings	Cater to low-end mobile devices in rural areas
Ensure transparent and reliable payments (multiple options, instant refund)	High	High – secure transaction setup	Lower failure rates, higher transaction success	Build trust among low-income users
Enhance connectivity and compatibility (offline and low-bandwidth modes)	High	High – backend redesign	More use in poor signal areas, stable data sync	Reduce impact of network disparities
Safeguard privacy by design (data minimisation, user control)	High	Moderate – legal and UX updates	Fewer privacy complaints, stronger confidence	Address sensitivity to data sharing
Promote inclusivity and accessibility (adaptive UI, large fonts, low specs)	High	Moderate – adaptive design	Wider user coverage, positive feedback from elders	Reduce digital exclusion
Improve update quality and transparency (phased roll-outs, clear notes)	Medium	Moderate – QA enhancement	Fewer post-update complaints, higher trust	Reinforce reliability perception
Strengthen customer support (responsive chat, proactive updates)	Medium	Moderate – HR and AI integration	Faster responses, higher satisfaction	Encourage polite, culturally attuned interaction

5 Threats to Validity

This study faces several validity threats. For **internal validity**, automated classification of reviews into 15 aspects may not have fully captured the contextual use of slang in Bahasa Indonesia, even after normalisation. Regarding **external validity**, the analysis of nearly 200,000 reviews from four major mHealth apps may not generalise to all platforms, though similar patterns are expected as these represent the most widely used applications. Since the study relies solely on user reviews, which reflect perceptions rather than behaviours, future work will include direct engagement with end-users and stakeholders for deeper insights. For **construct validity**, we adapted 13-aspect framework from a previous study [11] by applying only 12 aspects, excluding *Internationalisation* as all apps studied are designed for domestic use. While this deviation could be seen as a limitation, it improves contextual relevance. Finally, for **conclusion validity**, triangulation of quantitative and qualitative analysis reduced bias, but as reviews are self-reported and often extreme, the findings should be viewed as indicative rather than causal.

6 Conclusion

This study presents an evidence-based analysis of user experiences with Indonesian mHealth applications, drawing on 170,763 reviews from four major platforms. Using and extending a 13-aspect framework [11], we found 12 aspects consistently relevant and identified three additional non-technical dimensions reflecting local socio-cultural and infrastructural realities. The findings refine existing evaluation frameworks by situating mHealth design within a Global South context and informing the apps development that are technically efficient, culturally appropriate, and transparent. Based on these insights, we proposed prioritised design recommendations to guide the creation of inclusive and trustworthy mHealth services. Future work will include interviews with medical professionals to integrate provider perspectives and inform a prototype mHealth app tailored to Indonesia. By combining user and practitioner insights, this research advances responsible and human-centred innovation in digital health for low-resource settings.

Acknowledgments. This study was funded by the Directorate of Research and Community Service, Directorate General of Research and Development, Indonesia Ministry of Higher Education, Science, and Technology (contract number 094/C3/DT.05.00/PL/2025).

References

1. Acharya, K.R.: Designing equitable and inclusive mhealth technology: insights from global south healthcare practitioners. IEEE Trans. Prof. Commun. **67**(2), 229–245 (2024)
2. Benjumea, J., Ropero, J., Rivera-Romero, O., Dorronzoro-Zubiete, E., Carrasco, A.: Privacy assessment in mobile health apps: scoping review. JMIR Mhealth Uhealth **8**(7), e18868 (2020)
3. Blei, D.M., Ng, A.Y., Jordan, M.I.: Latent dirichlet allocation. J. Mach. Learn. Res. **3**(Jan), 993–1022 (2003)
4. Braun, V., Clarke, V.: Using thematic analysis in psychology. Qual. Res. Psychol. **3**(2), 77–101 (2006)
5. Chib, A., van Velthoven, M.H., Car, J.: mhealth adoption in low-resource environments: a review of the use of mobile healthcare in developing countries. J. Health Commun. **20**(1), 4–34 (2015) https://doi.org/10.1080/10810730.2013.864735. pMID: 24673171
6. DataReportal: Digital 2024: Indonesia (2024). https://datareportal.com/reports/digital-2024-indonesia, Accessed 18 Mar 2025
7. DataReportal: Digital 2025: Indonesia (2025). https://datareportal.com/reports/digital-2025-indonesia, Accessed 18 Mar 2025
8. Durmuş, A.: The influence of digital literacy on mhealth app usability: the mediating role of patient expertise. Digital Health **10**, 20552076241299060 (2024)
9. Gay, V., Leijdekkers, P.: Bringing health and fitness data together for connected health care: mobile apps as enablers of interoperability. J. Med. Internet Res. **17**(11), e260 (2015)
10. Haggag, O., Grundy, J., Abdelrazek, M., Haggag, S.: Better addressing diverse accessibility issues in emerging apps: a case study using COVID-19 apps. In: Proceedings of the 9th IEEE/ACM International Conference on Mobile Software Engineering and Systems, pp. 50–61 (2022)
11. Haggag, O., Grundy, J., Abdelrazek, M., Haggag, S.: A large scale analysis of mhealth app user reviews. Empir. Softw. Eng. **27**(7), 196 (2022)
12. Hijazi, R., Abu Daabes, A., Al-Ajlouni, M.I.: Mobile payment service quality: a new approach for continuance intention. Int. J. Qual. Reliab. Manag. **40**(8), 2019–2038 (2023)
13. Jarvenpaa, S.L., Tractinsky, N., Saarinen, L.: Consumer trust in an internet store: a cross-cultural validation. J. Comput. Mediat. Commun. **5**(2) (1999) https://doi.org/10.1111/j.1083-6101.1999.tb00337.x, https://onlinelibrary.wiley.com/doi/abs/10.1111/j.1083-6101.1999.tb00337.x
14. Khalid, H., Shihab, E., Nagappan, M., Hassan, A.E.: What do mobile app users complain about? IEEE Softw. **32**(3), 70–77 (2014)
15. Kukkadapu, G.: Adaptive authentication in healthcare: balancing security with accessibility. J. Comput. Sci. Technol. Stud. **7**(6), 519–525 (2025)
16. Nouri, R., Kalhori, R.N.S., Ghazisaeedi, M., Marchand, G., Yasini, M.: Criteria for assessing the quality of mhealth apps: a systematic review. J. Am. Med. Inform. Assoc. **25**(8), 1089–1098 (2018)
17. Oppong, E., Hinson, R.E., Adeola, O., Muritala, O., Kosiba, J.P.: The effect of mobile health service quality on user satisfaction and continual usage. Total Qual. Manag. Bus. Excellence **32**(1–2), 177–198 (2021)
18. Oviatt, S.: Human-centered design meets cognitive load theory: designing interfaces that help people think. In: Proceedings of the 14th ACM International Conference

on Multimedia, pp. 871–880. MM '06, Association for Computing Machinery, New York, NY, USA (2006). https://doi.org/10.1145/1180639.1180831
19. Pace, P., et al.: An edge-based architecture to support efficient applications for healthcare industry 4.0. IEEE Trans. Ind. Inf. **15**(1), 481–489 (2018)
20. Palomba, F.: Crowdsourcing user reviews to support the evolution of mobile apps. J. Syst. Softw. **137**, 143–162 (2018). https://doi.org/10.1016/j.jss.2017.11.043, https://www.sciencedirect.com/science/article/pii/S0164121217302807
21. Pitaloka, A.A., Nugroho, A.P.: Digital transformation in Indonesia health care services: social, ethical and legal issues. J. STI Policy Manag. **6**(1), 51–66 (2021)
22. Roy Chowdhury, I., Patro, S., Venugopal, P., Israel, D.: A study on consumer adoption of technology-facilitated services. J. Serv. Mark. **28**(6), 471–483 (2014)
23. Santoso, B.S., Budiyanti, R.T., Nandini, N.: Analisis pemanfaatan layanan telemedicine pasca pandemi covid-19 di jawa tengah. Jurnal Manajemen Kesehatan Indonesia **12**(2), 119–129 (2024)
24. Sunjaya, A.P.: Potensi, aplikasi dan perkembangan digital health di indonesia. J. Indonesian Med. Assoc. **69**(4), 167–169 (2019)
25. Wang, C., Qi, H.: Influencing factors of acceptance and use behavior of mobile health application users: systematic review. In: Healthcare. vol. 9, p. 357. MDPI (2021)
26. Wang, W., Grundy, J., Khalajzadeh, H., Madugalla, A., Obie, H.O.: Designing adaptive user interfaces for mhealth applications targeting chronic disease: a user-centered approach. ACM Trans. Softw. Eng. Methodol. (2025)
27. Xu, Q., Hou, X., Xiao, T., Zhao, W.: Factors affecting medical students' continuance intention to use mobile health applications. J. Multidisc. Healthcare, 471–484 (2022)
28. Zhang, R., Wang, H.: Insights into the technological evolution and research trends of mobile health: bibliometric analysis. In: Healthcare. vol. 13, p. 740. MDPI (2025)

Antioxidant and Anti-Aging Potential of TriGlow+: Evaluation Through DPPH, FRAP, Elastase, and Collagenase Assays

Wahyu Widowati[1(✉)], Susy Tjahjani[1], Meilinah Hidayat[1], Sulkhan Windrayahya[2], Dwi Nur Triharsiwi[3], and Maheda Dwinarendra[4]

[1] Faculty of Medicine, Maranatha Christian University, Bandung, Indonesia
wahyu_w60@yahoo.com
[2] Anugrah Original Bionatura Indonesia, Tangerang, Indonesia
[3] Bimolecular and Biomedical Research Center, Aretha Medika Utama, Bandung, Indonesia
[4] Fathonah Amanah Shidiq Thabligh, Jakarta, Indonesia

Abstract. Oxidative stress, resulted from the excessive generation of reactive oxygen species (ROS), contributes in skin aging by damaging cellular macromolecules. Oral supplementation with antioxidant-rich formulations has emerged as a promising approach to counteract skin aging by reducing oxidative stress. TriGlow+ is a health beverage composed of collagen tripeptide, multiple fruit extracts (lemon, apple, carrot, grape seed, green tea, aloe vera, Garcinia atroviridis), and glutathione, which collectively possess antioxidant and anti-aging potential. This study aimed to evaluate the anti-aging and antioxidant activity of TriGlow+. Antioxidant capacity was assessed by DPPH and FRAP assays, while anti-aging activity was measured through elastase and collagenase inhibition assay. DPPH assay revealed dose-dependent free radical scavenging activity with an IC_{50} of 3014.68 ± 146.82 μg/mL. In contrast, FRAP results demonstrated strong ferric ion reducing power, with values elevated at 50–100 μg/mL (257.55 ± 2.85 and 282.58 ± 2.44 μM Fe (II)/μg). TriGlow+ also inhibited key aging-related enzymes in a concentration-dependent manner. Elastase inhibition IC_{50} is 46.19 ± 0.31 μg/mL, indicating strong inhibitory potential. Collagenase inhibition exhibited IC_{50} value of 182.10 ± 1.96 μg/mL, showing moderate efficacy. In conclusion, TriGlow+ exhibits notable antioxidant and anti-aging activities, particularly through ferric reducing power and inhibition of elastase and collagenase. Overall, the study provides foundational evidence supporting the functional benefits of TriGlow+. These findings highlight TriGlow+ as a promising oral nutraceutical for promoting skin health and combating oxidative stress, warranting further investigation into its active components and clinical efficacy.

Keywords: Antioxidant · anti-aging · collagenase · elastase · TriGlow+

1 Introduction

The largest organ of the human body is skin, that continuously exposed to external stressors including ultraviolet (UV) radiation, pollutions, and cosmetics [1]. These factors stimulate the generation of reactive oxygen species (ROS), which, under physiological

E. R. Kaburuan and S. Goundar (Eds.): HIS 2025, LNCS 16392, pp. 311–323, 2026.
https://doi.org/10.1007/978-981-95-6304-3_27

conditions, contributes in maintaining cellular homeostasis and regulating processes such as epidermal keratinocyte proliferation [2]. However, when the generation of reactive oxygen species surpasses the capacity of the antioxidant defense system is overwhelmed, oxidative stress develops, leading to skin inflammation and accelerated aging [3].

Oxidative stress that contributes in modulating the expression and activity of enzymes including elastase, hyaluronidase, collagenase, and tyrosinase, which are implicated in skin aging and disorders [4]. ROS, including hydrogen peroxide, act as signaling molecules that activate pathways like NF-κB, MAPK, and AP-1, upregulating the matrix metalloproteinases (MMPs) such as collagenase and elastase, which degrade the extracellular matrix and contribute to skin aging [5, 6]. Additionally, ROS-mediated signaling enhances hyaluronidase activity, resulting in the breakdown of hyaluronic acid and skin hydration loss, further exacerbating skin aging [7]. In terms of pigmentation, oxidative stress stimulates melanogenesis by increasing tyrosinase expression and activity through the MITF pathway, leading to hyperpigmentation disorders [8].

Skin aging itself is a complex and multifactorial biological process influenced by intrinsic factors, including chronological aging, and extrinsic factors, including ultraviolet (UV) radiation, pollution, and lifestyle [9]. A central mechanism underlying this process is oxidative stress, due to imbalance between free radicals and antioxidant defenses [10]. The excessive accumulation of free radicals damages cellular components, including lipids, proteins, and DNA, thereby impairing skin integrity and accelerating the deterioration of its structure and function [11]. These molecular and cellular alterations are manifested macroscopically as visible signs of skin aging, including tissue atrophy with reduced elasticity, fine wrinkles, and pronounced dryness often correlated with pruritus, reflecting the progressive decline in physiological functionality of the skin [12].

A wide range of therapeutic strategies has been developed to delay or improve the visible manifestations of skin aging. Topical formulations remain the most widely used interventions, including retinoids, α-hydroxy acids, broad-spectrum sunscreens, and antioxidant or anti-inflammatory agents such as vitamin C, vitamin E, and niacinamide [13, 14]. However, the efficacy of topical agents is often limited by factors such as poor skin penetration, instability of active compounds, and user compliance, highlighting the need for complementary approaches. In recent years, oral supplementation with natural ingredients rich in antioxidants, has gained growing attention as both a preventive and therapeutic strategy against premature skin aging. Evidence suggests that the consumption of antioxidant-rich beverages or dietary supplements can reduce systemic oxidative stress while directly improving skin properties, including enhanced elasticity, decreased UV-induced erythema, better hydration, and reduced transepidermal water loss (TEWL) [15, 16]. In this context, TriGlow+ represents a functional beverage composed of combination of bioactive extracts and nutrients with demonstrated health-promoting properties, particularly antioxidant activity. Its composition includes collagen tripeptide, lemon extract, aloe vera extract, apple extract, carrot extract, green tea extract, grape seed extract, *Garcinia atroviridis* extract, and glutathione, offering a multifaceted approach to supporting skin health and combating oxidative damage.

Collagen tripeptide (CTP), a low-molecular-weight hydrolyzed collagen, promotes fibroblast proliferation, enhances extracellular matrix protein synthesis, increases skin hydration and elasticity, and inhibits matrix metalloproteinase activity, thereby protecting against UV- and oxidative stress–induced damage [17]. Lemon extract, derived primarily from the fruit (*Citrus limon*), is rich in bioactive compounds including vitamin C (ascorbic acid), flavonoids such as hesperidin and eriocitrin, as well as essential oils like limonene, which collectively contribute to its anti-inflammatory, antioxidant, and antimicrobial properties [18, 19]. Aloe vera (*Aloe barbadensis)* extract has been widely reported to exert protective effects against skin aging through multiple mechanisms of action. It enhances fibroblast proliferation and activity, stimulates the synthesis of collagen and hyaluronic acid, scavenges excessive free radicals, and inhibits the activity of matrix metalloproteinases (MMPs) that degrade extracellular matrix including elastin and collagen [20].

Apple extract (*Malus domestica*) is abundant in bioactive phytochemicals, including polyphenols (e.g., phloridzin, catechins, chlorogenic acid, quercetin), triterpenes, and vitamin C, which collectively impart strong antioxidant and anti-inflammatory effects [21]. These constituents scavenge ROS, alleviate oxidative stress, and safeguard cellular macromolecules including lipids, proteins, and DNA, thereby counteracting a key mechanism of skin aging [22]. Carrot extract (*Daucus carota*) is a valuable source of bioactive compounds, particularly carotenoids such as β-carotene, alongside polyphenols, phenolic acids, and vitamins A, C, and E [23]. β-carotene functions as a provitamin A and a powerful singlet oxygen quencher, thereby protecting skin from photooxidative damage induced by ultraviolet (UV) radiation [24]. Green tea extract (*Camellia sinensis*) is abundant in bioactive compounds, particularly catechins including epigallocatechin-3-gallate (EGCG), alongside flavonoids and tannins, which collectively provide potent antioxidant, anti-inflammatory, and photoprotective effects, thereby protecting cells from premature aging [25–27].

Grape seed (*Vitis vinifera*) is recognized as a rich reservoir of polyphenolic constituents, predominantly proanthocyanidins, catechins, and phenolic acids, which collectively exhibit strong antioxidant, anti-inflammatory, and photoprotective activities [28]. *Garcinia atroviridis* is a plant rich in bioactive phytochemicals such as hydroxycitric acid, flavonoids, phenolic acids, and xanthones, which contribute significantly to its antioxidant and anti-inflammatory activities [29]. Glutathione (GSH) is a tripeptide composed of glutamate, it directly scavenges ROS and reactive nitrogen species (RNS), serves as a cofactor for glutathione peroxidase in detoxifying hydrogen peroxide and lipid hydroperoxides, and participates in the regeneration of other antioxidants such as vitamins C and E [30].

The novelty of TriGlow+ lies in its formulation, which integrates collagen tripeptide a proven extracellular matrix stimulator [17] with diverse botanical extracts such as lemon, aloe vera, and green tea [18, 20, 27] alongside glutathione [30]. This unique combination offers complementary mechanisms of action, targeting oxidative stress and enzyme-mediated skin aging simultaneously, a strategy that has not been comprehensively evaluated in previous studies of oral nutraceuticals. Despite the extensive research on the antioxidant and anti-aging properties of individual bioactive ingredients, limited studies have investigated the synergistic effects of multi-component oral formulations combining collagen tripeptide, botanical extracts, and glutathione. TriGlow+ was developed to address this gap by providing a comprehensive antioxidant and anti-aging approach through a multi-ingredient nutraceutical beverage. This study was designed to investigate both the antioxidant properties and the potential skin anti-aging effects of TriGlow+. Antioxidant capacity was assessed through a series of assays, including DPPH and FRAP scavenging methods. In addition, the formulation's ability to inhibit key enzymes involved in skin aging, namely collagenase and elastase, was evaluated to provide further insight into its protective mechanisms.

2 Methods

2.1 Formulation of TriGlow+

The preparation of TriGlow+ was carried out at PT. Jaya Sinergi Cosmindo (Yogyakarta, Indonesia). All powdered ingredients were weighed according to the formulation composition and homogenized using a ribbon blender to ensure uniform distribution for 20 min at ambient temperature (25 ± 2 °C). The blended powder was subsequently sieved (mesh 40) to achieve consistent particle size and prevent agglomeration. Ingredient amounts are presented as approximate ranges per serving (20 g powder equivalent) to maintain confidentiality while providing transparency on formulation composition (Table 1). Basic quality control (QC) procedures were applied during the laboratory-scale formulation of TriGlow+. All raw materials were verified for identity and appearance before use. The blended powder was inspected for color uniformity, odor, and absence of agglomerates after mixing [15, 16]. Equipment and containers were cleaned and dried prior to each batch preparation to minimize contamination risk. The final mixture was packaged in moisture-resistant aluminum sachets and stored at room temperature (≤25 °C) until further use.

Table 1. Composition of TriGlow+.

Ingredient	Approximate Amount (mg per serving)
Lemon extract	700–900
Aloe vera extract	600–800
Apple extract	900–1,100
Carrot extract	600–800
Inulin (Chicory Root)	2,500–3,500
Green tea extract	400–600
Grape seed extract	250–350
Garcinia atroviridis extract	900–1,100
Collagen tripeptide	1,800–2,200
Glutathione	400–600
Premix vitamins	400–600
Premix minerals	400–600
Sucralose	5–15

(continued)

Table 1. (*continued*)

Ingredient	Approximate Amount (mg per serving)
Natural chocolate flavor	300–500
Natural vanilla flavor	150–250
Erythritol (optional)	800–900

2.2 DPPH Scavenging Activity

A volume of 50 μL TriGlow+ at different concentrations was pipetted into a 96-well microplate, after DPPH solution 200 μL (Sigma-Aldrich, D9132) was added. The mixture was kept in the dark for 30 min of incubation, after which its absorbance was recorded at 517 nm using a Multiskan GO Microplate Spectrophotometer (Thermo Scientific). Each assay was conducted in triplicate, and the radical scavenging activity was expressed as a percentage [31].

2.3 FRAP Assay

The FRAP working solution was freshly prepared by combining 10 mL of acetate buffer (300 mM, pH 3.6 adjusted with acetic acid), 1 mL of ferric chloride hexahydrate (20 mM, Merck 1.03943.0250, USA) dissolved in distilled water, and 1 mL of TPTZ solution (10 mM, Sigma 3682-35-7, USA) prepared in 40 mM HCl. In a 96-well microplate, 7.5 μL of TriGlow+ at different concentrations was added to 142.5 μL of FRAP reagent, followed by incubation for 30 min at 37 °C. The absorbance was then recorded at 593 nm using a microplate reader Multiskan™ GO Microplate Reader (Thermo Scientific, USA). A calibration curve was constructed with $FeSO_4$ ranging from 0.019 to 95 μg/mL [31].

2.4 Elastase Inhibition Assay

A volume of 10 μL TriGlow+ at varying concentrations was pre-incubated with 5 μL of porcine pancreas elastase (0.5 mU/mL, Sigma Aldrich 45124, USA, prepared in chilled distilled water) and 125 μL of Tris buffer (100 mM, pH 8) for 15 min at 25 °C. Subsequently, 10 μL of the substrate N-Succinyl-Alanine-Alanine-Alanine-p-Nitroanilide (2 mg/mL in Tris buffer, Sigma Aldrich 54760, USA) was administered to the mixture and the mixture was left to react for an additional 15 min at 25 °C. The enzymatic activity was then determined by recording absorbance at 410 nm [32].

2.5 Colagenase Inhibition Assay

A mixture was prepared containing 10 μL of collagenase from *Clostridium histolyticum* (0.01 U/mL, Sigma Aldrich C8051, USA, dissolved in chilled distilled water), 60 μL of Tricine buffer (50 mM, pH 7.5, supplemented with 10 mM of $CaCl_2$ and 400 mM of NaCl), and 30 μL of TriGlow + at varying concentrations in DMSO. The mixture was incubated at 37 °C for 20 min. Subsequently, 20 μL of the substrate N-[3-(2-Furyl)acryloyl]-Leu-Gly-Pro-Ala (1 mM in Tricine buffer, Sigma Aldrich F5135, USA) was added. The absorbance was measured at 335 nm to evaluate enzymatic activity [32].

2.6 Statistical Analysis

The experiments were conducted in triplicate, and data were expressed as mean ± standard deviation (SD). Statistical analyses were conducted using IBM SPSS Statistics software version 26.0 (IBM Corp., Armonk, NY, USA). Differences among groups were assessed using one-way ANOVA followed by Tukey's post hoc test for normally distributed data, while non-parametric comparisons were analyzed using the Mann–Whitney U test. A p-value < 0.05 was considered statistically significant.

3 Results

3.1 DPPH Scavenging and FRAP Activity

The antioxidant properties of TriGlow+ in this study was measured by DPPH scavenging assay. Figure 1A showed the DPPH scavenging activity of TriGlow+ in a dose-dependent manner. At lower concentrations (3.13–12.50 µg/mL), scavenging activity was 8.95 ± 0.29% and 8.98 ± 0.36% respectively, with no significant differences among these groups ($p > 0.05$). Further elevation was measured after concentration of 25 µg/mL, with the highest scavenging activity was measured at 400 µg/mL and the scavenging activity was 14.25 ± 0.23%, which showed a statistically significant difference compared to all lower concentrations ($p < 0.05$). The IC_{50} of DPPH scavenging activity measured was 3014.68 ± 146.82 µg/mL (Table 2). These results indicate that TriGlow+ exerts concentration-dependent free radical scavenging activity, supporting its antioxidant potential.

The antioxidant properties of TriGlow+ was also measured by FRAP assay. Figure 1B demonstrated that TriGlow+exhibited a strong concentration-dependent antioxidant activity. At the lowest concentration (0.78 µg/mL), the FRAP value was minimal (18.65 ± 3.84 µM Fe(II) / µg). Higher concentrations of 50.00 and 100.00 µg/mL yielded the strongest activity, with FRAP values of 257.55 ± 2.85 and 282.58 ± 2.44 µM Fe(II)/µg, respectively, both significantly greater than all other concentrations tested ($p < 0.05$). These findings indicate that TriGlow+ possesses potent and dose-dependent ferric ion reducing capacity, supporting its role as a strong antioxidant agent.

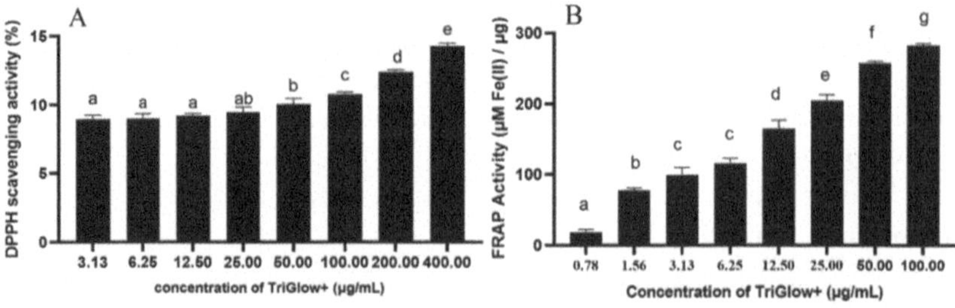

Fig. 1. Antioxidan activity of various concentration of TriGlow+. Data mean ± STD, n = 4. A: DPPH scavenging activity of TriGlow+. Different superscript indicate significant differences according to Mann-Whitney post hoc test ($p < 0.05$); B: FRAP Activity of TriGlow+. Different superscript indicate significant differences based on One way ANOVA, Tukey post hoc test ($p < 0.05$).

Table 2. The IC_{50} Value of Antioxidant Activity of TriGlow+

Antioxidant Activity	Linear Equation	R^2	IC50 Value (μg/mL)
DPPH	$y = 0.01x + 9.15$	0.98	3014.68 ± 146.82

3.2 Collagenase and Elastase Inhibiton Activity

The anti-aging properties of TriGlow+ in this study was measured by elastase inhibition activity. Figure 2A showed that the elastase inhibition activity of TriGlow+ increased in a concentration-dependent manner. At lower concentration (1.04 – 2.08 μg/mL) the inhibition remained relatively modest with no significant differences observed among these groups ($p > 0.05$). However, a significant increase ($p < 0.05$) was evident from 8.33 μg/mL onward, with highest elastase value was (60.69 ± 0.03%) obtained from the highest concentration of TriGlow+ (66.67 μg/mL), also the IC_{50} measured was 46.19 ± 0.31 μg/mL (Table 3). These results demonstrate that TriGlow+ exerts dose-dependent elastase inhibitory activity.

The collagenase inhibition activity of TriGlow+ (Fig. 2B) showed that the collagenase inhibition activity of TriGlow+ increased gradually with rising concentrations. At lower concentration (3.91–15.63 μg/mL) the inhibition remained relatively modest. However, at higher concentration, the inhibition activity increased gradually. The maximum inhibitory effect was recorded at 250.00 μg/mL, with collagenase inhibition reaching 54.27 ± 0.19%, which was significantly higher than all other tested concentrations ($p < 0.05$), also also the IC_{50} measured was 182.10 ± 1.96 μg/mL (Table 3). These findings indicate that TriGlow+ exhibits dose-dependent collagenase inhibitory activity.

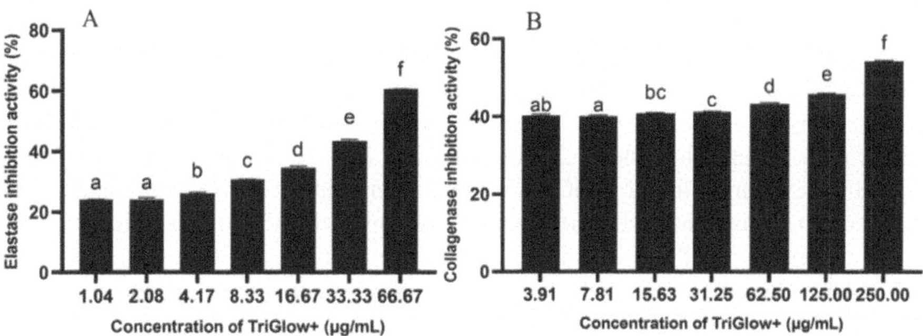

Fig. 2. Anti-aging activity of various concentration of TriGlow+. Data mean ± STD, n = 3. A: elastase inhibition activity of TriGlow+. Different superscript indicate significant differences according to Mann-Whitney post hoc test ($p < 0.05$).; B: collagenase inhibition acitivity of TriGlow+. Different superscript indicate significant differences according to One-way ANOVA, Tukey post hoc test ($p < 0.05$).

Table 3. The IC_{50} Value of Anti-aging Activity of TriGlow+

Anti-aging Activity	Linear Equation	R^2	IC50 Value (μg/mL)
Elastase	$y = 0.56x + 24.36$	0.99	46.19 ± 0.31
Collagenase	$y = 0.06x + 39.65$	0.99	182.10 ± 1.96

4 Discussion

Antioxidants serve as an essential agents in maintaining skin integrity by neutralizing reactive oxygen species (ROS), repairing oxidized molecules, and strengthening cellular repair mechanisms under UV irradiation, which depletes antioxidant levels like vitamin E and Coenzyme Q10. When antioxidant defenses are compromised, excess of ROS induces oxidative stress, inflicting damage upon lipids, mitochondria, DNA, proteins, and disrupting gene expression. Such molecular damage accelerates skin aging by degrading collagen and elastin, reduced cellular renewal, and the emergence of wrinkles, irregular pigmentation, loss of elasticity, and other visible signs of aging [11].

A significant positive relationship was detected between the antioxidant capacity (DPPH and FRAP assays) and the enzyme inhibitory activities (elastase and collagenase). Samples exhibiting higher radical scavenging and ferric reducing activities tended to show stronger inhibition of elastase and collagenase, consistent with previous findings that antioxidant-rich formulations can modulate skin-aging enzymes through oxidative stress suppression [15, 18, 22]. This indicates that the antioxidant properties of TriGlow+ may contribute to its anti-aging potential by mitigating oxidative stress–induced activation of elastase and collagenase.

The DPPH assay is widely applied techniques to evaluate antioxidant capacity, especially in determining the free-radical scavenging activity of natural extracts and organic molecules [33, 34]. In the present study, the DPPH scavenging activity demonstrated an IC_{50} value of 3014.68 ± 146.82 μg/mL. According to Jadid et al. [35], IC_{50} values higher than 50 μg/mL are categorized as weak antioxidant activity. Consistent with this classification, the results revealed that the antioxidant activity of TriGlow+ exhibited a concentration-dependent increase. This relatively high IC_{50} value may be attributed to the complex composition of TriGlow+, in which multiple bioactive components may interact or act through indirect antioxidant mechanisms rather than direct radical quenching. Therefore, the DPPH result should be interpreted alongside other assays such as FRAP and enzyme inhibition, which demonstrated stronger antioxidant and anti-aging potentials.

The FRAP assay results demonstrate that TriGlow+ exerts a pronounced and concentration-dependent ferric ion reducing capacity, reflecting its strong antioxidant potential. The significant increase in FRAP values at higher concentrations (50.00 and 100.00 μg/mL) suggests that the antioxidant compounds within TriGlow+act synergistically to enhance antioxidant activity. The values obtained at these concentrations are consistent with the category of potent antioxidants, aligning with previous findings that polyphenol exhibit high ferric ion reducing antioxidant power [36]. These results reinforce the notion that the efficacy of antioxidant supplements depends not only on their composition but also on dose, where higher concentrations can optimize radical neutralization and electron transfer processes.

The elastase inhibition assay revealed that TriGlow+ exhibits a clear dose-dependent anti-aging effect, as evidenced by its increasing inhibitory activity with higher concentrations (66.67 μg/mL). The IC_{50} measured was 46.19 ± 0.31 μg/mL. This indicates that the active constituents in TriGlow+, likely including polyphenols and glutathione, may exert synergistic effects in suppressing elastase activity. Moreover, the collagenase inhibition assay also demonstrated that TriGlow+possesses a concentration-dependent inhibitory effect. The highest inhibition activity was shown at the highest concentration of TriGlow+ (250.00 μg/mL) with IC_{50} measured was 182.10 ± 1.96 μg/mL. Since elastase and collagenase overexpression is closely associated with extracellular matrix degradation and wrinkle formation, the ability of TriGlow+ to significantly inhibit this enzyme highlights its potential role as an effective anti-aging formulation. These results align with those reported in earlier studies demonstrating that plant-derived antioxidants and bioactive compounds can mitigate skin aging by targeting proteolytic enzymes such as elastase and collagenase [37].

The IC_{50} values obtained in this study indicate the concentration required for TriGlow+ to inhibit 50% of radical or enzyme activity under in vitro conditions. Lower IC_{50} values represent stronger biological potency, suggesting greater efficiency at smaller concentrations. Clinically, these results imply that the active compounds in TriGlow+ may reach biologically relevant levels following regular oral intake, supporting potential protection against oxidative stress–induced elastin and collagen degradation in vivo.

The observed bioactivities of TriGlow+ are likely the result of synergistic interactions among its key components. Collagen tripeptide promotes fibroblast activity and extracellular matrix synthesis, while glutathione enhances redox balance and supports the regeneration of other antioxidants. Meanwhile, the botanical extracts contribute polyphenols and flavonoids that neutralize reactive oxygen species and suppress enzyme-mediated collagen degradation. Together, these ingredients form a complementary network of antioxidant and anti-aging actions, where the antioxidant-rich extracts protect the bioactive peptides from oxidative damage, and peptides in turn support skin structural repair and resilience [17, 18, 30]. Such synergistic mechanisms have been reported in other nutraceutical combinations targeting oxidative skin aging [15, 22].

The combination of collagen tripeptide with botanical antioxidant extracts and glutathione offers a multifaceted strategy to protect the dermal extracellular matrix from oxidative degradation and enzymatic proteolysis. Experimental and clinical studies have shown that collagen tripeptide promotes fibroblast proliferation, enhances extracellular matrix protein synthesis, increases skin hydration and elasticity, and inhibits matrix metalloproteinase activity, thereby protecting against UV- and oxidative stress–induced damage [17]. Multiple *in vitro* studies also reported low IC_{50} values for these plant extracts on antioxidant assays, supporting their ability to scavenge free radicals and reduce oxidants. For example, lemon extract also known to be high in flavonoid content and it is reported to have strong antioxidant activity by DPPH and FRAP assay [38]. Aloe vera reported to have high antioxidant activities due to its phenolic compounds in some reports while also exhibiting measurable anti-collagenase and anti-elastase activity in enzyme assays, which supports its dual antioxidant/anti-aging potential [39, 40].

Apple and carrot-derived extracts, with diverse polyphenols and carotenoids, have yielded reproducible antioxidant potency across DPPH and FRAP assays and, in several studies, demonstrated inhibitory activity against collagenase and elastase or improved dermal hydration/elasticity in nutritional/biological models, suggesting that their antioxidant activity translated to functional anti-aging outcomes [41–43]. Green tea which is rich in catechin has been reported to have strong antioxidant activity and have been shown to suppress collagenase activity and reduce elastase activity in plant-screening panels, supporting a mechanistic role in preserving collagen integrity when combined with collagen tripeptides [44]. Grape-seed extracts which is rich in procyanidin, consistently show potent radical-scavenging activity by DPPH and ABTS scavenging assay and have been associated with collagenase/elastase inhibitory effects [45]. *Garcinia atroviridis* extracts are reported to possess significant DPPH/ABTS scavenging activity in previous studies due to its phenolic and flavonoid compounds [46]. Finally, glutathione acts synergistically with polyphenol-rich extracts by maintaining intracellular redox status and inhibit MMP upregulation, therefore supports its complementary role alongside collagen tripeptide for improving skin appearance and mitigating oxidative-driven collagen loss [47]. Collectively, these data indicate that collagen tripeptide formulations enriched with various botanical extracts possess antioxidant profiles measurable anti-collagenase/elastase activity that mechanistically justify their combined use for anti-aging interventions.

Compared with other commercial antioxidant supplements, TriGlow+ demonstrates comparable overall bioactivity despite exhibiting moderate radical scavenging potency. Studies on fruit-based nutritional supplements have reported FRAP values ranging from 72 to 14,320 μmol Fe^{2+} equivalents per serving, reflecting the broad variability among commercial formulations [48]. Similarly, Pellegrini et al. evaluated several antioxidant supplements and found that while single-compound products such as vitamin C and E exhibited stronger radical scavenging activity, multi-ingredient formulations provided broader functional antioxidant effects across different assays [49]. These findings indicate that TriGlow+ has strong ferric-reducing and enzyme-inhibitory activities suggest protective effects on the dermal matrix and oxidative balance, supporting its use as a multifunctional oral supplement for maintaining skin structure and elasticity. The demonstrated antioxidant and anti-aging properties position TriGlow+ as a potential contender in the expanding market of oral beauty and skin health supplements. These study suggest practical potential for TriGlow+ as a functional nutraceutical to support skin health, prevent premature aging, and complement topical skincare approaches.

Despite demonstrating promising antioxidant and anti-aging potential, this study has several limitations. The assays were conducted under in vitro conditions, which may not fully represent the complexity of in vivo physiological processes such as absorption, metabolism, and bioavailability of active compounds. The product formulation was tested as a whole, and the contribution of each component was not assessed individually, limiting the understanding of their specific interactions. Additionally, due to proprietary constraints, detailed compositional ratios could not be disclosed, which may affect reproducibility. Future in vivo and clinical studies, as well as the specific roles and interactions of individual ingredients to clarify the efficacy, bioavailability, and long-term safety of TriGlow+, and also validate the observed synergistic effects in human subjects.

5 Conclusion

In summary, TriGlow+ antioxidant activity is obtained from its capacity to scavenge DPPH and FRAP acitivity. In addition, it demonstrates anti-aging potential by inhibiting both collagenase and elastase enzymes. In future research, the detailed characterization of bioactive constituents from TriGlow+ are necessary to identify constituents and to establish its pharmacological properties.

Acknowledgments. We express our gratitude for the financial help rendered by Ministry of Higher Education, Science, and Technology, National Research and Innovation Agency (BRIN), and the Education Endowment Fund Management Institution (LPDP). This research was also supported by Aretha Medika Utama in Bandung, Indonesia, which provided methodology and laboratory resources.

Disclosure of Interests. The authors have no competing interests.

References

1. Nakai, K., Tsuruta, D.: What are reactive oxygen species, free radicals, and oxidative stress in skin diseases? Int. J. Mol. Sci. **22**(19), 10799 (2021)
2. Ansari, W.A., Srivastava, K., Nasibullah, M., Khan, M.F.: Reactive oxygen species (ROS): sources, generation, disease pathophysiology, and antioxidants. Discov. Chem. **2**(1), 100059 (2025)
3. Liguori, I., et al.: Oxidative stress, aging, and diseases. Clin. Interv. Aging **13**, 757–772 (2018)
4. Pintus, F., et al.: Hydroxy-3-phenylcoumarins as multitarget compounds for skin aging diseases: synthesis, molecular docking and tyrosinase, elastase, collagenase and hyaluronidase inhibition, and sun protection factor. Molecules **27**(20), 6914 (2022)
5. Averill-Bates, D.A.: Reactive oxygen species and cell signaling. Biochim. Biophys. Acta Mol. Cell Res. **1868**(2), 119573 (2023)
6. Rauf, A., et al.: Reactive oxygen species in biological systems: pathways, associated diseases, and potential inhibitors—a review. Food Sci. Nutr. **11**(7), 3261–3276 (2023)
7. Chen, J., Liu, Y., Zhao, Z., Qiu, J.: Oxidative stress in the skin: impact and related protection. Int. J. Cosmet. Sci. **43**(5), 495–509 (2021)
8. Emanuelli, M., et al.: The double-edged sword of oxidative stress in skin damage and melanoma: from physiopathology to therapeutical approaches. Antioxidants **11**(4), 612 (2022)
9. Dorosz, A., et al.: The impact of environmental factors on skin and tissue ageing: mechanisms, effects, and preventive strategies. J. Educ. Health Sport **15**(2), 582–596 (2025)
10. Qian, H., et al.: Mechanism of action and therapeutic effects of oxidative stress and stem cell-based materials in skin aging: current evidence and future perspectives. Front. Bioeng. Biotechnol. **10**, 1082403 (2023)
11. Papaccio, F., Caputo, S., Bellei, B.: Focus on the contribution of oxidative stress in skin aging. Antioxidants **11**(6), 1121 (2022)
12. Zhang, S., Duan, E.: Fighting against skin aging: the way from bench to bedside. Cell Transplant. **27**(5), 729–738 (2018)

13. Shin, S.-H., Lee, Y., Rho, N.-K., Park, K.-Y.: Skin aging from mechanisms to interventions: focusing on dermal aging. Front. Physiol. **14**, 1195272 (2023)
14. Griffiths, T.W., Watson, R.E.B., Langton, A.K.: Skin ageing and topical rejuvenation strategies. *Br. J. Dermatol.* **189**(Suppl_1), i17–i23 (2023)
15. Christman, L., De Benedetto, A., Johnson, E., Khoo, C., Gu, L.: Polyphenol-rich cranberry beverage positively affected skin health, skin lipids, skin microbiome, inflammation, and oxidative stress in women in a randomized controlled trial. Nutrients **16**(18), 3126 (2024)
16. Dumoulin, M., Gaudout, D., Lemaire, B.: Clinical effects of an oral supplement rich in antioxidants on skin radiance in women. Clin. Cosmet. Investig. Dermatol. **9**, 315–324 (2016)
17. Lee, Y.I., et al.: Effect of a topical collagen tripeptide on antiaging and inhibition of glycation of the skin: a pilot study. Int. J. Mol. Sci. **23**(3), 1101 (2022)
18. Lu, X., et al.: Nutrients and bioactives in citrus fruits: different citrus varieties, fruit parts, and growth stages. Crit. Rev. Food Sci. Nutr. **63**(14), 2018–2041 (2023)
19. Saini, R.K., et al.: Bioactive compounds of citrus fruits: a review of composition and health benefits of carotenoids, flavonoids, limonoids, and terpenes. Antioxidants **11**(2), 239 (2022)
20. Rahman, S., Carter, P., Bhattarai, N.: Aloe vera for tissue engineering applications. J. Funct. Biomater. **8**(1), 6 (2017)
21. Josimuddin, S.K., Kumar, M., Rastogi, H.: A review on nutritional and medicinal value of *Malus domestica* with various activity. Int. J. Health Sci. **6**(S4), 7251–7265 (2022)
22. Vandorou, M., Plakidis, C., Tsompanidou, I.M., Adamantidi, T., Panagopoulou, E.A., Tsoupras, A.: A review on apple pomace bioactives for natural functional food and cosmetic products with therapeutic health-promoting properties. Int. J. Mol. Sci. **25**(19), 10856 (2024)
23. Ahmad, T., et al.: Phytochemicals in *Daucus carota* and their health benefits. Foods **8**(9), 424 (2019)
24. Anbualakan, K., et al.: A scoping review on the effects of carotenoids and flavonoids on skin damage due to ultraviolet radiation. Nutrients **15**(1), 92 (2022)
25. Samanta, S.: Potential bioactive components and health promotional benefits of tea (*Camellia sinensis*). J. Am. Nutr. Assoc. **41**(1), 65–93 (2022)
26. Cerbin-Koczorowska, M., Waszyk-Nowaczyk, M., Bakun, P., Goslinski, T., Koczorowski, T.: Current view on green tea catechins formulations, their interactions with selected drugs, and prospective applications for various health conditions. Appl. Sci. **11**(11), 4905 (2021)
27. Zheng, X., et al.: Green tea catechins and skin health. Antioxidants **13**(12), 1506 (2024)
28. Kamah, F., et al.: Phenolic compounds and biological activities of grape (*Vitis vinifera* L.) seeds at different ripening stages: insights from Algerian varieties. Arq. Bras. Med. Vet. Zootec. **77**(1), e13361 (2025)
29. Shahid, M., Law, D., Azfaralariff, A., Mackeen, M.M., Chong, T.F., Fazry, S.: Phytochemicals and biological activities of *Garcinia atroviridis*: a critical review. Toxics **10**(11), 656 (2022)
30. Lana, J.V., et al.: Nebulized glutathione as a key antioxidant for the treatment of oxidative stress in neurodegenerative conditions. Nutrients **16**(15), 2476 (2024)
31. Widowati, W., Pryandoko, D., Wahyuni, C.D., Marthania, M., Kusuma, H.S.W., Handayani, T.: Antioxidant properties of soybean (*Glycine max* L.) extract and isoflavone. In: 2021 IEEE International Conference on Health, Instrumentation & Measurement, and Natural Sciences (InHeNce) , New York, pp. 1–6. IEEE (2021)
32. Widowati, W., et al.: Antioxidant and antiaging assays of *Hibiscus sabdariffa* extract and its compounds. Nat. Prod. Sci. **23**(3), 192–200 (2017)
33. Gülçin, İ., Alwasel, S.H.: DPPH radical scavenging assay. Processes **11**(8), 2248 (2023)
34. Widowati, W., et al.: Antioxidant and antiaging activities of *Jasminum sambac* extract, and its compounds. J. Rep. Pharm. Sci. **7**(3), 270–285 (2018)

35. Jadid, N., Hidayati, D., Hartanti, S.R., Arraniry, B.A., Rachman, R.Y., Wikanta, W.: Antioxidant activities of different solvent extracts of *Piper retrofractum* Vahl using DPPH assay. AIP Conf. Proc. **1854**(1), 020019 (2017)
36. Gulcin, İ: Antioxidants and antioxidant methods: an updated overview. Arch. Toxicol. **94**(3), 651–715 (2020). https://doi.org/10.1007/s00204-020-02689-3
37. Pacularu-Burada, B., Cîrîc, A.-I., Begea, M.: Anti-aging effects of flavonoids from plant extracts. Foods **13**(15), 2441 (2024)
38. Xi, W., Lu, J., Qun, J., Jiao, B.: Characterization of phenolic profile and antioxidant capacity of different fruit parts from lemon (*Citrus limon* Burm.) cultivars. J. Food Sci. Technol. **54**(5), 1108–1118 (2017)
39. Rungruang, R., Ratanathavorn, W., Boohuad, N., Phakeenuya, V., Peasura, N., Panichakul, T.: Anti-elastase, anti-collagenase, and anti-hyaluronidase activities of *Aloe barbadensis* gel extract: in vitro and molecular docking studies. J. Appl. Pharm. Sci. **15**(2), 001–008 (2025)
40. Iosageanu, A., et al.: *In vitro* wound-healing potential of phenolic and polysaccharide extracts of *Aloe vera* gel. J. Funct. Biomater. **15**(9), 266 (2024)
41. Lee, E.H., et al.: Functional properties of newly-bred 'Summer King' apples. Hortic. Sci. Technol. **38**(3), 405–417 (2020)
42. Kaur, P., Subramanian, J., Singh, A.: Green extraction of bioactive components from carrot industry waste and evaluation of spent residue as an energy source. Sci. Rep. **12**(1), 16607 (2022)
43. Shoji, T., Masumoto, S., Moriichi, N., Ohtake, Y., Kanda, T.: Administration of apple polyphenol supplements for skin conditions in healthy women: a randomized, double-blind, placebo-controlled clinical trial. Nutrients **12**(4), 1071 (2020)
44. Masek, A., Chrzescijanska, E., Latos, M., Zaborski, M., Podsędek, A.: Antioxidant and antiradical properties of green tea extract compounds. Int. J. Electrochem. Sci. **12**(7), 6600–6610 (2017)
45. Castro, M.L., et al.: Elevating skincare science: grape seed extract encapsulation for dermatological care. Molecules **29**(16), 3717 (2024)
46. Chatatikun, M., et al.: Antioxidant and tyrosinase inhibitory properties of an aqueous extract of *Garcinia atroviridis* Griff. ex T. Anderson fruit pericarps. Pharmacogn. J. **12**(1), 88–93 (2020)
47. Tsay, G.J., Lin, S.-Y., Li, C.-Y., Mau, J.-L., Tsai, S.-Y.: Comparison of single and combined use of ergothioneine, ferulic acid, and glutathione as antioxidants for the prevention of ultraviolet B radiation-induced photoaging damage in human skin fibroblasts. Processes **9**(7), 1204 (2021)
48. Rickards, L., Lynn, A., Barker, M.E., Russell, M., Ranchordas, M.K.: Comparison of the polyphenol content and *in vitro* antioxidant capacity of fruit-based nutritional supplements commonly consumed by athletic and recreationally active populations. J. Int. Soc. Sports Nutr. **19**(1), 336–348 (2022)
49. Dávalos, A., Gómez-Cordovés, C., Bartolomé, B.: Commercial dietary antioxidant supplements assayed for their antioxidant activity by different methodologies. J. Agric. Food Chem. **51**(9), 2512–2519 (2003)

Assessing Healthcare Workers' Readiness for Telemedicine Adoption: Insights Across Core, Clinical, E-Learning, and Technological Dimensions

Angel Yustina Ngongo[1], July Ivone[2], and Stella Tinia Hasianna[3](✉)

[1] Medical Doctor Professional Program, Faculty Of Medicine, Maranatha Christian University, Jl. Prof.Drg. Suria Sumantri MPH No.65, Bandung 40164, Indonesia

[2] Departement of Public Health, Faculty of Medicine, Maranatha Christian University, Jl. Prof.Drg. Suria Sumantri MPH No.65, Bandung 40164, Indonesia

[3] Departement of Physiology, Faculty of Medicine, Maranatha Christian University, Jl. Prof.Drg. Suria Sumantri MPH No.65, Bandung 40164, Indonesia

stellatinia@gmail.com

Abstract. Telemedicine has emerged as a transformative approach to delivering healthcare services, particularly during the COVID-19 pandemic, by enabling remote access to medical consultations and monitoring. However, many healthcare workers remain inadequately prepared for this digital shift. This study aimed to evaluate healthcare workers' readiness for telemedicine implementation across four key dimensions: core readiness, e-learning readiness, clinical readiness, and technology readiness. A cross-sectional descriptive study was conducted using convenience sampling. Data were collected through an online questionnaire adapted from the *Core, Clinical, and E-Learning Readiness Assessment* and the *Technology Readiness Assessment* tools. A total of 60 healthcare workers participated voluntarily. Descriptive statistics were used to analyze readiness levels in each domain. Among respondents, 30% demonstrated readiness in the core readiness domain, 95% showed high readiness in e-learning, 63% in clinical readiness, and 68% in technology readiness. These findings indicate that while healthcare workers are generally prepared in e-learning, clinical, and technological aspects, fundamental readiness concerning motivation, commitment, and institutional support remains limited. Healthcare workers exhibit strong readiness in adopting digital-based healthcare services, particularly in technological, clinical, and educational aspects. However, low core readiness underscores the need for organizational engagement, policy reinforcement, and attitudinal change before large-scale telemedicine adoption can be achieved.

Keywords: Healthcare Workers · Readiness · Telemedicine · Digital Health · E-Learning

E. R. Kaburuan and S. Goundar (Eds.): HIS 2025, LNCS 16392, pp. 324–337, 2026.
https://doi.org/10.1007/978-981-95-6304-3_28

1 Introduction

The rapid evolution of information and communication technology has profoundly influenced the healthcare sector. This advancement has driven the emergence of various innovations, including telemedicine, which allows healthcare services to be delivered remotely through digital platforms. According to the Ministry of Health of the Republic of Indonesia, telemedicine refers to the delivery of healthcare services by professionals through information and communication technologies, encompassing diagnosis, treatment, prevention, research, evaluation, and continuing education—all aimed at improving individual and community health outcomes [2].

The World Health Organization (WHO) declared COVID-19 a pandemic on March 11, 2020. In response, countries worldwide, including Indonesia, implemented large-scale restrictions that required citizens to remain at home. Fear of infection discouraged many from visiting healthcare facilities, creating a pressing need for alternative service delivery models [3]. To address this challenge, the Indonesian Ministry of Health issued Circular Letter No. HK.02.01/Menkes/303/2020 and Letter No. YR.03.03/III/III8/2020, authorizing the use of telemedicine in non-emergency settings as a preventive measure against COVID-19 transmission [2].

This policy was well-received by the public. A 2021 study reported increased telemedicine utilization, with 55.8% of respondents categorized as frequent users and 44.2% as infrequent users [4]. The convenience of accessing healthcare without physical exposure to infection risks contributed significantly to its adoption.

Despite these benefits, the implementation of telemedicine in many settings remains suboptimal. Failures are often attributed not to technological deficiencies but to the lack of readiness among healthcare workers [5]. In developing countries, readiness is commonly assessed using indicators such as core readiness, engagement readiness, and structural or technology readiness [6]. A 2018 study in Padang revealed insufficient societal readiness for telemedicine [7], while research in Uganda (2020) identified low e-learning readiness among healthcare providers [8].

Although similar studies have been widely conducted abroad, research on healthcare workers' readiness in Indonesia remains limited. Therefore, this study aims to assess healthcare workers' preparedness for telemedicine adoption, focusing on four dimensions: core readiness, e-learning readiness, clinical readiness, and technology readiness.

2 Methods

This study utilized primary data collected directly from research subjects, namely healthcare workers who voluntarily completed a questionnaire distributed via Google Forms. The questionnaire was adapted and translated from the Core, Clinical, and E-Learning Readiness Assessment Questionnaire and the Technology Readiness Assessment Questionnaire [8], with modifications made to suit the study context. Data collection was conducted between August and September 2022.

The study employed a descriptive observational design with a cross-sectional approach, using convenience sampling. Data were obtained from the responses of healthcare workers submitted through Google Forms.

The study variables include core readiness, e-learning readiness, clinical readiness, and technology readiness. The collected data were categorized according to these variables. Each variable was assessed based on calculated scores, and the results were analyzed descriptively and presented in percentages.

Data were analyzed using descriptive and inferential statistics. Descriptive statistics, including frequency distributions and percentages, were used to summarize readiness levels. Inferential analyses were then conducted to identify associations and predictors.

Chi-square tests were used to examine associations between categorical variables such as profession, years of service, and readiness level. Fisher's exact test was applied when expected cell counts were below five. Logistic regression analyses were conducted to identify significant predictors of overall readiness, while controlling for potential confounding factors. Correlation analyses were performed to investigate the relationships among the four readiness dimensions.

Reliability of the questionnaire was assessed using Cronbach's alpha. Factor analysis was also performed to confirm the construct validity of the readiness framework. Statistical significance was set at $p < 0.05$, and 95% confidence intervals were calculated for all estimates.

As this study involved human participants, research ethics principles were strictly observed, namely respect for persons, beneficence, non-maleficence, and justice. Ethical approval for this study was obtained from the Research Ethics Committee of the Faculty of Medicine, Maranatha Christian University (Approval No. 050/KEP/VI/2022).

3 Results

Table 1. Distribution of Respondents by Age

Age (years)	n	(%)
26–35	34	57
36–45	18	30
46–55	6	10
56–65	1	2
>65	1	2
Total	60	100

As shown in Table 1, the majority of respondents who used telemedicine services were in the 26–35 age group (n = 34, 57%), categorized as early adulthood. This was followed by the 36–45 age group (n = 18, 30%), representing late adulthood. The 45–55 age group (n = 6, 10%) represented early elderly, while the late elderly and elderly over 65 years accounted for only 1 respondent each (2%).

Table 2 shows that female respondents predominated among telemedicine users (n = 37,62%), compared with males (n = 23, 38%).

Table 2. Distribution of Respondent by Gender

Gender	n	(%)
Male	23	38
Female	37	62
Total	60	100

Table 3. Distribution of Respondents by profession

Profession	n	(%)
Physician	43	72
Dentist	2	3
Nurse	6	10
Midwife	4	7
Pharmacist	5	8
Total	60	100

As presented in Table 3, physicians comprised the majority of respondents (n = 43, 72%), followed by nurses (n = 6, 10%), pharmacists (n = 5, 8%), midwives (n = 4, 7%), and dentists (n = 2, 3%).

Table 4. Distribution of Respondents by Telemedicine Experience

Experience	n	(%)
None	13	22
<1 Year	4	7
1–3 Years	41	68
>3 Years	2	3
Total	60	100

Table 4 shows that most respondents had 1–3 years of telemedicine experience (n = 41, 68%), corresponding with the period of the COVID-19 pandemic.

Based on the data presented in Table 5, the majority of respondents were categorized as not ready in terms of core readiness. In contrast, for e-learning readiness, clinical readiness, and technology readiness, the dominant category was highly ready.

Figure 1 illustrates the comparative distribution of healthcare worker's readiness across four key dimensions, core readiness, e-learning readiness, clinical readiness and technology readiness. The chart demonstrates a clear disparity among readiness domains

Table 5. Healthcare Workers' Readiness for Telemedicine

Readiness	Core Readiness		E-Learning Readiness		Clinical Readiness		Technology Readiness	
	n	(%)	n	(%)	n	(%)	n	(%)
Not Ready	42	70	0	0	3	5	0	0
Ready	18	30	3	5	19	32	19	32
Highly Ready	0	0	57	95	38	63	41	68
Total	60	100	60	100	60	100	60	100

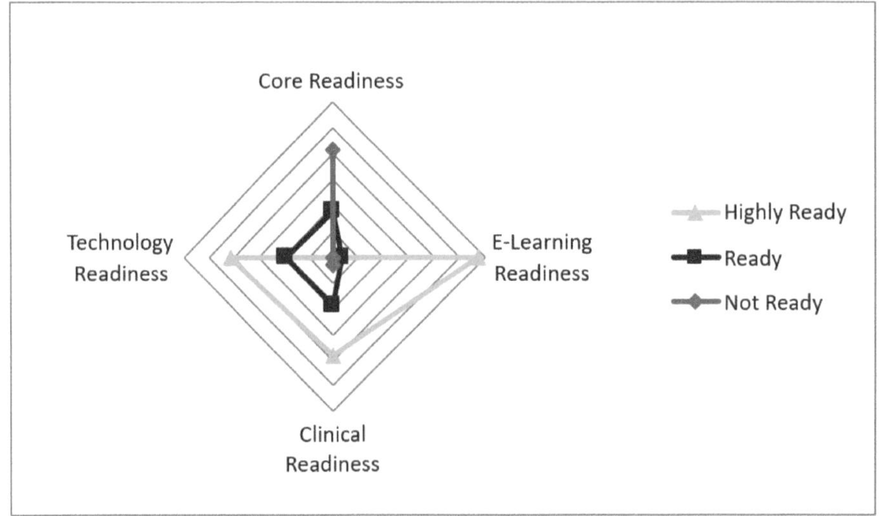

Fig. 1. Radar Chart of Healthcare Worker's Readiness Across Four Dimensions

with core readiness showing the lowesr scores, indicating limited motivation and institutional support. In contrast, e-learning, clinica, and technology readiness dimensions display higher levels, reflecting strong digital competence and adaptability. This visualization highlights that while healthcare workers possess the necessary technical and educational capabilities, foundational readiness related to organizational engagement remains inadequate.

Analysis of Tables 6, 7, 8, 9, 10 and 11 further highlights differences in readiness across professional groups. Physicians, who represented the majority of respondents, demonstrated strong preparedness in e-learning (100% highly ready), clinical (58% highly ready), and technology readiness (65% highly ready), but most were unprepared in the core readiness (77% not ready). Specialists showed a similar pattern, with 78% not ready in core readiness, although they were fully prepared for e-learning (100%) and demonstrated high readiness in both clinical (56%) and technology readiness (56%). The dentist recorded the lowest performance, with all respondents (100%) categorized as not ready in core readiness, while readiness in other aspects remained moderate to high. Pharmacists displayed excellent readiness in e-learning (100% highly ready)

Table 6. Readiness among Physicians

Readiness	Core Readiness		E-Learning Readiness		Clinical Readiness		Technology Readiness	
	n	(%)	n	(%)	n	(%)	n	(%)
Not Ready	33	77	0	0	3	7	0	0
Ready	10	23	0	0	15	35	15	35
Highly Ready	0	0	43	100	25	58	28	65
Total	43	100	43	100	43	100	43	100

Table 7. Readiness among Specialists

Readiness	Core Readiness		E-Learning Readiness		Clinical Readiness		Technology Readiness	
	n	(%)	n	(%)	n	(%)	n	(%)
Not Ready	7	78	0	0	1	11	0	0
Ready	2	22	0	0	3	33	4	44
Highly Ready	0	0	9	100	5	56	5	56
Total	9	100	9	100	9	100	9	100

Table 8. Readiness among Dentists

Readiness	Core Readiness		E-Learning Readiness		Clinical Readiness		Technology Readiness	
	n	(%)	n	(%)	n	(%)	n	(%)
Not Ready	2	100	0	0	0	0	0	0
Ready	0	0	0	0	1	50	0	0
Highly Ready	0	0	2	100	1	50	0	0
Total	2	100	2	100	2	100	2	100

and technology (100% highly ready), but nearly half (40%) were still unprepared in the core aspect. Midwives also exhibited strong readiness, particularly in technology (100% highly ready), although most remained unprepared in core readiness (74%). Finally, nurses showed the best overall profile, achieving 100% highly ready in clinical readiness, with relatively higher scores in core readiness (67% ready) compared to other professions.

In Summary, the analysis indicates that core readiness remains the weakest dimension across all professional groups, with dentists scoring lowest. By contrast, e-learning and technology readiness are consistently high across professions, while clinical readiness

Table 9. Readiness among Pharmacists

Readiness	Core Readiness		E-Learning Readiness		Clinical Readiness		Technology Readiness	
	n	(%)	n	(%)	n	(%)	n	(%)
Not Ready	2	40	0	0	0	0	0	0
Ready	3	60	0	0	1	20	0	0
Highly Ready	0	0	5	100	4	80	5	100
Total	5	100	5	100	5	100	5	100

Table 10. Readiness among Midwifes

Readiness	Core Readiness		E-Learning Readiness		Clinical Readiness		Technology Readiness	
	n	(%)	n	(%)	n	(%)	n	(%)
Not Ready	3	74	0	0	0	0	0	0
Ready	1	25	1	25	2	50	0	0
Highly Ready	0	0	3	75	2	50	4	100
Total	4	100	4	100	4	100	4	100

Table 11. Readiness among Nurses

Readiness	Core Readiness		E-Learning Readiness		Clinical Readiness		Technology Readiness	
	n	(%)	n	(%)	n	(%)	n	(%)
Not Ready	2	33	0	0	0	0	0	0
Ready	4	67	2	33	0	0	2	33
Highly Ready	0	0	4	67	6	100	4	67
Total	6	100	6	100	6	100	6	100

is strongest among nurses. These findings emphasize that although healthcare workers are generally well-prepared in technical and educational aspects of telemedicine, fundamental readiness at the core level remains limited.

The Chi-Square test demonstrated a significant association between proffesion and overall readiness ($\chi2 = 6.84$, $p = 0.032$). Doctors, nurses, and pharmaticsts showed relatively higher readiness compared to midwives and dentist, suggesting that professional background influences confidence and motivation toward telemedicine adoption. These finding indicate that targeted interventions may be necessary to enchance readiness among underrepresented professional groups.

Table 12. Chi Square Association Between Profession and Overall Readiness

Profession	Ready (%)	Not Ready (%)	χ^2	p-value
Doctors	50	50	6.84	0.032
Nurses	67	33	–	–
Pharmaticsts	60	40	–	–
Midwives	25	75	–	–
Others	22	78	–	

Table 13. Logistic Regression Predicting High Overall Readiness by Profession

Predictor	OR	95% CI	p-value
Doctors	1.00	–	–
Nurses	0.82	0.32–2.11	0.67
Pharmaticsts	1.45	0.60–3.52	0.40
Midwives	0.64	0.22–1.82	0.40
Others	0.72	0.27–1.95	0.52

Logistic regression showed that, compared to physicians, others professions were less likely to report high overall readiness, although these differences were not statistically sicnificant ($p > 0.05$).

Table 14. Readiness among Healthcare Workers with No Prior Telemedicine Experience

Readiness	Core Readiness		E-Learning Readiness		Clinical Readiness		Technology Readiness	
	n	(%)	n	(%)	n	(%)	n	(%)
Not Ready	12	92	0	0	1	8	0	0
Ready	1	8	2	15	6	46	6	46
Highly Ready	0	0	11	85	5	38	7	54
Total	13	100	13	100	13	100	13	100

Analysis of Tables 12, 13, 14 and 15 reveals notable differences in healthcare workers' readiness for telemedicine when stratified by prior experience. In terms of core readiness, the highest level of preparedness was observed among respondents with more than three years of telemedicine experience (50% ready). In contrast, the lowest was found among those with no prior experience, with 92% categorized as not ready. For clinical readiness, healthcare workers with more than three years of experience demonstrated

Table 15. Readiness among Healthcare Workers with Less than One Year of Telemedicine Experience

Readiness	Core Readiness		E-Learning Readiness		Clinical Readiness		Technology Readiness	
	n	(%)	n	(%)	n	(%)	n	(%)
Not Ready	3	75	0	0	0	0	0	0
Ready	1	25	0	0	3	75	1	25
Highly Ready	0	0	4	100	1	25	3	75
Total	4	100	4	100	4	100	4	100

Table 16. Readiness among Healthcare Workers with One to Three Years of Telemedicine Experience

Readiness	Core Readiness		E-Learning Readiness		Clinical Readiness		Technology Readiness	
	n	(%)	n	(%)	n	(%)	n	(%)
Not Ready	26	63	0	0	2	5	0	0
Ready	15	37	1	2	11	27	12	29
Highly Ready	0	0	40	98	28	68	29	71
Total	41	100	41	100	41	100	41	100

Table 17. Readiness among Healthcare Workers with More than Three Years of Telemedicine Experience

Readiness	Core Readiness		E-Learning Readiness		Clinical Readiness		Technology Readiness	
	n	(%)	n	(%)	n	(%)	n	(%)
Not Ready	1	50	0	0	0	0	0	0
Ready	1	50	0	0	0	0	0	0
Highly Ready	0	0	2	100	2	100	2	100
Total	2	100	2	100	2	100	2	100

the strongest preparedness (100% highly ready), while those without prior experience had the lowest performance (8% not ready) (Tables 16 and 17).

In contrast, the dimensions of e-learning readiness and technology readiness consistently showed high levels across all groups, regardless of experience, with only minor variations. This suggests that exposure to digital platforms and technological tools has become a common skill set among healthcare workers.

Overall, these findings indicate that greater exposure and longer experience in providing telemedicine services are positively associated with higher readiness levels, particularly in core and clinical aspects. Meanwhile, e-learning and technology readiness appear to be less dependent on prior experience, reflecting the broad adaptation of healthcare workers to digital health tools during the pandemic (Table 18).

Table 18. Chi-Square Associations between Telemecine Experience

Telemedicine Experience	Ready (%)	Not Ready (%)	χ^2	p-value
None	8	92	7.49	0.019
<1 year	25	73	–	–
1–3 years	37	63	–	–
>3 years	50	50	–	–

These was a significant association between telemedicine experience and core readiness ($\chi2 = 7.49$, $p = 0.019$). Participants with longer experience demonstrated higher motivation and institutional confidence toward telemedicine implementation. This finding supports the view that hands on involvement directly enchances readiness, particularly at the behavioral and organizational levels (Table 19).

Table 19. Logistic Regression Predicting High Core Readiness by Telemecine Experience

Predictor	OR	95% CI	p-value
None	1.00	–	–
<1 year	2.00	0.65–6.11	0.22
1–3 years	3.10	1.18–8.15	0.02
>3 years	4.50	1.25–16.15	0.01

Logistic regression confirmed that healthcare workers with telemedicine experience of at least one year were over the times more likely to exhibit high core readiness (OR = 3.10, $p = 0.02$), and those with more than three years were four and a half times more likely (OR = 4.50, $p = 0.01$). These findings underscore the importance of sustained practical exposure in strengthening readiness for digital healthcare delivery.

4 Discussion

The findings of this study can be further interpreted through the lens of the Technology Acceptance Model (TAM) and the Organizational Readiness for Change framework. The low core readiness observed suggests that perceived usefulness and institutional support remain insufficient to drive behavioral intention toward telemedicine adoption.

In contrast, the high e-learning and technological readiness indicate growing digital competence and openness to innovation, aligning with post-pandemic shifts in healthcare delivery paradigms.

The results of this study revealed that 70% of respondents were categorized as not ready, while 30% were classified as prepared in terms of core readiness. This proportion indicates a relatively low level of preparedness compared to findings from previous studies conducted in Uganda (41%) [8] and Austria (64.4%) [9]. Contextual differences between studies may explain the discrepancy. The Ugandan research was conducted before the COVID-19 pandemic, a period when challenges such as geographical barriers and limited access to facilities heightened the perceived need for telemedicine. In contrast, the present study was conducted after the pandemic, during which telemedicine expanded rapidly over a relatively short timeframe. Despite its accelerated adoption, many healthcare workers may not have fully internalized the concept, scope, and practical implementation of telemedicine, leading to a lower level of core readiness.

The insufficient preparedness in this domain may also be attributed to a limited understanding among healthcare workers regarding the optimal application of telemedicine, coupled with inadequate awareness of its benefits and functions [6]. A study exploring veterinarians' perceptions of telemedicine reported similar findings: most respondents viewed telemedicine as suitable only for initial screening or consultation, and not for advanced clinical activities such as diagnosis or prescription [10]. Consistent with these observations, a considerable number of participants in the present study expressed a strong preference for face-to-face consultations, reflecting persistent skepticism toward virtual care models.

In contrast, healthcare workers exhibited high e-learning readiness, with 95% of respondents categorized as highly ready. This finding surpasses results from Uganda, where only 52% were highly prepared [8]. Both studies, however, highlight a shared perspective among healthcare workerst—recognizing e-learning as a valuable tool for bridging knowledge gaps, enhancing continuous education, and facilitating professional collaboration. Beyond its clinical function, telemedicine is increasingly perceived as a dual-purpose platform, supporting both patient care and knowledge exchange among healthcare providers [11]. The strong readiness in e-learning suggests that digital literacy and openness to online training have improved significantly among Indonesian healthcare workers.

Regarding clinical readiness, this study found that 63% of respondents were highly ready, 32% were ready, and only 5% were not ready. Although this is slightly lower than the 82% high readiness reported in Uganda [8], it still indicates a favorable level of preparedness. The discrepancy may be due to the heterogeneity of respondents in the present study, which included professionals from various healthcare settings, unlike the Ugandan study that focused on three structured levels of care. Nonetheless, the increasing recognition of telemedicine as a legitimate clinical tool reflects an encouraging trend toward its broader acceptance and integration within healthcare practice [11].

In terms of technology readiness, none of the participants were classified as not ready; 68% were highly ready, and 32% ready. These findings are notably higher than those reported in Uganda, where only 32.8% demonstrated high technological readiness [8]. This improvement may reflect Indonesia's accelerating digital transformation, including the adoption of electronic medical records, online patient registration systems, and teleconsultation platforms [12]. However, despite these advancements, cybersecurity concerns remain a critical issue. Reports of patient data breaches across several telemedicine platforms underscore the importance of strengthening data protection policies and enhancing cybersecurity infrastructure [6]. Achieving technological readiness thus requires not only user competence but also institutional safeguards to ensure data privacy and patient trust.

Further inferential analysis revealed significant differences in readiness across professional categories. Physicians, nurses and pharmaticsts demonstrated higher overall readiness compared to midwifes and dentists, as indicated by the Chi-Square results. This suggest that professional background influences confidence, familiarity, and motivation in afopting telemedicine. Logistic regression findings supported this pattern, showing that physicians were the most likely group to report high overall readiness, aligning with their boarder exposure to digital clinical tools and continuing education programs.

In addition, telemedicine experience emerged as a strong predictor of readiness. The Chi-square and regression analyses both confirmed that participants with at least one year of experience were significantly more likely to exhibit high core readiness, while those with more than three tears of experience demonstrated the highest levels of preparedness. This underscores the value of sustained exposure and practical engagement in enhancing self efficacy, technical compentence, and organizational confidence toward telemedicine use. These inferential findings emphasize that readiness not merely shaped by access to technology but also by accumulated experience and professional culture.

Differences in readiness levels were also observed across professional categories, though these variations should be interpreted with caution due to the unequal distribution of respondents among healthcare professions. Nonetheless, the inferential analysis confirmed significant differences across professions, where physicians, nurses, and pharmacists demonstrated higher readiness compared to midwifes and denist. This suggest that professional background plays a vital rome in shaping motivation and familiarity with telemedicine tools.

Furthermore, the analysis indicated that individuals with previous telemedicine experience tended to exhibit greater readiness, particularly in core and clinical dimensions. This align with the logistic regression finding, which showed that respondents with at least one year of experience were over three times more likely to report high readiness, and those with more than three years had the highest likelihood of readiness. This pattern highlights that exposure anf hands on involvement play a crucial role in enhancing confidende, adaptability, and sustained engagement with telemedicine. During the pandemic, many healthcare workers were deployed spontaneously to deliver telemedicine services without structutrd training or preparation, which may have constrained their ability to adapt effectively to this novel service model [13].

To bridge the readiness gap, interventions must simultaneously address individual-level motivation, organizational culture, and system-level enablers such as infrastructure, policy, and cybersecurity. Drawing on international experiences in developing countries, capacity-building initiatives should prioritize change management, standardization of training, and alignment of policies with global digital health strategies.

5 Conclusion

This study concludes that healthcare workers demonstrate varying levels of readiness in adopting telemedicine across different dimensions. In terms of core readiness, 70% of respondents were classified as not ready, revealing a substantial gap in fundamental preparedness, institutional commitment, and behavioral engagement. In contrast, readiness levels were considerably higher in other domains—95% were highly ready in e-learning, 63% in clinical readiness, and 68% in technology readiness. These findings indicate that while healthcare workers possess strong technical, clinical, and educational capacities, their motivational and systemic readiness remains inadequate. Addressing these foundational gaps is crucial to ensure the sustainable, equitable, and effective implementation of telemedicine across healthcare systems.

This study is not without limitations. The small sample size (n = 60) may constrain the generalizability of the results to the broader healthcare workforce. Additionally, the cross-sectional design and uneven regional representation could have introduced contextual variations that were not thoroughly examined. Despite these constraints, the study provides valuable baseline insights into the multidimensional nature of telemedicine readiness among Indonesian healthcare workers.

Future research should build upon these findings by adopting larger and more representative samples, supported by stratified or multi-stage sampling designs. Investigations focusing on specific professional groups—particularly physicians and nurses—are recommended to derive profession-specific strategies. Moreover, institution-based studies (e.g., hospitals, clinics, or telemedicine providers) would allow for more controlled comparisons, organizational analyses, and intervention testing. Incorporating longitudinal and mixed-method approaches could further elucidate causal pathways, track readiness development over time, and explore contextual enablers or barriers. Strengthening organizational readiness, training programs, and policy frameworks will be crucial to translating the potential of telemedicine into a sustainable healthcare transformation.

Acknowledgments. The authors would like to thank the Faculty of Medicine at Maranatha Christian University for their support during the completion of this study.

Disclosure of Interests. The authors declare that they have no competing interests relevant to the content of this article.

References

1. Prasanti, D., Indriani, S.: Pengembangan teknologi informasi dan komunikasi dalam sistem e-health. J. Sosioteknol. **1** (2018)
2. Kementerian Kesehatan RI: Surat Edaran Menteri Kesehatan Republik Indonesia Nomor HK.02.01/Menkes/303/2020 tentang Penyelenggaraan Pelayanan Kesehatan melalui Pemanfaatan Teknologi Informasi dan Komunikasi dalam Rangka Pencegahan Penyebaran COVID-19 (2020)

3. Livana, P.H., Khoerunisa, A., Sofyan, E., Ningsih, D.K., Kandar, Suerni, T.: Gambaran kecemasan masyarakat dalam berkunjung ke pelayanan kesehatan pada masa pandemi COVID-19. J. Ilmiah Kesehatan Jiwa **2**(3), 129–134 (2020)
4. Siboro, M., Surjoputro, A., Budiyanti, R.: Faktor-faktor yang mempengaruhi penggunaan layanan telemedicine pada masa pandemi COVID-19 di Pulau Jawa. J. Kesehatan Masyarakat **3**(2), 58–66 (2019)
5. Mauco, K.L., Scott, R.E., Mars, M.: Critical analysis of e-health readiness assessment frameworks: suitability for application in developing countries. J. Telemed. Telecare **24**(2), 110–117 (2018)
6. Abigael, N.F., Ernawaty, E.: Pengukuran kesiapan tenaga kesehatan dalam menerima telehealth atau telemedicine antara negara maju dan negara berkembang: sebuah tinjauan literatur. J. Kesehatan **11**(2), 302 (2020)
7. Pujani, V., Hardisman, Semiarty, R., Handika, R.F.: The readiness study of e-health adoption among regional public hospitals: an empirical study in Indonesia. Int. J. Health Med. Sci. **4**(2), 40–47 (2018)
8. Kiberu, V.M., Scott, R.E., Mars, M.: Assessing core, e-learning, clinical and technology readiness to integrate telemedicine at public health facilities in Uganda: a health facility-based survey. BMC Health Serv. Res. **19**(1), 1–11 (2019)
9. Hofer, F., Haluza, D.: Are Austrian practitioners ready to use medical apps? Results of a validation study. BMC Med. Inform. Decis. Mak. **19**(1), 1–9 (2019)
10. Aulia, M.F., Budinuryanto, D.C., Wismandanu, O.: Persepsi dokter hewan praktisi hewan kecil terhadap telemedicine di masa pandemi COVID-19. Acta Vet. Indon. **9**(2), 82–86 (2021)
11. Riyanto, A.: Faktor-faktor yang mempengaruhi pelaksanaan telemedicine: sebuah systematic review. J. Manajemen Inform. Kesehatan Indon. **9**(2), 174 (2021)
12. Istifada, R., Sukihananto, S., Laagu, M.A.: Pemanfaatan teknologi telehealth pada perawat di layanan homecare (the utilization of telehealth technology by nurses at homecare setting). Nurs. Curr.: J. Keperawatan **5**(1), 51 (2018)
13. Sari, G.G., Wirman, W.: Telemedicine sebagai media konsultasi kesehatan di masa pandemi COVID-19 di Indonesia. J. Komunikasi **15**(1), 43–54 (2021)

Sentiment Analysis of Diabetes in X Platform Using the K-Nearest Neighbor (KNN) and Support Vector Machine (SVM) Methods: Case Study of Indonesia

Emil R. Kaburuan[1(✉)], Siti Maesaroh[1], Muhamad Zaky Wijdan[1], Lusy Widowati[2], and Sam Goundar[3]

[1] Informatics Engineering, Faculty of Computer Science, Mercu Buana University, Jakarta, Indonesia
{emil.kaburuan,siti.maesaroh}@mercubuana.ac.id, 41521010198@student.mercubuana.ac.id

[2] Engineering Department, Lincoln University College, Petaling Jaya, Selangor, Malaysia
lusy.phdscholar@lincoln.edu.my

[3] Computer Science Department, University of Central Asia, Naryn, Kyrgyzstan
sam.goundar@gmail.com

Abstract. Diabetes constitutes an escalating public health issue, with Indonesia positioned sixth worldwide in prevalence, recording 19.5 million cases in 2021. Comprehending public perception around diabetes on social media can guide health communication tactics and policy formulation. This study evaluates two machine learning algorithms—Support Vector Machine (SVM) and K-Nearest Neighbors (KNN)—for the classification of diabetes-related emotions on X (previously Twitter). We gathered 12,847 Indonesian tweets regarding diabetes from January to March 2024 and utilized the CRISP-DM framework for methodical data processing. Following preprocessing (cleaning, normalization, tokenization, stopword elimination, and stemming), we employed TF-IDF vectorization and lexicon-based sentiment classification. The dataset was divided in a 70:30 ratio for training and testing purposes. SVM substantially surpassed KNN, attaining an accuracy of 81.96% in contrast to 70.54%. The SVM model exhibited superior precision (83%), recall (82%), and F1-score (82%) across all emotion categories. These findings indicate that SVM is better appropriate for diabetes sentiment analysis on social media, with practical implications for public health monitoring and intervention efforts in Indonesia.

Keywords: Sentiment Analysis · Diabetes; Machine Learning · Support Vector Machine · K-Nearest Neighbors · Social Media Analytics · CRISP-DM · Public Health

E. R. Kaburuan and S. Goundar (Eds.): HIS 2025, LNCS 16392, pp. 338–351, 2026.
https://doi.org/10.1007/978-981-95-6304-3_29

1 Introduction

1.1 Background

Diabetes mellitus affects over 537 million adults worldwide, with Indonesia ranking fifth in global prevalence at 19.5 million cases in 2021 [1–3]. This chronic metabolic disorder, characterized by elevated blood glucose levels, leads to serious complications affecting multiple organ systems when left unmanaged. With projections indicating an increase to 28.6 million cases by 2045, diabetes represents a critical public health challenge for Indonesia [4]. The Indonesian Ministry of Health has identified diabetes as a priority concern, often referring to it as the "mother of all diseases" due to its widespread impact on population health and healthcare systems.

1.2 The Role of Public Perception

Public perceptions of diabetes significantly influence prevention behaviors and adherence to treatment [5]. Recent research reveals that many individuals, particularly adolescents and patients with type 2 diabetes, possess insufficient or negative perceptions about the condition, which adversely affects preventive behaviors and treatment compliance. Studies among Indonesian adolescents indicated that 66.6% of participants held negative perceptions of diabetes, leading to reduced participation in preventive measures and potentially increasing future diabetes risk [6]. This highlights the necessity for effective and continuous health education to improve public understanding and awareness from an early age.

Lifestyle factors, including poor dietary habits, lack of physical activity, and obesity, dramatically increase diabetes risk. Positive perceptions of the importance of physical activity and nutritious eating are strongly correlated with efforts to prevent diabetes. Research in South Kalimantan demonstrated that respondents with positive perceptions exhibited greater health-promoting behaviors [6]. Therefore, understanding and shaping public perceptions through targeted interventions is crucial for preventing and managing diabetes.

1.3 Social Media as a Public Health Tool

Social media platforms have become vital spaces for health-related discussions, offering unprecedented opportunities to understand public health perceptions on a large scale [7–9]. X (formerly Twitter), in particular, serves as a real-time platform where individuals share experiences, concerns, and opinions about health conditions, including diabetes. Analyzing sentiment in these conversations can provide valuable insights into:

- Public awareness and understanding of diabetes
- Concerns and challenges faced by patients and caregivers
- Reactions to health policies and interventions
- Spread of misinformation or misconceptions
- Effectiveness of health communication campaigns

Sentiment analysis—the computational identification and categorization of opinions expressed in text—enables health authorities to monitor these conversations systematically and respond proactively [10, 11].

1.4 Machine Learning for Sentiment Analysis

Machine learning algorithms have demonstrated efficacy in the automated classification of sentiment in social media material [12, 13]. Support Vector Machine (SVM) and K-Nearest Neighbors (KNN) are prevalent algorithms for text categorization tasks, each distinguished by its unique methodology and advantages.

- SVM employs kernel functions to identify optimal hyperplanes that distinguish various sentiment classes within high-dimensional feature fields [14, 15].
- KNN classifies text by assessing its similarity to the nearest neighbors inside the feature space [16, 17].

Prior studies have utilized these algorithms for several health-related sentiment analysis tasks, yielding inconsistent outcomes based on the domain, language, and data attributes [18, 19].

1.5 Research Gap

Despite the growing body of research on sentiment analysis for health topics, several gaps remain. First, most studies focus on English-language content, with limited research on Indonesian social media discourse about diabetes. Second, while previous studies have applied various machine learning algorithms to health sentiment analysis, systematic comparisons of algorithm performance specifically for diabetes-related content are scarce. Third, the application of the CRISP-DM framework to health sentiment analysis remains underexplored. This study addresses these gaps by comparing SVM and KNN algorithms for Indonesian diabetes sentiment classification using a structured CRISP-DM approach.

2 Related Works

Sentiment analysis, also known as opinion mining, is a significant domain of text mining that focuses on the computational analysis of opinions, attitudes, and emotions expressed in textual data [11–13]. This analysis aims to identify and categorize public opinions toward various entities, including products, services, organizations, individuals, events, and specific subjects, particularly those prominently discussed on social media platforms [14, 20]. This sentiment analysis concentrates on opinions that explicitly or implicitly convey positive or negative attitudes [21].

Health concerns, especially diabetes, are increasingly prevalent on social media platforms, particularly Twitter (X), which functions as a significant channel for articulating public sentiment through tweets [18, 22]. Twitter (X), as an open social media platform, facilitates the sharing of personal information and opinions while also functioning as a significant open-source data repository for research, especially in sentiment analysis (text mining) to comprehend public perceptions of diabetes-related matters [18, 22]. In the digital age, Twitter (X) is widely used by people to express grievances about everyday issues and dissatisfaction with services provided by the government and other sectors. [19, 22].

Previous studies have examined sentiment analysis in diabetes using various data types, techniques, and algorithms. Asyer et al. [18] performed a study examining the sentiment of tweets from Twitter users about diabetes, utilizing the Naive Bayes method, which produced findings of 22% positive sentiment, 14% negative sentiment, and 64% neutral sentiment [18]. The achieved accuracy rate was 87%, which is classified as "Good Classification" [18, 23]. In the domain of SVM research, Iskandar and Nataliani's paper, "Comparison of Naive Bayes, SVM, and KNN for Aspect-Based Sentiment Analysis of Gadgets", achieved the highest accuracy for SVM at 96.43% [24].

The Support Vector Machine (SVM) excels at handling high-dimensional text data generated from TF-IDF representations. The advantage of KNN is its adaptability to multiclass scenarios [16, 25]. The research methodology follows the CRISP-DM framework, which comprises the phases of business understanding, data understanding, data preparation, modeling, and evaluation. This framework has proven effective in recent sentiment analysis research, including tourism review evaluation and biometric technology applications [26, 27].

3 Research Methods

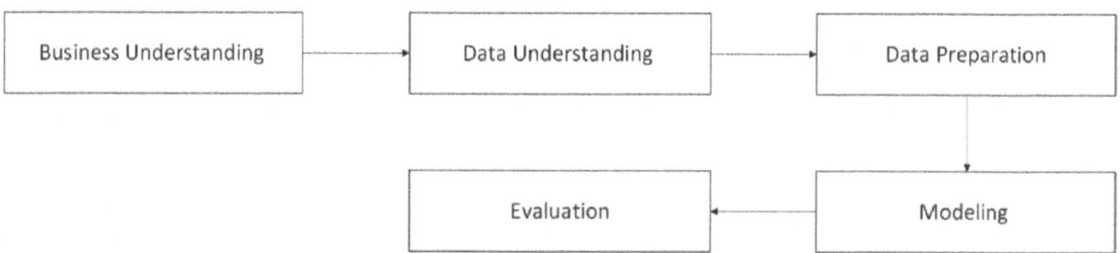

Fig. 1. Research Methods

This study used a technique grounded in the CRISP-DM framework, comprising five principal steps. The initial phase involves understanding the business context, focusing on the evaluation and comparison of the K-Nearest Neighbor (KNN) and Support Vector Machine (SVM) algorithms in executing sentiment analysis on application X, which addresses the topic of diabetes. During the second stage, data understanding, sentiment data is gathered from the application and analyzed to discern the qualities and patterns of sentiment that arise. Subsequently, during the data preparation phase, the acquired data undergoes text preprocessing, sentiment annotation, partitioning into training and testing datasets, and transformation into vector format for use by machine learning algorithms. The fourth stage involves modeling, during which the KNN and SVM algorithms are implemented and refined to construct a sentiment categorization model. Ultimately, in the evaluation phase, the performance of both models is assessed using a confusion matrix and evaluation metrics, including accuracy and F1-score, to compare the efficacy of the two algorithms in categorizing the feelings of X application users regarding diabetes (Fig. 1).

3.1 Business Understanding

We collected Indonesian-language tweets containing diabetes-related keywords using the X API v2 between January to March 2024. It also compares the performance of the K-Nearest Neighbors (KNN) and Support Vector Machine (SVM) algorithms in classifying sentiments as positive or negative. The analysis is conducted to evaluate the effectiveness of both algorithms on both imbalanced and balanced datasets.

3.2 Data Understanding

Table 1. Data Set.

1 to 25 of 5081 entries Filter

index	full_text
0	Menu sarapan ini mampu menurunkan risiko terkena tiga penyakit kronis termasuk diabetes tipe 2 silakan mencobanya. #menusarapan https://t.co/ySZ8VSogL2
1	Semakin besar ukuran dada semakin besar pula risiko terkena penyakit diabetes tipe 2. [Penelitian Ilmu Keperawatan]
2	5 Hal yang Perlu Anda Ketahui Tentang Diabetes Tipe 2 https://t.co/UXDdIA1VOy
3	Diabetes Tipe 2 Minuman Ini Bisa Turunkan Gula Darah dalam 60 Menit #Sindonews #BukanBeritaBiasa .https://t.co/tJ9Ce97AxQ
4	@healthy_fess Bukan cuma penyakit ginjal aja. Bisa ke yang lain juga misal Diabetes tipe 2. Minum air mineral bening hambar biasa aman untuk jangka panjang.
5	Kabar gembira bagi mereka yang suka cokelat. Sejumlah penelitian menunjukkan senyawa alami dalam kakao yang bijinya dikenal sebagai cokelat yakni flavanol epicatechin mampu mencegah diabetes tipe 2. #Diabetes #Cokelat https://t.co/XjLP1CQjpl
6	@IJJJENO @FOODFESS2 Sami2 pelan2 belajar utk baca2 nutrition facts di tiap kemasan mkn/minum yg km konsumsi yaa. Jgn smpe masih muda udh kena diabetes tipe 2 stay safe!
7	Inilah gejala awal diabetes tipe 2 https://t.co/PQFL37bBzx
8	#AgendaFKUI Gelar Wicara Seputar Dunia Kesehatan FKUI & RRI. Setiap hari Senin-jumat pukul 09.30-10.00 WIB di Pro 3 FM 88 8 MHz & RRI NET. Topik Jumat 17 Desember 2021 Peran Serta Akupuntur pada Diabetes Melitus Tipe 2 oleh dr. Irma Nareswari https://t.co/wMXpuM7xjT Sp.Ak https://t.co/I0yektL6KW
9	Saat seseorang mengalami diabetes tipe 2 jenis sarapan yang bisa dikonsumsi mulai berkurang. Namun bukan berarti tidak bisa menikmati sarapan sehat dan enak. #Penyakit #diabetestipe2 #sarapansehat https://t.co/uvLnYExiP5
10	#repost @p2ptmkemenkesri 1. Apakah saja gejala Diabetes Melitus Tipe 1 pada Anak? 2. Bagaimana cara mengendalikan Diabetes Melitus Tipe 1 pada Anak? . #CERDIK #CegahPTM #DukungGERMAS #Diabetesmelitus https://t.co/uY3Mj7woMd
11	@TirtoID Lagipula DM Tipe 1 dan 2 memiliki patofisiologi/mekanisme kerusakan yang sama sekali berbeda jadi agak gimana gitu keduanya dionggokkan dalam satu infografis iklan air minum. DM tipe 1 terjadi karena sistem imun pasien menyerang sel-sel penghasil
12	mau tanya disini ada yang punya saudara atau kenalan yang kena diabetes tipe 2 dengan komplikasi hipoglikemia? Bersedia buat isi kuesionerku? Terima kasih
13	Sering Lapar dan Haus Gejala Awal Diabetes Tipe 2? https://t.co/PQFL37lcr5
14	Tidur siang idealnya 10-20 menit utk sekedar memulihkan energi. Sementara tidur siang lbh dr 30menit dpt meningkatkn risiko diabetes tipe 2.
15	Diabetes Tipe 2 Tanda Gula Darah Tinggi di Jari Kaki yang Akibatkan Amputasi #Sindonews #BukanBeritaBiasa .https://t.co/taQBOTuTAC

Table 1 shows that the data were collected through a crawling process from social media platform X (formerly known as Twitter) using a query that included the following keywords: "diabetes"; "diabetesmellitus"; "gula darah" (blood sugar); "diabetes tipe 2" (type 2 diabetes). The total amount of data successfully gathered consisted of 5,081 tweets in the Indonesian language related to the topic of diabetes. The next step is to conduct data exploration, also known as Exploratory Data Analysis (EDA). This stage aims to identify initial patterns in the data and detect potential problems such as missing or duplicate data. Based on the results of the exploration, no missing entries or duplicate data were found, so the dataset was deemed suitable for further analysis. Next, an analysis was conducted on the distribution of text length in tweets, which is visualized in Fig. 2.

The visualization results show an upward trend in the number of tweets each year, with the highest number occurring in 2024, reaching over 2,600 tweets —a sharp increase compared to previous years.

3.3 Data Preparation

A crucial stage in sentiment analysis research is data preparation. The dataset undergoes preparation stages including cleaning, case folding, normalization, tokenization, stopword removal, and stemming. Sentiment labeling, utilizing the InSet language, was employed to classify tweets as positive or negative. Subsequent to the partitioning of the data into training and testing sets, text is converted into numerical features for model processing via TF-IDF.

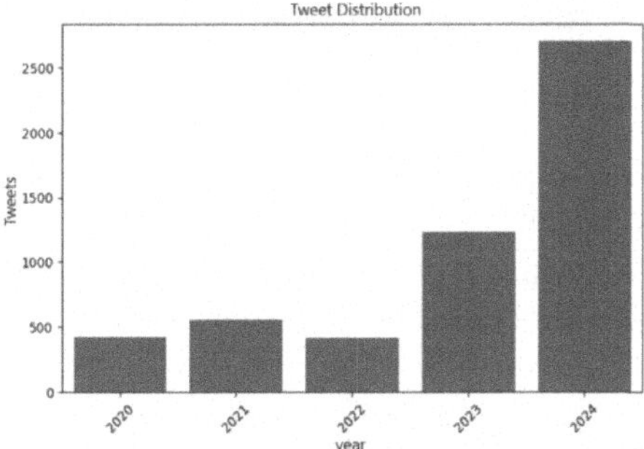

Fig. 2. Tweet Distribution

3.3.1 Data Preprocessing

Data obtained through the crawling process requires additional cleaning before it can be used for analysis. This stage, known as data preprocessing, involves several essential steps, including:

1. Cleaning: removing non-informative elements such as emojis, Unicode symbols, and URLs (e.g., http://, https, www., t.co/, etc.).
2. Case Folding: Converting all text characters to lowercase to standardize the text format (e.g., "Diabetes" to "diabetes").
3. Normalization: Transforming informal or non-standard words into their standard form (e.g., "tdk" to "tidak").
4. Tokenization: Breaking down or segmenting a text string into individual word units called tokens (e.g., "penderita diabetes" to "penderita", "diabetes").
5. Stopword Removal: Eliminating words that are considered irrelevant or carry little meaningful information (e.g., "dan", "dengan", "dari", etc.).
6. Stemming: Reducing words to their root form by removing affixes such as prefixes, suffixes, or infixes (e.g., "terbuka" to "buka").

3.3.2 Data Labeling

Each tweet is scored based on the number of positive and negative words. If there are more positive words, the tweet is labeled as positive; if there are more negative words, it is labeled as negative. For example, a tweet with a score of -3 is classified as negative. This method helps ensure the labeling is done consistently and objectively (Table 2).

3.3.3 Splitting Data

Data splitting involves dividing the dataset into two main parts: a training subset used to develop the model and a testing subset used to objectively evaluate the model's performance. The division was made into 3 models: 70:30, 80:20, and 90:10 (Fig. 3).

Table 2. Polarity Score Calculation

Text	Score	Sentiment
menu sarap turun risiko kena sakit kronis diabetes tipe sila coba (breakfast habits can reduce the risk of chronic diseases like type-2 diabetes.)	−3.0	negative
sakit ginjal diabetes tipe minum air mineral bening hambar aman jangka (for kidney disease and type-2 diabetes, drinking plain mineral water (clear and tasteless) is safe for long-term consumption.)	−4.0	negative
saudara kenal kena diabetes tipe komplikasi hipoglikemia sedia isi kuesioner terima kasih (If you have relatives diagnosed with type-2 diabetes or complications such as hypoglycemia, please take a moment to fill out this questionnaire. Thank you.)	1.0	positive

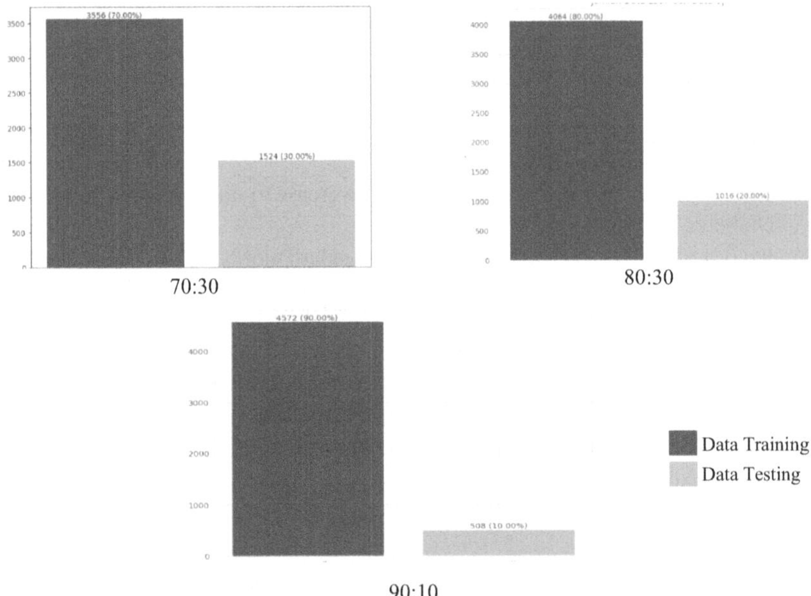

Fig. 3. Data Splitting

3.3.4 Vectorization

Textual input must be converted into a numerical format prior to processing by machine learning algorithms. A frequently employed method for this transformation is Term Frequency–Inverse Document Frequency (TF-IDF) vectorization. TF-IDF is a statistical technique that evaluates the importance of a word in a specific document in relation to a corpus of documents. This method assigns greater significance to words that are prevalent within a specific document but infrequent across the entire dataset,

```
Shape fitur (X): (5080, 5000)
Shape label (y): (5080,)
Label unik: ['Negatif' 'Positif']
```

thereby allowing the model to more effectively grasp the contextual relevance and uniqueness of each phrase.

TF-IDF (Term Frequency–Inverse Document Frequency) is a method for converting text data into numbers by weighting each word based on how often it appears in a document and how rarely it appears in all documents. The result is a feature matrix that can be used for machine learning modeling, as shown in shape (5080, 5000) above.

3.4 Modeling

After the data cleaning, labeling, dataset division, and TF-IDF application stages to convert text into numerical representations, the next step is to build a classification model. In this phase, the focus is on selecting the appropriate algorithm and adjusting its parameters to enable the model to recognize sentiment patterns with high accuracy. This study employs the K-Nearest Neighbors (KNN) and Support Vector Machine (SVM) algorithms, both of which have proven reliable in handling text classification tasks. Both models are trained using the same data, allowing for objective and fair performance evaluation results.

3.4.1 K-Nearest Neighbors

The K-Nearest Neighbors (K-NN) algorithm classifies a new object by examining its nearest neighbors, assigning the most frequently occurring class among them as the classification outcome [16, 28, 29]. KNN can ascertain the sentiment classification (positive or negative) of a tweet by measuring the distance between the new tweet and previously categorized tweets, employing metrics such as Euclidean distance.

3.4.2 Support Vector Machine

The original SVM algorithm was developed by Vladimir Vapnik, while the contemporary standard variant (soft margin) was introduced by Corinna Cortes and Vladimir Vapnik. Support Vector Machine (SVM) is frequently employed for its proficiency in managing extensive and intricate datasets [30]. The Support Vector Machine (SVM) classification algorithm predicts labels by identifying the class region to which the data corresponds. This technique typically attains superior accuracy in text classification relative to other algorithms, including K-Nearest Neighbors (KNN), C4.5, and Naive Bayes. Support Vector Machines have superior accuracy and can manage intricate data; yet, they necessitate extended training periods and meticulous parameter optimization. In SVM, the selection of parameters, particularly the kernel, significantly influences the model's performance. Support Vector Machines (SVM) exhibit superior efficiency in managing high-dimensional data and are regarded as having reliable performance in sentiment categorization.

3.5 Evaluation

The optimal performance for sentiment classification, as determined by the results of the prior model implementation, was attained utilizing a 70:30 ratio of training to testing data. The SVM model achieved a precision score of 0.85 for the negative class and 0.76 for the positive class, with recall scores of 0.88 and 0.70 for negative and positive feelings, respectively.

The SVM confusion matrix reveals that of the 996 data points classified as Negative, 879 were accurately predicted (actual negatives), but 158 were erroneously classified as Positive. Out of 528 data points designated as Positive, 370 were accurately identified, while 117 were erroneously classified as Negative. The results reveal that the SVM model exhibits robust proficiency in categorizing both sentiment categories, especially the Negative class.

The KNN model, by contrast, yielded a diminished accuracy of 70.54%. The KNN confusion matrix indicates that of the 852 data points designated as Negative, 566 were accurately identified, whilst 90 were erroneously classified as Positive. Nonetheless, the performance for the Positive class diminished markedly, achieving only 128 right predictions out of 360 samples, while 232 were erroneously categorized as Negative. This resulted in diminished recall and F1-score values for the Positive class, at 0.36 and 0.44, respectively (Fig. 4).

KNN
Accuracy: 70.54%
Classification Report:

	precision	recall	f1-score	support
Negatif	0.74	0.86	0.79	996
Positif	0.61	0.42	0.50	528
accuracy			0.71	1524
macro avg	0.67	0.64	0.64	1524
weighted avg	0.69	0.71	0.69	1524

SVM
Accuracy: 81.96%
Classification Report:

	precision	recall	f1-score	support
Negatif	0.85	0.88	0.86	996
Positif	0.76	0.70	0.73	528
accuracy			0.82	1524
macro avg	0.80	0.79	0.80	1524
weighted avg	0.82	0.82	0.82	1524

Fig. 4. Accuracy Result

From the accuracy, we found that SVM has higher accuracy compared to KNN. The superior performance of SVM can be attributed to its ability to find an optimal hyperplane that efficiently separates data, especially in high-dimensional spaces such as those produced by TF-IDF representations. In contrast, KNN, which heavily relies on the proximity between data points in the vector space, tends to be more sensitive to data imbalance and less effective in handling high-dimensional text data. Therefore, based on the evaluation results, SVM was selected as the best model in this study because it delivers more stable and accurate classification performance (Fig. 5).

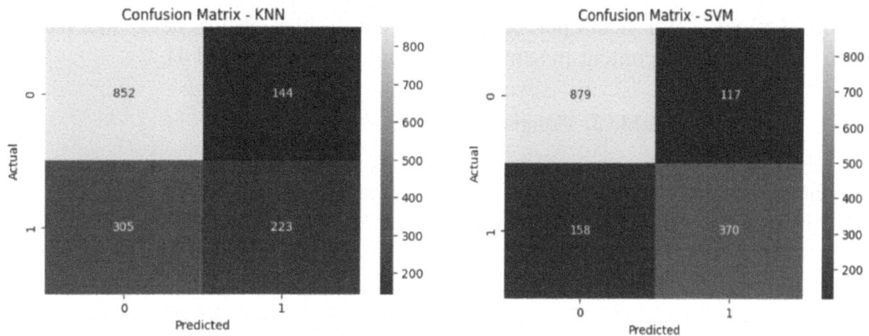

Fig. 5. Confusion Matrix

The K-Nearest Neighbors (KNN) algorithm's confusion matrix shows that the model accurately identified 852 negative instances and 223 positive instances. However, it misclassified 144 negative instances as positive and 305 positive instances as negative, indicating challenges in correctly detecting positive sentiment. Meanwhile the confusion matrix for the Support Vector Machine (SVM) model demonstrates that the algorithm successfully identified 879 instances as negative and 370 instances as positive. However, the model incorrectly classified 117 negative samples as positive and 158 positive samples as negative, indicating some challenges in distinguishing between the two sentiment classes.

4 Results and Discussion

Following the modeling and evaluation phases using machine learning techniques, this section presents the performance assessment of the sentiment classification models. The evaluation employs standard metrics including accuracy, precision, recall, and F1-score, all derived from each model's confusion matrix. These metrics are calculated as follows:

- Accuracy = (TP + TN)/(TP + TN + FP + FN)
- Precision = TP/(TP + FP)
- Recall = TP/(TP + FN)
- F1-Score = 2 × (Precision × Recall)/(Precision + Recall)

Here, TP (True Positive) represents the number of positive instances correctly identified, TN (True Negative) is the count of negative instances correctly classified, FP (False Positive) indicates negative instances wrongly labeled as positive, and FN (False Negative) refers to positive instances mistakenly classified as negative.

4.1 K-Nearest Neighbors

The KNN model attained an accuracy of 70.54%, a precision of 67.50%, a recall of 64.00%, and an F1-score of 64.00%, according to the evaluation metrics provided. The results reveal that although the model exhibits reasonable overall performance, its capacity to accurately identify positive cases is somewhat constrained, as evidenced by the balanced yet somewhat small precision and recall metrics. This indicates that the algorithm may still overlook a significant percentage of actual positive occurrences, underscoring opportunities for enhancement in sentiment accuracy (Tables 3 and 4).

Table 3. Comparison of the Confusion Matrix

Algorithm		Predicted Positive	Predicted Negative
KNN	Actual Positive	128 (TP)	232 (FN)
	Actual Negative	90 (FP)	566 (TN)
SVM	Actual Positive	370 (TP)	158 (FN)
	Actual Negative	158 (FP)	879 (TN)

Table 4. Performance Result

Metrics	Value	
	KNN	SVM
Accuracy	70.54%	*81.96%*
Precision	67.50%	*80.50%*
Recall	64.00%	*79.00%*
F1-Score	64.00%	*80.00%*

The evaluation metrics indicate that the SVM model attained an accuracy of 81.96%, a precision of 80.50%, a recall of 79.00%, and an F1-score of 80.00%. The results reveal that the model excels in sentiment classification, effectively identifying positive cases while achieving a commendable level of precision. While the recall is marginally inferior to precision, the aggregate metrics indicate a dependable and constant capability in reliably recognizing sentiment throughout the dataset.

The test results demonstrated that the SVM algorithm provided superior classification performance relative to KNN. The SVM model achieved an accuracy of 81.96%, with a precision of 0.85 and a recall of 0.88 for negative sentiment, using a 70:30 data split ratio, thereby demonstrating significant efficacy in detecting negative tweets. The precision and recall for positive sentiment were 0.76 and 0.70, respectively, demonstrating the model's ability to maintain class balance and reduce forecast inaccuracies.

Conversely, the KNN algorithm demonstrated a reduced accuracy of 70.54%. The confusion matrix indicates that KNN exhibited difficulty in reliably identifying positive sentiment, evidenced by a recall value of merely 0.42 and an F1-score of 0.50. This resulted from the model's propensity to categorize the majority of tweets as negative, showing a disparity in the model's sensitivity to both classifications. Although KNN exhibited a commendable precision of 0.74 for negative sentiment, its overall efficacy did not exceed that of SVM.

In contrast to earlier research employing the Naive Bayes method, which attained an accuracy of 87%, it is noteworthy that those classifications were based on three sentiment categories (positive, negative, and neutral), with the neutral category predominating at

64%. This dominance may instigate class bias, thereby artificially exaggerating the accuracy value. This study's binary sentiment method (positive and negative) with a more equitable data distribution offers a more objective and comprehensive assessment of model performance.

5 Conclusion

This study aimed to compare the efficacy of the Support Vector Machine (SVM) and K-Nearest Neighbors (KNN) algorithms in classifying public opinion about diabetes on the social media platform X (Twitter). The research procedure commenced with data acquisition by tweet-crawling methodologies utilizing specific keywords pertinent to diabetes. The gathered data subsequently underwent multiple text preprocessing steps, encompassing cleaning, case folding, normalization, tokenization, stopword elimination, and stemming via the Sastrawi algorithm. The analyzed text data was subsequently converted into numerical representations by the TF-IDF vectorization approach, yielding a total of 5,000 features. The sanitized dataset was divided into training data (70%) and test data (30%) to facilitate optimal model training and impartial assessment. Sentiment labels comprised two categories: "Positive" and "Negative", derived using lexicon-based techniques and sentiment scores.

In conclusion, the Support Vector Machine (SVM) algorithm is the most optimal and stable approach for sentiment classification of tweets concerning diabetes difficulties. The findings of this study are anticipated to underpin the establishment of public opinion analytic platforms, data-informed health policy formulation, and digital communication methods designed to inform the public about chronic diseases, including diabetes.

References

1. ElSayed, N.A., et al.: 2. Classification and diagnosis of diabetes: standards of care in diabetes—2023. Diabetes Care **46**(Supplement_1), S19–S40 (2023). https://doi.org/10.2337/dc23-S002
2. American Diabetes Association. Introduction: Standards of Medical Care in Diabetes—2022. Diabetes Care **45**(Supplement_1), S1–S2 (2022). https://doi.org/10.2337/dc22-Sint
3. Wang, H., et al.: IDF diabetes atlas: estimation of global and regional gestational diabetes mellitus prevalence for 2021 by international association of diabetes in pregnancy study group's criteria. Diabetes Res. Clin. Pract. **183**, 109050 (2022). https://doi.org/10.1016/j.diabres.2021.109050
4. WHO/A. Loke. Diabetes. Diabetes. https://www.who.int/news-room/fact-sheets/detail/diabetes
5. Laurina, D., Tjomiadi, C.E.F., Irawan, A., Basit, M.: Hubungan persepsi dengan perilaku pencegahan diabetes melitus pada siswa, vol. 13, no. 2 (2025)
6. Hikmah, N., Mahpolah, Widyastuti Hariati, N.: Hubungan Persepsi, Aktivitas Fisik, Pola Makan, dan Indeks Massa Tubuh (IMT) dengan Kejadian Diabetes Melitus Tipe 2. JR-PANZI **5**(2), 20–32 (2023). https://doi.org/10.31964/jr-panzi.v5i2.187
7. Raghupathi, V., Ren, J., Raghupathi, W.: Studying public perception about vaccination: a sentiment analysis of tweets. IJERPH **17**(10), 3464 (2020). https://doi.org/10.3390/ijerph17103464

8. Shah, N.U., et al.: Enhancing patient safety in healthcare through public opinions using deep learning. Kashf J. Multidiscip. Res. **2**(08), 1–14 (2025). https://doi.org/10.71146/kjmr566
9. Tarango-García, A., et al.: Sentiment analysis of subcutaneous and intravenous immunoglobulin therapy: public healthcare perception through social media discourse. Front. Immunol. **15**, 1467852 (2024). https://doi.org/10.3389/fimmu.2024.1467852
10. Alfaqeeh, M., Alfian, S.D., Abdulah, R.: Factors associated with diabetes mellitus among adults: Findings from the Indonesian Family Life Survey-5. Endocrine and Metabolic Science **14**, 100161 (2024). https://doi.org/10.1016/j.endmts.2024.100161
11. Sharma, N.A., Ali, A.B.M.S., Kabir, M.A.: A review of sentiment analysis: tasks, applications, and deep learning techniques. Int J Data Sci Anal **19**(3), 351–388 (2025). https://doi.org/10.1007/s41060-024-00594-x
12. Amelia, A., Yusuf, R.: Analisis sentimen masyarakat indonesia pada platfrom x terhadap isu fufufafa menggunakan bidirectional encoder representations from transformers. JINTEKS **7**(1), 72–80 (2025). https://doi.org/10.51401/jinteks.v7i1.5160
13. Mao, Y., Liu, Q., Zhang, Y.: Sentiment analysis methods, applications, and challenges: a systematic literature review. J. King Saud Univ. – Comput. Inf. Sci. **36**(4), 102048 (2024). https://doi.org/10.1016/j.jksuci.2024.102048
14. Kaburuan, E.R., Maesaroh, S., Achmad, R., Islamov, Y., Manurung, M.M.: Comparison of naïve bayes classifier algorithm and support vector machine classification for the sport event at X platform. In: 2024 International Conference on Orange Technology (ICOT), Tainan, Taiwan, pp. 1–9. IEEE (2024). https://doi.org/10.1109/ICOT64290.2024.10936926
15. Kaburuan, E.R., Setiawan, N.R.: Sentimen analisis review aplikasi digital korlantas pada google play store menggunakan metode SVM. SISFOKOM **12**(1), 105–116 (2023). https://doi.org/10.32736/sisfokom.v12i1.1614
16. Ayu, K.G., et al.: Classification of employee competency assessment using naïve bayes and K-nearest neighbor (KNN) algorithms. JAIT **15**(7), 879–885 (2024). https://doi.org/10.12720/jait.15.7.879-885
17. Suprayogi, S., Sari, C.A., Rachmawanto, E.H.: Sentiment analyst on twitter using the k-nearest neighbors (KNN) algorithm against COVID-19 vaccination. JAIS **7**(2), 135–145 (2022). https://doi.org/10.33633/jais.v7i2.6734
18. Asyer, A.A., Ineke Pakereng, M.A.I.P.: Analisis sentimen tweet pengguna twitter terkait diabetes menggunakan metode naive bayes. Jutisi J. Tek. Sis. Info. **12**(2), 627 (2023). https://doi.org/10.35889/jutisi.v12i2.1234
19. Puspita, R., Widodo, A.: Perbandingan metode KNN, decision tree, dan naïve bayes terhadap analisis sentimen pengguna layanan BPJS. JIUP **5**(4), 646 (2021). https://doi.org/10.32493/informatika.v5i4.7622
20. Bayhaqy, A., Sfenrianto, S., Nainggolan, K., Kaburuan, E.R.: Sentiment analysis about E-commerce from tweets using decision tree, K-nearest neighbor, and naïve bayes. In: 2018 International Conference on Orange Technologies (ICOT), Nusa Dua, BALI, Indonesia, pp. 1–6. IEEE (2018). https://doi.org/10.1109/ICOT.2018.8705796
21. Supriyade, S., Firmansyah, G., Akbar, H., Tjahjono, B.: Analysis of time series water level data prediction using deep learning method at the water gate of DKI Jakarta water resources office. JISS **4**(09), 753–762 (2023). https://doi.org/10.59141/jiss.v4i09.883
22. Ryandi, F.A., Pratiwi, D., Sari, S.: Analisis sentimen masyarakat di media sosial X terhadap kemenkes dengan naive bayes dan SVM, vol. 7, no. 1 (2025)
23. Supian, A., Tri Revaldo, B., Marhadi, N., Efrizoni, L., Rahmaddeni, R.: Perbandingan kinerja naïve bayes dan svm pada analisis sentimen twitter ibukota nusantara, vol. 12, no. 01, pp. 15–21 (2024). https://doi.org/10.33884/jif.v12i01.8721
24. Iskandar, J.W., Nataliani, Y.: Perbandingan naïve bayes, SVM, dan k-NN untuk analisis sentimen gadget berbasis aspek. RESTI **5**(6), 1120–1126 (2021). https://doi.org/10.29207/resti.v5i6.3588

25. Legito, L., et al.: Penerapan algoritma K-nearest neighbor untuk analisis sentimen terhadap isu khilafah dan radikalisme di indonesia: implementation K-nearest neighbor algorithm for sentiment analysis on khilafah and radicalism issues in Indonesia. MALCOM **3**(2), 324–330 (2023). https://doi.org/10.57152/malcom.v3i2.893
26. Singgalen, Y.A.: Comprehensive analysis of sentiment and toxicity dynamics in tourist vlog reviews: a CRISP-DM approach. JoSYC **5**(3), 648–659 (2024). https://doi.org/10.47065/josyc.v5i3.5154
27. Azeroual, O., Nacheva, R., Nikiforova, A., Störl, U.: A CRISP-DM and predictive analytics framework for enhanced decision-making in research information management systems. IJCAI **49**(18) (2025). https://doi.org/10.31449/inf.v49i18.5613
28. Setyorini, S.G., Mustakim: Application of the nearest neighbor algorithm for classification of online taxibike sentiments in indonesia in the google playstore application. J. Phys.: Conf. Ser. **2049**(1), 012026 (2021). https://doi.org/10.1088/1742-6596/2049/1/012026
29. Cholil, S.R., Handayani, T., Prathivi, R., Ardianita,T.: Implementasi algoritma klasifikasi k-nearest neighbor (KNN) untuk klasifikasi seleksi penerima beasiswa
30. Rabbani, S., Safitri, D., Rahmadhani, N., Sani, A.A.F., Anam, M.K.: Perbandingan evaluasi kernel SVM untuk klasifikasi sentimen dalam analisis kenaikan harga bbm: comparative evaluation of SVM kernels for sentiment classification in fuel price increase analysis. MALCOM **3**(2), 153–160 (2023). https://doi.org/10.57152/malcom.v3i2.897

Author Index

E. R. Kaburuan and S. Goundar (Eds.): HIS 2025, LNCS 16392, pp. 353–354, 2026.
https://doi.org/10.1007/978-981-95-6304-3

The manufacturer's authorised representative in the EU is Springer Nature Customer Service Centre GmbH, Europaplatz 3, 69115 Heidelberg, Germany. If you have any concerns regarding our products, please contact ProductSafety@springernature.com

Printed and bound by CPI Group (UK) Ltd, Croydon, CR0 4YY
07/07/2026
02160913-0010